G.R. Williams
St. Thomas's Hosp.

OXFORD MEDICAL PUBLICATIONS

GADDUM'S PHARMACOLOGY

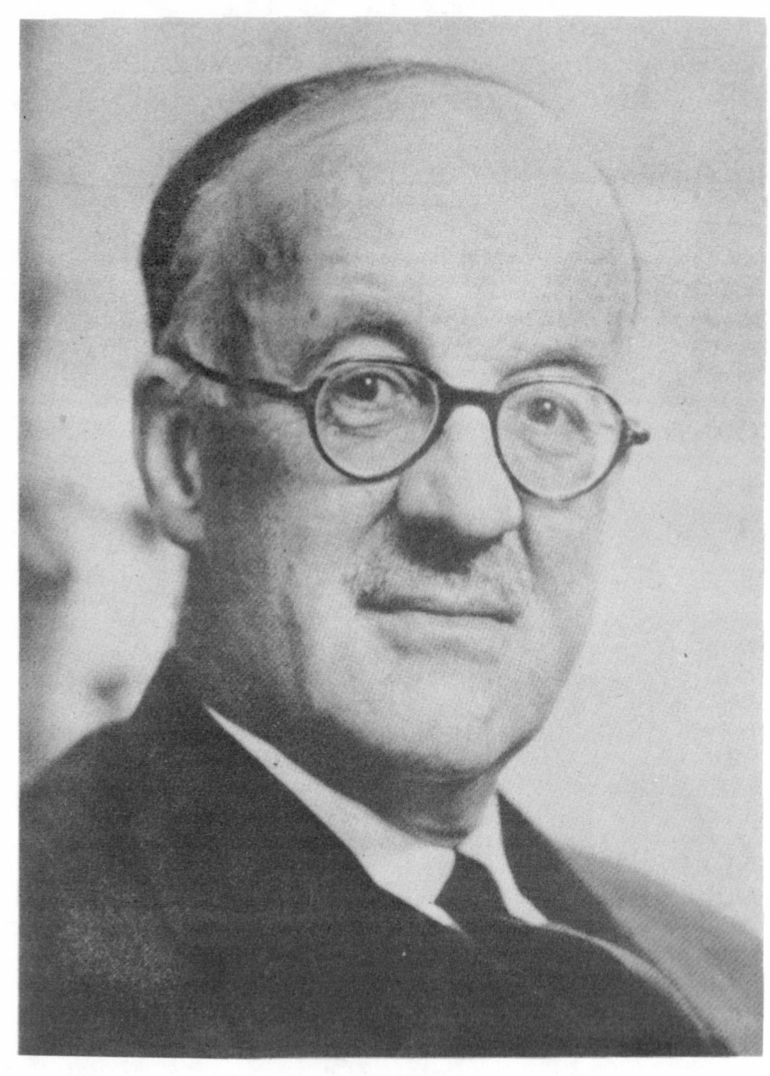

SIR JOHN GADDUM, F.R.S

GADDUM'S PHARMACOLOGY

EIGHTH EDITION

REVISED BY

A. S. V. BURGEN, M.D., F.R.C.P., F.R.S.

Director, National Institute for Medical Research, Mill Hill
Formerly Shield Professor of Pharmacology, University of Cambridge

AND

J. F. MITCHELL, M.A., B.SC., PH.D. F.I. BIOL.

Professor of Pharmacology, University of Bristol

LONDON

OXFORD UNIVERSITY PRESS

NEW YORK TORONTO

Oxford University Press, Walton Street, Oxford OX2 6DP

OXFORD LONDON GLASGOW

NEW YORK TORONTO MELBOURNE WELLINGTON

IBADAN NAIROBI DAR ES SALAAM LUSAKA CAPE TOWN

KUALA LUMPUR SINGAPORE JAKARTA HONG KONG TOKYO

DELHI BOMBAY CALCUTTA MADRAS KARACHI

ISBN 0 19 261307 3

First Edition 1940
Eighth Edition 1978

TYPE SET BY THE UNIVERSITIES PRESS, BELFAST
PRINTED IN GREAT BRITAIN
BY RICHARD CLAY (THE CHAUCER PRESS) LTD,
BUNGAY, SUFFOLK

PREFACE TO THE EIGHTH EDITION

In the period since the last edition appeared the advances in pharmacology have been so rapid and extensive that a great deal of new material has needed to be included.

Pharmacokinetics has become an important area which is having a major impact on the rational administration of drugs, and now merits a chapter on its own. The area covered by Chapter 9, including prostaglandins, peptides, and histamine H_2 antagonists, is perhaps the most rapidly growing area of pharmacology. But important advances are occurring in the central nervous system, especially in relation to the role of dopamine and the action of opiates and elsewhere. It has also been a period when many phenomena which were curiosities of one area of pharmacology have been found to have a general relevance to many drug actions. Altogether we hope that this new edition conveys to the reader the excitement which this rapid evolution of pharmacology has engendered.

As with previous editions, this book is intended primarily for preclinical medical students and for students of science and pharmacy to give them an introduction to the ideas of pharmacology, with an emphasis on the mechanisms of drug action and on the relationship of the chemical structure of drugs to their action. The book is not intended to cover clinical pharmacology but rather to provide a sound foundation on which the use of drugs in human therapeutics can be built.

June 1977

A.S.V.B.
J.F.M.

CONTENTS

1. GENERAL PHARMACOLOGY 1
   What are drugs? Drug action on isolated tissues

2. DRUG KINETICS 13
   Distribution of drugs after intravenous injection. Absorption of drugs when injected into the tissues. Administration by mouth. Administration by inhalation. Bioavailability. Excretion of drugs. Drug metabolism.

3. CENTRAL NERVOUS SYSTEM TRANSMITTERS 24
   Experimental methods for the study of centrally acting drugs on transmitter mechanisms. The neurotransmitters. Other possible central transmitters.

4. CENTRAL NERVOUS SYSTEM DEPRESSANTS 33
   Anaesthetics. Hypnotics and sedatives. Anticonvulsants. Tranquillizing drugs. Analgesics.

5. CENTRAL NERVOUS SYSTEM STIMULANTS 57
   Antidepressants. Convulsants and analeptics. Hallucinogens.

6. LOCAL ANAESTHETICS 67

7. CHOLINERGIC SYSTEM 72
   Methods of studying the cholinergic system. Nicotinic responses. Muscarinic responses. Mixed receptor sites. Individual cholinergic drugs and their antagonists.

8. ADRENERGIC SYSTEM 96
   The effects of sympathetic nerve stimulation and of noradrenaline and adrenaline. α-Blockers. β-Blockers. Drugs affecting noradrenaline release.

9. PEPTIDES, HISTAMINE, AND PROSTAGLANDINS 110
   Pharmacologically active peptides. Histamine. Antihistamines. Prostaglandins.

10. CIRCULATION 122
    Noradrenaline and related compounds. Hypotensive drugs. Angina pectoris. The cardiac glycosides. Antiarrhythmic drugs.

11. BODY TEMPERATURE AND THE ANTIPYRETIC-ANALGESICS 132

12. ALIMENTARY CANAL 137
    Gastric secretion. Antacids. Vomiting. Drugs which relieve motion sickness. Bile. Purgatives. Protectives, demulcents, and astringents.

13. VITAMINS 144
    The water-soluble vitamins. The fat-soluble vitamins.

14. BLOOD 154

Oral iron preparations. Macrocytic anaemias. Polycythaemia vera. Blood coagulation.

15. HORMONES 161

The pituitary gland. The thyroid. The parathyroids. The pancreas. The adrenal steroids. The sex hormones.

16. RENAL PHARMACOLOGY 188

Normal functions of the kidney. Action of drugs.

17. CHEMOTHERAPY I: BACTERIA, FUNGI, VIRUSES 196

Historical. Principles of chemotherapeutic action. Resistance. Chemotherapeutic spectra. Antibacterial agents. Antifungal agents. Antiviral agents. Antiseptics.

18. CHEMOTHERAPY II: PROTOZOA AND METAZOA 214

Malaria. Leischmariasis. Trypanosomiasis. Trichomonas. Amoebiasis. Helminthiasis. Filaria. Schistosomiasis.

19. CHEMOTHERAPY III: CANCER 221

General principles of cancer chemotherapy. Antimetabolites. Alkylators. Immunosuppression.

20. QUANTITATIVE AND HUMAN PHARMACOLOGY 229

Biological assay. Sequential analysis. Qualitative pharmacological analysis. The discovery of new drugs. The development of new drugs.

ADDITIONAL GENERAL READING IN PHARMACOLOGY 249

UNITS OF MEASUREMENT 250

AQUEOUS SOLUTIONS 251

INDEX OF CHEMICAL RINGS 252

INDEX 255

1

GENERAL PHARMACOLOGY

WHAT ARE DRUGS?

DRUGS are chemical substances which, by interacting with biological systems, change them. They may cause contraction of muscles, secretion of glands, change the metabolism of tissues, and cause or prevent growth or division of cells. They may also act on the central nervous system so as to alter the pattern of behaviour, to relieve pain, or to affect some neuronal disorder such as in epilepsy or Parkinson's disease.

The fact that drugs differ in their actions means that they must be selective in the tissues with which they interact and indeed in the way that they affect different cells. Since there is no known way in which drugs can act other than by a direct combination with one or more components of the tissues, the selective action of a drug must depend on forming a combination with certain tissue components and not others.

In a few cases the selectivity of a drug for a single combining site is so great that we can call the drug *specific*; much more frequently the drug may combine with more than one site and hence produce more than one action. We talk of a drug as being highly selective if one action predominates and the other actions are not intensive.

When a drug has more than one action, the actions are often classified in a rather arbitrary fashion, with a *main action*—i.e. one that we wish to use therapeutically or pharmacologically—and *side actions*—those that are undesirable in the particular application. This division may just serve the needs of the particular situation. For instance, when we are using morphine to relieve pain, it may be a nuisance that morphine causes constipation by its action on the intestine. When we wish to reduce gut motility in the relief of diarrhoea, this action becomes our main action and the other actions of morphine become side actions.

In earlier times, drugs were mostly plant or animal substances that had been found by practical, daily experience to be toxic—eating the berries of the belladonna plant caused dilation of the pupils, a bright red flush, and convulsions, or the beans of the cascara caused violent purging—and these, together with some minerals such as arsenic trioxide or mercuric chloride, became the stock-in-trade of the pharmacist until early in the nineteenth century when pure drugs were first isolated (e.g. morphine from dried opium) and synthetic organic chemicals began to be made. Since that time most new drugs have been prepared by synthesis, although natural products have continued to be important notably for hormones (e.g. insulin) and antibacterial substances (e.g. penicillin, streptomycin, tetracycline).

DRUG ACTION ON ISOLATED TISSUES

Since the action of drugs in the body may be complicated by many factors, including distribution, metabolism, and the interaction between different systems, it is easier to investigate some of the basic actions of drugs on a simplified system such as a piece of tissue isolated from the body. One of the simplest tissues to use in this way is the small intestine. The procedure for using it was first introduced by Magnus. If a short piece of small intestine (2–5 cm) is placed in a salt solution whose ionic composition is similar to

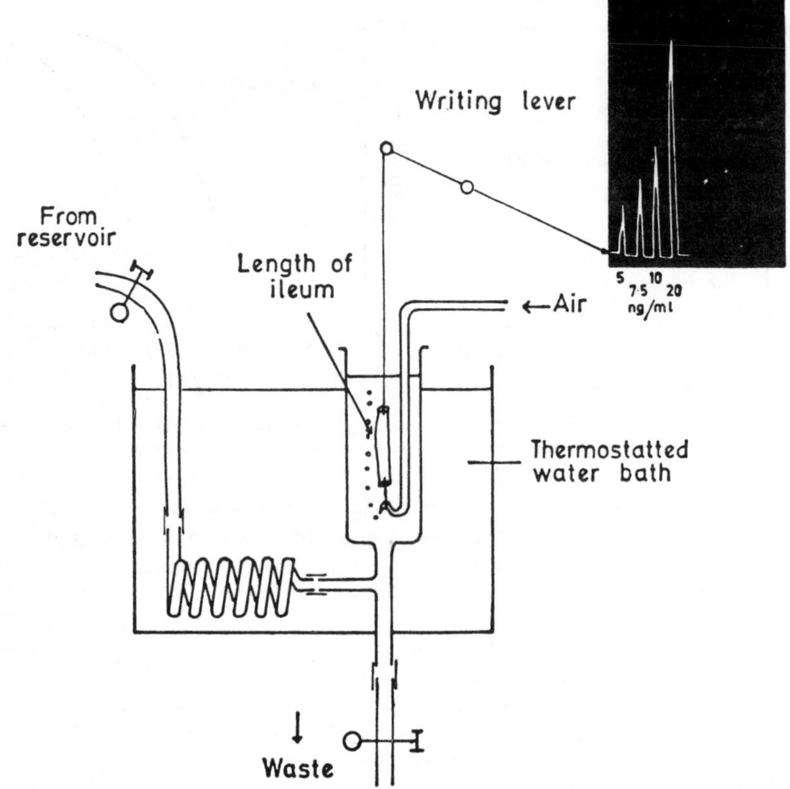

Fig 1.1. Arrangements for recording the contractions of the longitudinal muscle of the small intestine. The water bath is usually kept at about 35° C.

that of blood plasma, and the solution is kept warm and oxygen is blown through it, then the gut will survive and respond to suitable drugs for many hours. Such a piece of gut can be set up so that one end is anchored and the other is connected to a lever so that the length of the intestine is recorded (Fig. 1.1). The length of the intestine is determined by the tone of the longitudinal muscle coat, so that the addition of substances that contract this muscle will be registered as a shortening of the piece of intestine. *In vivo* this muscle layer contracts in response to activity in nerve fibres originating in the myenteric plexus. These nerves release the chemical mediator, acetylcholine (Fig. 1.2) from their terminals and it is the acetylcholine that produces the contraction rather than any direct action of the nerves. By adding a solution of acetylcholine to the bath in which the intestine is immersed we can produce a similar response. On adding the acetylcholine the muscle begins to contract within a few seconds. The muscle may be relaxed back to its original length by removing the bath fluid and replacing it by fresh fluid; the relaxation occurs rapidly and a further test may be made in a few minutes.

If we reduce the concentration of acetylcholine sufficiently we will eventually reach a

$$CH_3COOCH_2CH_2\overset{+}{N}(CH_3)_3$$

Fig. 1.2. Acetylcholine

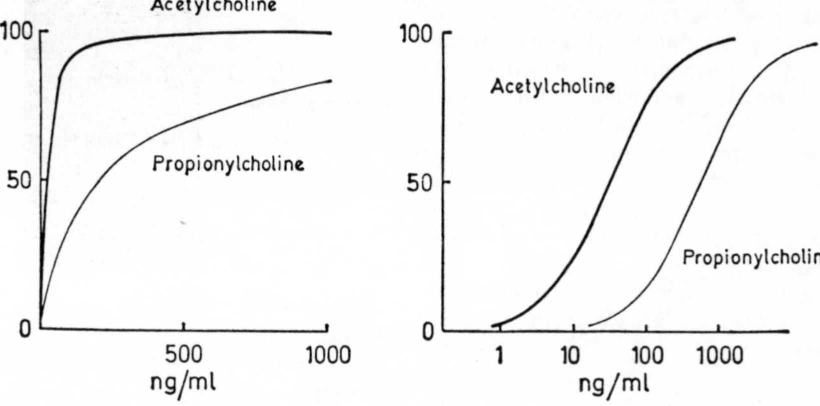

Fig. 1.3. Dose–response curves obtained on the guinea-pig ileum. The abscissa shows the contraction as a percentage of the maximum obtainable. In the left-hand graph the dose of drug is shown on a *linear* scale; in the right-hand graph on a *logarithmic* scale.

concentration that is ineffective; if we systematically increase the dose from this level we will find that the degree of contraction increases with dose until a maximum is produced, and further increase in acetycholine concentration does not produce a greater effect. The curve relating dose to response is called a *dose–response curve* and the type of curve obtained is shown in Fig. 1.3.

This graded response to drugs is the most common behaviour studied but there are, of course, cases where this cannot occur. For instance, if one is trying to find the dose of drug that kills an animal, the effect is quantal, that is, the animal either dies or survives and no intermediate category of 'half dead' exists. The way such responses can be examined is discussed in detail in Chapter 20.

Although acetylcholine is the natural excitant agent for the longitudinal muscle, it is not necessarily the case that the chemical structure of this substance is unique in being able to produce this action. If we look at the structure of acetylcholine we see that it is the ester of the quarternary ammonium base choline with acetic acid. One of the simplest and most informative ways of finding out how specific a chemical structure is needed for a biological action is by preparing a homologous series. This is done by modifying a particular chemical group by the addition or removal of carbon atoms. In the present case we can do this by preparing esters of choline with the series of normal aliphatic acids—formic, acetic, propionic, butyric, valeric, etc. (Fig. 1.4).

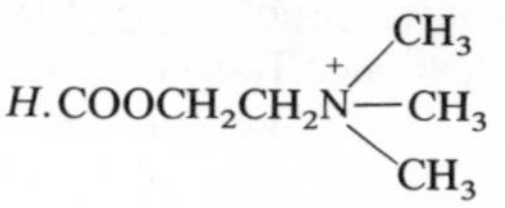

$$H.COOCH_2CH_2\overset{+}{N}(CH_3)_3$$

formylcholine

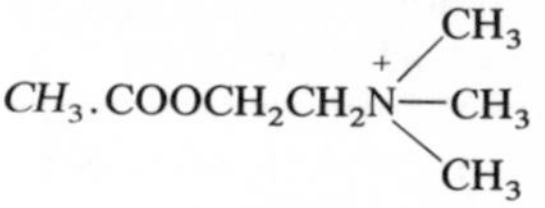

$$CH_3.COOCH_2CH_2\overset{+}{N}(CH_3)_3$$

acetylcholine

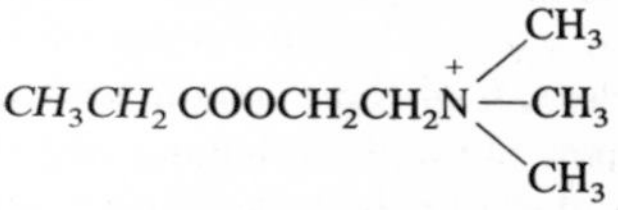

$$CH_3CH_2\,COOCH_2CH_2\overset{+}{N}(CH_3)_3$$

propionylcholine

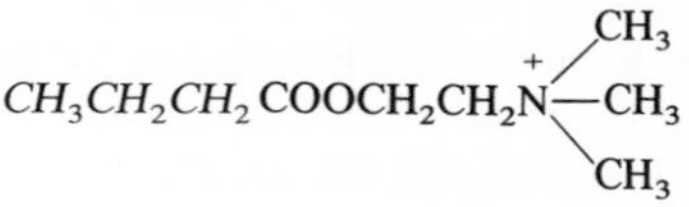

$$CH_3CH_2CH_2\,COOCH_2CH_2\overset{+}{N}(CH_3)_3$$

butyrylcholine

$$CH_3CH_2CH_2CH_2\,COOCH_2CH_2\overset{+}{N}(CH_3)_3$$

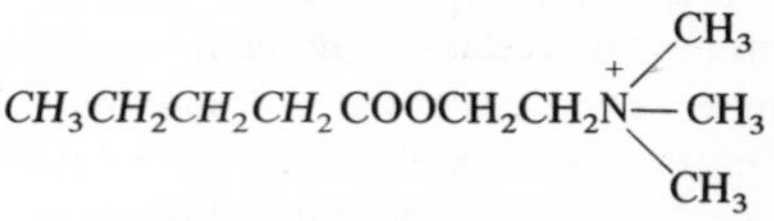

valerylcholine

Fig. 1.4.

Let us now test *propionylcholine* in the same way that we did acetylcholine on the intestine. It also produces a contraction that is graded with dose and when sufficient propionycholine is added to the bath a maximum contraction is produced that is exactly the same as that produced by acetylcholine. The form of the dose–response curve is shown in Fig. 1.3. The only difference is that about twenty times as much propionylcholine is needed to produce any level of response as is needed for acetylcholine. We can say that propionylcholine is a *full agonist* (an agonist is a drug producing a directly observable physiological effect; it is *full* because it produces the same maximum as a related drug) but its *potency* is 5 per cent of that of acetylcholine. If we now test butyrylcholine we find that it is about ten times weaker than propionylcholine and that the maximum response produced is not as great as that of acetylcholine or propionylcholine; it is therefore called a *partial agonist,* its potency is only 0·5 per cent of acetylcholine. The next member of the series, valerylcholine, produces no effect at all and is not an agonist. At the other end of the scale formylcholine is active, is a full agonist, and has about 25 per cent of the potency of acetylcholine.

We have learned from these experiments that acetylcholine is not unique amongst the normal aliphatic esters of choline in being able to contract intestinal smooth muscle but that it is the *most potent* of the series. We find that small changes of chain length are tolerable but give reduced potency, and that lengthening by more than two carbon atoms leads to complete loss of ability to cause contraction.

Similar homologous changes can be made in the length of the alcohol group and in the methyl groups or the nitrogen. The results are similar i.e. acetylcholine is the optimal structure. Small changes can be made with retention of reduced activity, and larger changes cause loss of agonist activity.

We can next look at whether the particular chemical groupings in acetylcholine are essential for activity. Apart from the methylene and methyl groups, the acetylcholine molecule consists of a carbonyl, an ester oxygen, and the positively charged onium. In Table 1.1 the effects of changing some of these groups can be seen. Replacement of the carbonyl by a methylene reduces potency by a factor of twelve, the replacement of the ester oxygen has a larger effect. However, when the side chain is replaced by a normal paraffin with the same number of backbone atoms, (n-pentyl) activity still remains, as it does even in the very simple compound tetramethylammonium.

Table 1.1.

	Relative activity
$CH_3—CO—O—CH_2CH_2\overset{+}{N}(CH_3)_3$ Acetylcholine	*100*
$CH_3—\mathit{CH_2}—O—CH_2CH_2\overset{+}{N}(CH_3)_3$ Choline ethylether	8
$CH_3—CO—\mathit{CH_2}—CH_2CH_2\overset{+}{N}(CH_3)_3$ 4-ketopentyl trimethylammonium	0·5
$CH_3—\mathit{CH_2}—\mathit{CH_2}—CH_2CH_2\overset{+}{N}(CH_3)_3$ Pentyl trimethylammonium	0·5
$CH_3\overset{+}{N}(CH_3)_3$ Tetramethylammonium	0·1

Up to this point we have applied simple chemical reasoning to the study of a structure activity series, but new drugs are often found as a result of *screening,* i.e. new chemical compounds are tested empirically on a biological system to see if they have activity and by this means activity may be found in quite unexpected structures. Table 1.2 shows the structure of five such compounds and in the case of three of them the activity is greater than that of acetylcholine. Muscarine and arecoline are natural compounds obtained from toadstools and betel nuts respectively. The other three compounds were prepared synthetically. The first three compounds show obvious structural resemblances to acetylcholine: they all have a terminal methyl group connected through a carbon–oxygen–carbon linkage to a final $—CH_2\overset{+}{N}(CH_3)_3$. In the case of arecoline the resemblance is not nearly so obvious, and in the case of oxotremorine it is really rather remote. When the resemblance to the parent compound is so slight we must bear in mind

Table 1.2.

Compound	*Relative activity*
$CH_3-C(=O)-O-CH_2-CH_2-\overset{+}{N}(CH_3)_3$ Acetylcholine	100
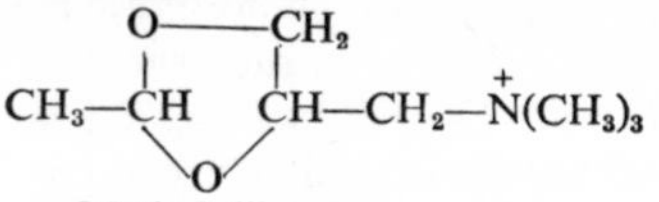 CH_3-CH … $CH-CH_2-\overset{+}{N}(CH_3)_3$ (ring: O—CH_2, O) Methyl dilvasene	1000
OH, CH—CH_2, CH_3-CH … $CH-CH_2-\overset{+}{N}(CH_3)_3$ (ring O) Muscarine	300
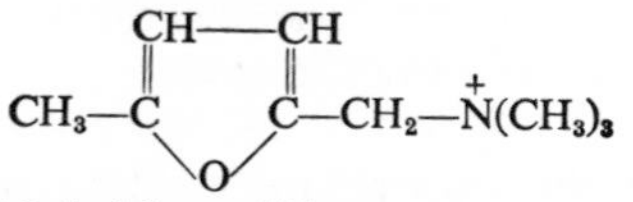 CH═CH, CH_3-C … $C-CH_2-\overset{+}{N}(CH_3)_3$ (ring O) Methyl furmethide	300
$CH_3OC(=O)$–, ring $\overset{+}{N}$ with CH_3 and H Arecoline	100
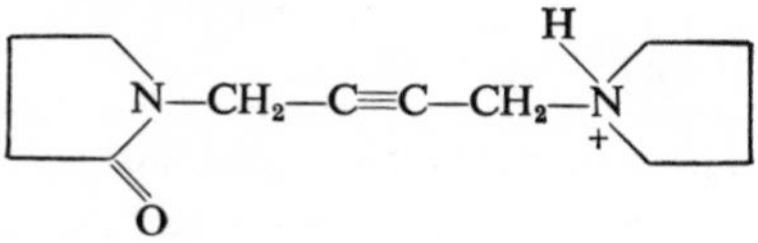 (ring, =O) $N-CH_2-C{\equiv}C-CH_2-\overset{+}{N}$(H)(ring) Oxotremorine	50

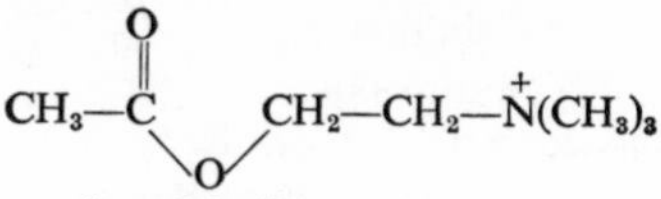

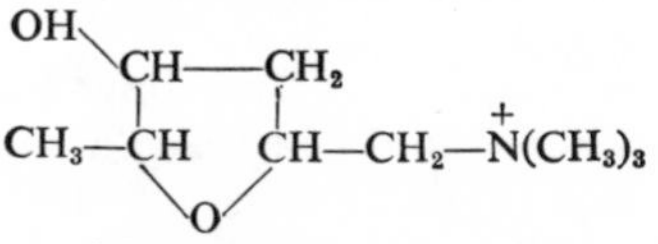

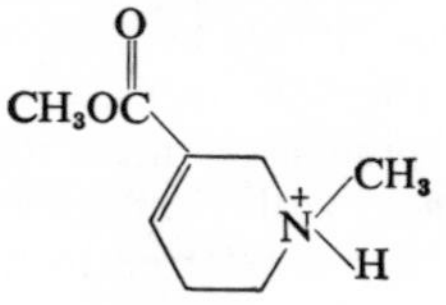

the possibility that this drug is not acting by the same mechanism. We will return to this point later.

What we have shown then is that the chemical structure of acetylcholine is not a unique requirement for the type of action it produces on smooth muscle. This fact gives great scope to the synthetic chemist and is the philosophical basis of new drug development. The principle is a general one that applies to all drug types, although the variety of structure permissible with retention of activity varies widely.

DOSE–RESPONSE CURVES

In Fig. 1.3 the dose–response curves for acetylcholine and propionylcholine have been plotted in two ways. In the left-hand panel the dose has been plotted along the abscissa on an arithmetical scale. The form of the curve is that of a rectangular hyperbola. In the case of acetylcholine the values corresponding to the main part of the curve are compressed at the left side of the graph. On the other hand, with the less potent propionylcholine the main part of the curve is displayed but the upper values cannot be included. To the unpractised eye the resemblances between the shape of the two curves is not obvious.

In the right-hand curve of Fig. 1.3 the doses on the abscissa have been placed on a logarithmic scale. The effect is to turn the curve into a symmetric S-shape which accommodates all the values for acetylcholine. It is equally effective at accommodating all the values for propionylcholine and gives a curve identical in form but displaced to the right (i.e. to higher doses) because of its lower potency. It is now obvious that at all doses the potency of propionylcholine is lower than that of acetylcholine by a fixed ratio (20) corresponding to 1·3 log units shift along the abscissa. We can refer to the curves as *parallel.*

Log dose–response curves are almost invariably used for plotting the results of pharmacological measurements for the following reasons:

1. Most commonly, substances acting on the same biological system give curves of the same form; on a log scale this is easy to see, and the parallelism of the curves can be observed.
2. Ratios of potencies are easily estimated.
3. A logarithmic scale gives an equal weighting to all dose levels and so allows a wide range of doses to be plotted on a single graph without compression of any part of the curve. It allows accurate plotting of the responses to substances even when they differ in potency by a large ratio.
4. The middle part of the response range is very nearly linear. If responses between 20 per cent and 80 per cent of the

maximum are obtained, a straight line may be drawn through these points; this is very useful when the curve must be defined from only two or three observations.

ANTAGONISTS

Up to this point we have taken as evidence of drug action a contraction of the longitudinal muscle which we have called an agonist response. We have not considered the possibility that the drug might be interacting with the tissue in such a way that it does not produce an *observable response* directly but might be able to modify the response of the tissue to an agonist.

An example of this is shown in Fig. 1.5. The dose–response relationship for acetylcholine was established and then atropine sulphate was added to the Ringer solution bathing the intestine. No direct effect was produced by atropine but when, after a few minutes, the response to acetylcholine was retested, the response to the lowest dose of acetylcholine was barely perceptible. However, when increased doses of acetylcholine were used, larger responses were obtained

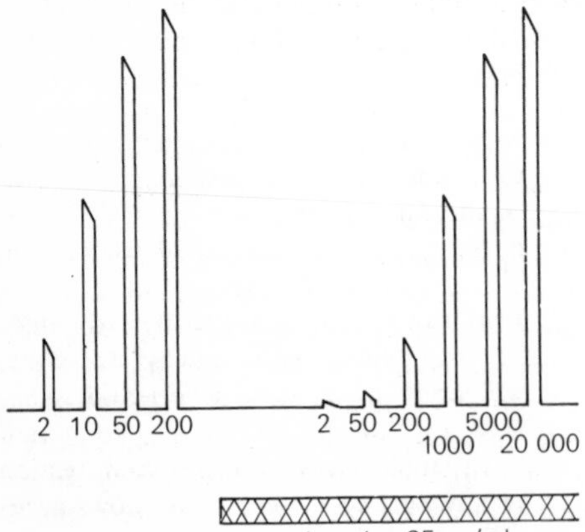

Fig. 1.5. The contractions of the ileum shown on the left part of the curve were produced by the concentrations of acetylcholine marked under each curve. After adding atropine, 25 ng/ml, to the fluid bathing the intestine larger doses of acetylcholine were required to produce effects equal to those produced before atropine was added.

and indeed with a large enough dose a maximum response was obtainable that was not smaller than before atropine was applied. When the muscle was immersed again in Ringer solution containing no atropine the normal sensitivity to acetylcholine gradually becomes restored, i.e. the antagonism is reversible. If we look carefully at Fig. 1.5 we will see that to obtain matching sizes of response, one hundred times the concentration of acetylcholine is needed in the presence of atropine. If we plot the log dose–response curve of acetylcholine in the presence of atropine it is shifted to the right and the effect is to make acetylcholine appear to be one hundred times less potent as an agonist (Fig. 1.6). If a lower concentration of atropine is used, the shift to the right is less, and with a higher concentration the shift is greater; the degree of antagonism is thus dose dependent. The degree of antagonism can be conveniently characterized by the ratio of the dose of agonist needed to produce a matching response in the presence of the antagonist to that in its absence, thus is referred to as the *dose ratio* (d); the rule governing the relationship of d to concentration of antagonist is that

$$(d-1) \propto \text{concentration of antagonist.}$$

It is well to note that with the antagonist action studied here, where the antagonism can be overcome by increased concentration of agonist, the antagonist action is often referred to as *competitive*.

The simplest explanation of the results with atropine is that, if acetylcholine combines with an 'acetylcholine receptor' to produce its action, then atropine combines with the same receptor *without* producing an action but denies access to the receptor by acetylcholine. The antagonistic effect of atropine is thus due to its ability to compete with acetylcholine for the acetylcholine receptor. Our earlier discussion of structure activity of acetylcholine congeners emphasized points of chemical resemblance, yet atropine at first sight (Fig. 1.7) has little resemblance to acetylcholine. Certainly there is an ester grouping and a basic nitrogen, but

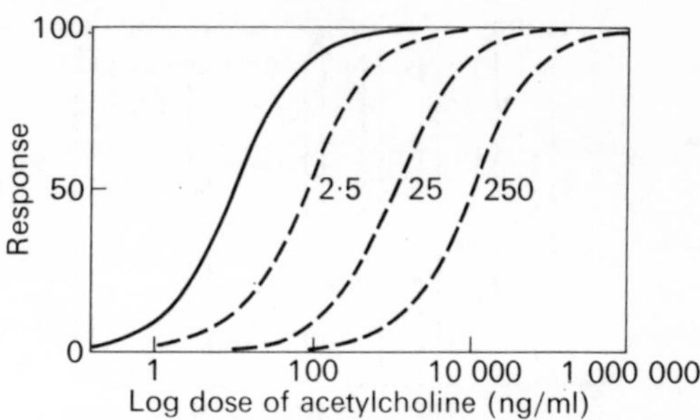

Fig. 1.6. Antagonism of acetylcholine by atropine on the isolated guineapig ileum. The *solid curve* is the dose response curve in the absence of atropine. The hatched curves are the atetylcholine dose response curves in the presence of the concentration of atropine indicated (ng/ml).

beyond that the similarity is less obvious. However, the hypothesis gains ground when we reconsider the longer-chain esters of choline of which valerylcholine is an example. We noted earlier that this substance was not an agonist. However, in appropriate concentration it will reduce the response to acetylcholine and behaves just like atropine, although it is much less potent. In fact we

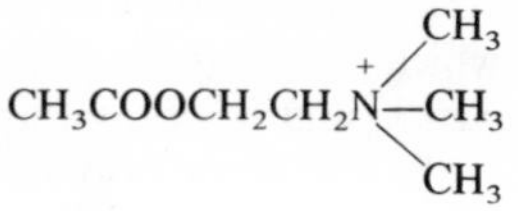

$CH_3COOCH_2CH_2\overset{+}{N}(CH_3)_3$

acetylcholine

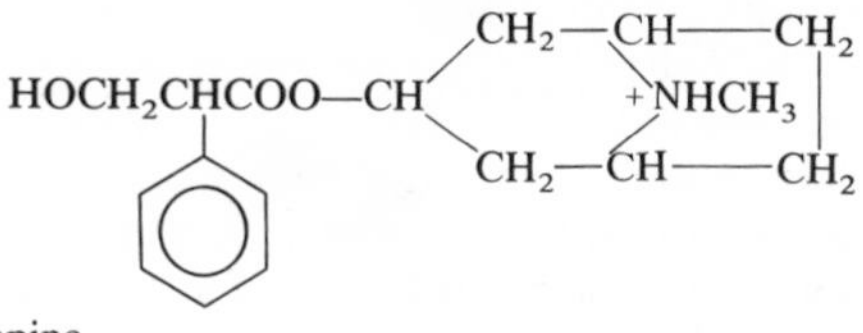

$HOCH_2CH(C_6H_5)COO{-}CH\langle(CH_2{-}CH{-}CH_2)(CH_2{-}CH{-}CH_2)\rangle\overset{+}{N}HCH_3$

atropine

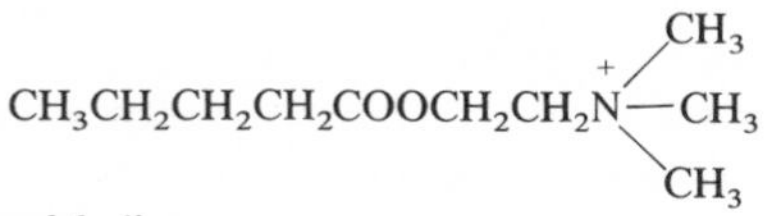

$CH_3CH_2CH_2CH_2COOCH_2CH_2\overset{+}{N}(CH_3)_3$

valerylcholine

$(C_6H_5)_2C(OH){-}COO{-}CH_2CH_2\overset{+}{N}(CH_3)_3$

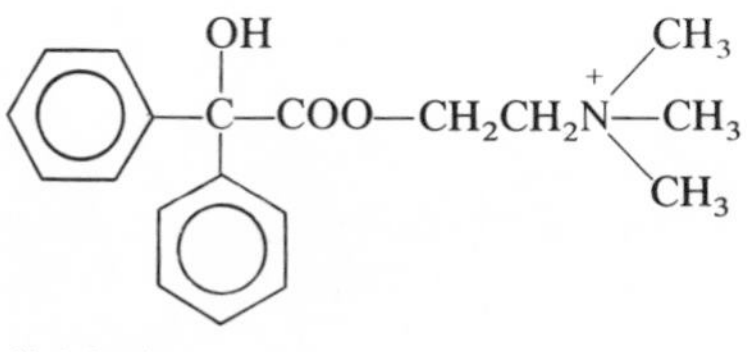

benzilylcholine

Fig. 1.7.

find that it is a general rule that when the acyl part of acetylcholine is substituted by bulky residues, particularly aromatic groups, potent antagonists are produced; for instance, the choline ester of benzilic acid has about the same potency as atropine.

Since the resemblance to acetylcholine is more obvious in these compounds, it becomes more plausible that they might be combining with the same receptor.

It is apparent that this proposal also makes the assumption that atropine and related antagonists should not only antagonize the actions of acetylcholine itself but should also antagonize the actions of *all other agonists interacting with the same receptor.* This is indeed found to be the case and, for instance, it confirms that oxotremorine, in spite of its unusual chemical structure, also combines with this receptor. Indeed, with few exceptions the quantitative nature of the antagonism applies to all the agonists so that the *same dose ratio* is found for a given concentration of antagonist.

Suppose, however that one of the agonists we had included in our structure–activity series was not producing contraction of the ileum by combining with the acetylcholine receptor but really belonged to a totally different class of drugs and reacted with a *different receptor*; in this case we would expect that an acetylcholine antagonist such as atropine would not antagonize it.

Among the substances that contract the smooth muscle of the guinea-pig ileum is histamine; it has a similar potency to acetylcholine, produces the same maximum response, and gives a similar log dose–response

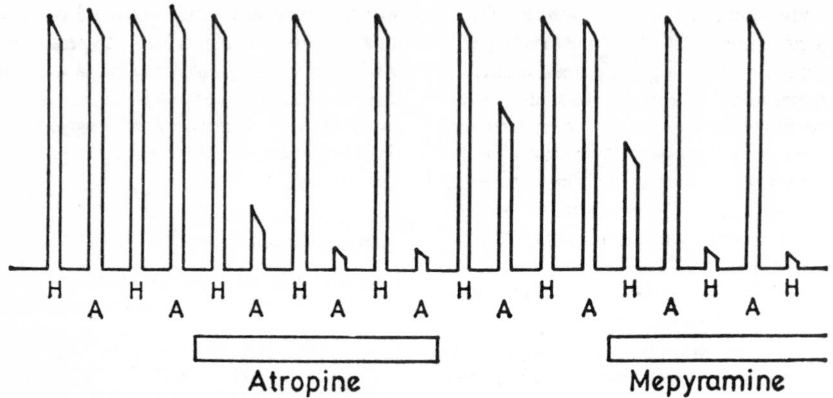

Fig. 1.8. The ileum was made to contract by addition of alternate doses of acetylcholine (A) and histamine (H). Atropine selectively antagonizes the acetylcholine effects and mepyramine the histamine effects.

curve. Its structure (p. 117) is not very similar to acetylcholine, but we have learnt to treat this lack of similarity with some caution. Let us apply the antagonist test. The test procedure is shown in Fig. 1.8. Doses of acetylcholine and histamine are chosen which give responses of similar size and are applied alternately. Atropine is then added to the bath, the acetylcholine response rapidly declines in size but the histamine response remains unchanged. This suggests that histamine is not combining with the same receptor as acetylcholine (and atropine). It might be possible to find an antagonist that is selective for the histamine receptor. In fact many such **antihistamines** are known of which mepyramine (p. 117) may be used as an example. If a suitable concentration of mepyramine is now added to the Ringer solution in the organ bath, the histamine response is reduced rapidly without any effect on the acetylcholine response. This experiment shows how in the use of selective antagonists we have a very satisfactory and discriminating criterion for distinguishing between types of receptors and hence between groups of drugs.

So far we have considered the action of acetylcholine on one tissue, the smooth muscle of the ileum. We need now to ask the question, whether the characteristics of acetylcholine action on other tissues are the same. Acetylcholine also acts on skeletal muscle being in addition the chemical mediator at motor nerve terminals. We can conveniently study structure–activity relationships by using the rectus abdominis muscle of the frog which responds to acetylcholine by a contraction and can be set up in an isolated organ bath in a similar way to the ileum. When we look at the potency of the acetylcholine series on this tissue we find that propionylcholine is four times as active as acetylcholine, not one twentieth as active as on the ileum (Table 1.3) and that butyrylcholine is also more active than acetylcholine, and that even valerylcholine retains about one third of the activity of acetylcholine. It is evident that acetylcholine is not the optimum structure on this tissue and that the *structure–activity relationships*

Table 1.3. Activity relative to acetylcholine
The relative potencies of a homologous series of choline esters in causing contractions of the guinea-pig ileum and the frog rectus abdominis muscle.

	Ileum	Rectus abdominis
Formylcholine	25	10
Acetylcholine	*100*	*100*
Propionylcholine	5	400
Butyrylcholine	0·5	150
Valerylcholine	0	30

are not the same as for the ileum. This is prima facie evidence that we are dealing with a different receptor and we would expect to find confirmation of this by the use of antagonists. Sure enough, atropine in concentrations that are strongly antagonistic in the ileum is totally without effect on the rectus. On the other hand, *d*-tubocurarine and gallamine are potent antagonists for acetylcholine on the rectus but are ineffective on the ileum. The existence of two distinct receptors for acetylcholine was first envisaged by Dale when he described two actions which he referred to as muscarine-like and nicotine-like. Dale was in fact comparing the kind of actions we have seen on the ileum with muscarine, a drug that is higly selective for this acetylcholine receptor and inactive on skeletal muscle, whereas nicotine is active on skeletal muscle but inactive on smooth muscle.

In fact, using the criteria that we have now established, i.e. structure—activity relationships in agonists and selective antagonists, we can show that **muscarinic receptors** for acetylcholine seem to be very similar whether they are in intestinal smooth muscle, the heart, blood vessels, salivary glands, or central nervous system. The **nicotinic type** of receptor is found only in skeletal muscle, autonomic ganglia, and to a minor extent, in the central nervous system. The existence of a receptor that is distributed in many tissues of course defines the basic spectrum of activity of the drug when administered systemically; it is no use expecting atropine to have a selective effect on the intestine, since it will also produce a drying of the mouth, increase in heart rate, and defective focusing of the eye, due to its action on the muscarinic receptors in these tissues.

Although receptors may have similar properties, as indicated by sensitivity to agonists and antagonists, this does not necessarily indicate that the *effects* produced by activating the receptor are the same.

For instance the action of acetylcholine on the muscarinic receptor in the intestinal muscle is to depolarize it and to cause it to contract, whereas in the auricle it causes hyperpolarization and reduced contractility, and in the salivary gland hyperpolarization and secretion. Therefore, it is evident that the muscarinic receptor is in some way coupled to a variety of *effector* mechanisms that initiate the physiological responses that are produced.

WHAT ARE DRUG RECEPTORS?

Our analysis of drug action has been related to a specific tissue component with which the agonist and antagonist interact. Is this simply a useful concept or can we isolate an actual receptor substance and purify and characterize it? Until recently little success had been achieved in dealing with this problem, but methods now exist for studying many pharmacological receptors and in one case the nicotine receptor structural studies have made substantial progress.

The simplest way of studying drug receptors directly is by measuring the binding of radioactively-labelled antagonists and agonists to whole tissue and to purified components of the tissues. These permit the measurement of the concentration of the receptors as well as a binding constant. Fig. 1.9 shows such a study in which the binding of *N*-methylatropine to muscarinic receptors in rat brain was measured. In this case the binding capacity was 1·2 nmol/g protein which would correspond to a few thousand receptor sites per cell. The binding constant is tested by the simple theory of formation of a bimolecular complex (called the law of mass action). The equilibrium

$$\mathrm{D}+\mathrm{R} \overset{K}{\rightleftharpoons} \mathrm{DR}$$

is governed by the affinity constant *K*. The proportion of the receptor complexed by the drug is

$$p=\frac{\mathrm{D}K}{\mathrm{D}K+1}$$

where the function *p* is known as the *occupancy*. When the product $\mathrm{D}K=1$ then $p=0{\cdot}5$ and hence we can conclude that the *reciprocal* of the concentration that produces half occupancy of the receptor gives the *affinity constant* of the drug for the receptor.

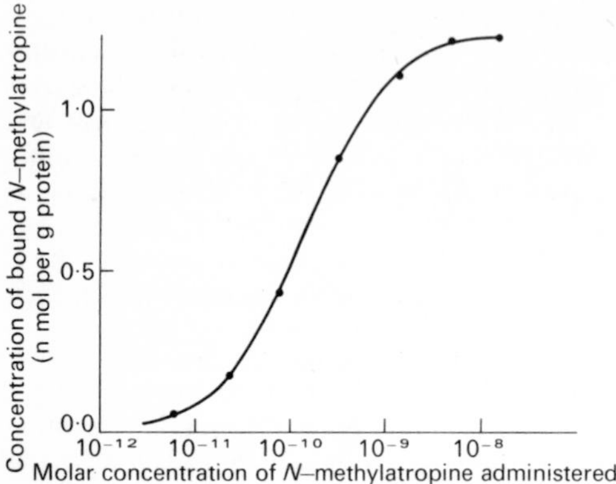

Fig. 1.9. The binding of tritium-labelled *N*-methylatropine to a cell membrane preparation from rat brain. The maximum amount bound corresponds to the amount of receptor present and is 1·2 nmol/g of protein.

In this case the affinity constant is $7 \times 10^9\,\text{M}^{-1}$. In our discussion of antagonists we suggested that antagonists acted by competing with agonists for the receptor, and in fact a minor reformulation of the quantitative relationship discussed earlier gives

$$(d-1) = \text{D}K$$

so that an apparent affinity constant of the antagonist can be derived in this way from the pharmacological experiment. The affinity constants of antagonists derived pharmacologically and by direct binding studies agree very well with each other. In addition, the predicted competitative behaviour between pairs of antagonists or between antagonists and agonists occur.

As yet the only membrane-binding receptor that has been characterized chemically is the nicotinic receptor in the electric organ of electric fishes (the nicotinic receptor in skeletal muscle appears to be very similar). In this case the binding site for the drugs is a protein of molecular weight ~250 000. From their properties it seems likely that other membrane receptors will have a similar constitution and it appears that probably all such receptors will be protein-like molecules.

The part of the receptor sensitive to drugs is on the outside of the cell; this has been shown most elegantly by applying acetylcholine from a micropipette. When the application is made to the outside of the cell depolarization occurs, but no effect is seen when the application is made to the inside of the cell. It is also possible to locate the receptors by a histochemical method (Fig. 1.10).

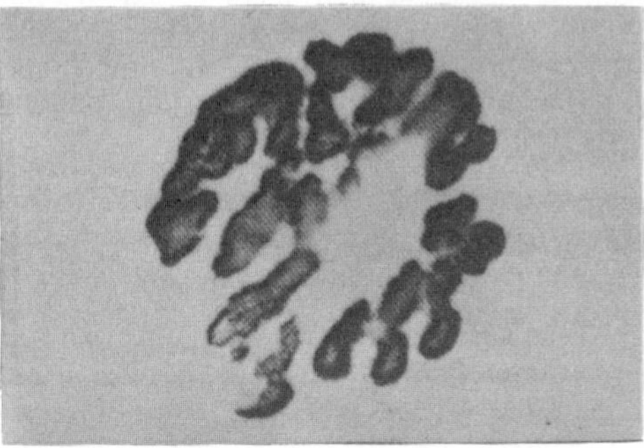

Fig. 1.10. Distribution of nicotinic acetylcholine receptors at the neuromuscular junction. The receptor has been localized by immersing the muscle fragment in α-bungarotoxin tagged with fluorescein. The picture was obtained by fluorescence microscopy. (Photograph by the courtesy of M. W. Cohen).

HOW DO DRUG RECEPTORS WORK?

When agonists act on cells they may lead to a change in ionic permeability. The best studied of these changes is at the motor end-plate where activation of the nicotinic receptors leads to a large increase in passive permeability for sodium and potassium ions. The effect appears to be a direct one since it is very rapid. Permeability changes can also be detected in fragments of electroplax in which metabolic activity has ceased. It appears that the nicotinic receptor is directly coupled to an ion **permease** in the membrane whose properties are changed when acetylcholine combines with the receptor.

In other tissues receptor activation seems to lead to activation of enzymes so that metabolic changes ensue. The best examples of this are found in the adrenergic system where catecholamines cause the activation of the membrane enzyme adenylcyclase. This is discussed in detail in Chapter 8.

How does the interaction of an agonist with a receptor activate either a permease or an enzyme? The explanation that seems most plausible is that the receptor undergoes a change of shape (conformation) which is communicated to the permease or enzyme, and by changing their shape makes them active. Regulation of conformation of this sort is well established with soluble multisubunit enzymes. It is presumed that antagonists combine with the receptor without being able to induce the appropriate conformation changes.

GENERAL CONSIDERATIONS OF RECEPTORS AND SPECIFICITY

We have so far concentrated on a consideration of acetylcholine and its receptors because both the chemistry and pharmacology are rather straightforward. The principles that we have uncovered are quite general. In order that drugs may have a specific effect they must combine with receptors. Receptors may be membrane-bound neuroreceptors, or hormonal receptors, they may be enzyme catalytic or control sites, or concerned with the tertiary structure of a protein (e.g. colchicine and the intracellular protein tubulin) or nucleic acid.

The combination of the drug with its receptor depends on the operation of weak intermolecular forces; these may be due to ion–ion interactions, hydrogen bonds, long-range dispersion forces, or to a minimization of the effects of the solvent (hydrophobic interaction). Since each of these forces is weak, the overall interaction depends on the co-operation of many component forces, the number and strength of which will depend on how appropriate the fit of the drug is for the receptor. This topology of the fit is what lies behind structure–activity relationships and the selective interaction of a drug with one receptor rather than another. It is perfectly possible for a drug to combine with more than one receptor and hence have actions that belong to more than one class of drug, and it is comparatively uncommon for a drug to show complete specificity. For instance, atropine *does* combine with histamine receptors at a concentration some thousand times greater than that needed to inhibit muscarinic receptors, but on the other hand diphenhydramine shows rather little discrimination between these two receptors. It is thus possible to build specificity or a broader sensitivity into drug structures.

WHAT IS THE NORMAL FUNCTION OF DRUG RECEPTORS?

In the case of the muscarinic and nicotinic receptors, the physiological function in both cases is associated with the action of acetylcholine at the relevant synapses. Drugs here can be regarded as chemical analogues of the physiological material. In other cases, a similar analogy is equally clear. For instance the antifolic methotrexate is an analogue of the normal substrate of the enzyme dihydrofolic reductase, namely dihydrofolic acid. As knowledge of the targets of drug action becomes elucidated it becomes clearer that there are likely to be few exceptions to the rule that **drugs act by combining with receptors for which there is a physiological substrate or mediator**. This rule may be restated in the form that drugs owe their activity to the fact that they are analogues of natural mediators, hormones, or biochemical substrates.

This way of looking at drugs has practical consequences. The classical way of discovering a drug was to make a new chemical and then test it empirically for actions on biological systems. Later, through further understanding of the biological system it became possible to provide a rational explanation for why the drug produced its actions. With our greater understanding of biological systems it is now frequently possible to consider the physiological system and *design* an analogue to mimic or interfere with the physiological mediator. The scope of drug development can be seen to be extremely wide and whereas only a few hundred classes of drugs are at present known, potentially there are many thousands more waiting to be discovered.

FURTHER READING

Ariëns, E. J. and Rossum, J. M. van (1964). *Molecular pharmacology*, London.

Barlow, R. B. (1964). *Introduction to chemical pharmacology*, London.

Burgen, A. S. V. (1970). Drug receptors. *Ann. Rev. Pharmacol.*

Burger, A. (1970). *Medicinal chemistry*, New York.

Clark, A. J. (1933). *The mode of action of drugs on cells*, London.

Cuatrecasas, P. and Hollenberg, M. D. (1976). Membrane receptors and hormone action. *Adv. Protein Chem.* **30**.

Goldstein, A., Aronow, L., and Kalman, S. M. (1974). *Principles of drug action*, New York.

Korolkovas, A. (1970). *Essentials of molecular pharmacology*, New York.

Porter, R. and O'Connor, M. (1970). *Molecular properties of drug receptors*, London.

Triggle, D. J. (1965). *Chemical aspects of the autonomic nervous system*, London.

2

DRUG KINETICS

THE term drug kinetics (or **pharmacokinetics**) refers to the processes concerned with the distribution of drugs in the body, their absorption, excretion, and metabolism. In short it is concerned with the processes that determine the concentration of drug that is attained at its site of action.

DISTRIBUTION OF DRUGS AFTER INTRAVENOUS INJECTION

When a drug is injected into the blood stream it will become evenly distributed in the plasma within two or three circulation times (~1 minute) provided it is unable to leave the circulation. The volume of distribution (in man) corresponds to 40 ml/kg body weight, so that if the dose of drug is 1 g/kg the concentration achieved will be 25 g/l in the plasma. Drugs stay within the plasma compartment either if they are macromolecules comparable in size to the plasma proteins or if they are rapidly and strongly bound to the plasma protein. The plasma proteins do slowly exchange with protein in the tissue fluid over a period of a day or two, so that even under these circumstances the plasma concentration of the drug will slowly fall to about half of its initial value.

If the drug is of low molecular weight (say under 1000) and not bound to protein it will be rapidly distributed in the water space between the cells which has a volume of 140 ml/kg—i.e. at equilibrium the drug concentration following the injection of 1 g/kg will be 5·5 g/l. Exchange with the extracellular fluid occurs relatively quickly and will be effectively complete in 10–60 minutes.

The further movement of the drug into the intracellular water depends on the ease with which the drug can penetrate cell membranes. Drugs that are insoluble in lipids penetrate cell membranes only very slowly and hence are effectively excluded. This applies, for example, to the quaternary ammonium ganglion-blocking drugs, such as hexamethonium. Lipid-soluble drugs such as anaesthetics will penetrate rapidly and the concentration in the intracellular water will be one equilibrated with that in the extracellular space. Since the volume of intracellular water is 400 ml/kg, the equilibrium plasma concentration after a dose of 1 g/kg will be ~1·7 g/l (Table 2.1).

Lipid-soluble drugs will also dissolve in the body fat so that the effective volume of distribution for these drugs will be increased considerably beyond that available in the body water.

The picture we have considered so far is essentially an equilibrium one, but the kinetics of the drug concentrations have important consequences for drug action. Let us consider now the kinetics of a low molecular weight drug, which is not plasma bound and which has a distribution coefficient of *one* between lipids and water.

The drug will equilibrate very rapidly in the tissues, so that the concentration in the tissues will equal that in the *venous blood* leaving the tissue. Therefore the rate at which the concentration of drug in each tissue will increase depends on the blood flow to the tissue—this process is called *blood-flow limited access*. If all the tissues were perfused at the same rate, the concentration in the tissues would increase at the same rate, but this is not the case. Some tissues—notably the brain, heart, kidneys, and liver—are perfused at high rates, whereas the subcutaneous fat and bones are perfused at very low rates, and skin and muscle are perfused at intermediate rates (Table 2.2) but depend very much on activity and the ambient temperature. The rapidly perfused organs contribute only a small fraction of the body mass but rapidly acquire a drug concentration equal to

Table 2.1. Concentration of drugs when distributed in body compartments

	Volume (ml/kg)	1 g/kg distributed in	
Plasma water	40	40 ml/kg	= 25 g/kg
Extracellular water	140	140 + 40 ml/kg	= 5·5 g/kg
Intracellular water	400	400 + 140 + 40 ml/kg	= 1·7 g/kg

that in the *arterial plasma*. The concentration in the slowly perfused organs rises more slowly and, as it does so, the concentration in the plasma and rapidly perfused organs falls due to the redistribution of the drug. This redistribution occurs with a half-life of 20–40 minutes and is effectively complete in 2 hours (Fig. 2.1). This phenomenon has important consequences; for instance, if an intravenous anaesthetic is given quickly it will produce rapid effects on the central nervous system that will start to wane within a few minutes and will reach a steady level only after 2 hours. The evanescent effects of intravenous anaesthetics are largely as a result of this. It can be seen that after intravenous injection the rapidly perfused tissues are exposed to very high concentrations of the drug, and for this reason this mode of administration can be very dangerous, particularly if the drug has actions on the *heart or brain.*

If the drug has only a low solubility in lipids it will not be able to enter the intracellular space so rapidly, and the tissue concentration will not come into equilibrium with the plasma concentration in one passage, the result will be that there will be much less difference in the concentrations of drug in the rapidly and slowly perfused tissues; this is called a *diffusion-limited access.* On the other hand, when the drug is much more soluble in lipids than in water, the subcutaneous fat acts as a very large reservoir into which the drug is slowly transported and from which it is only slowly released as drug removal from the plasma occurs by other processes, such as excretion and metabolism. The adipose tissue thus acts as a reservoir whose size is in-

Table 2.2. Blood flow in various parts of the body

	Mass (kg)	% Body weight	Blood flow 1/min	% Cardiac output	Turnover time (minutes)
Well perfused					
Kidneys	0·3	0·5	1·25	23	0·25
Heart	0·3	0·5	0·25	5	1
Brain	1·4	2·2	0·75	14	2
Liver	2·6	4·1	1·50	28	2
		7·3		70	
Poorly perfused					
Skin	4	6·3	0·45	8	9
Muscle	30	48	0·83	16	35
Skeleton	13	21	0·2	4	65
Fat	11	17	0·15	3	70
Total	63		5·4		

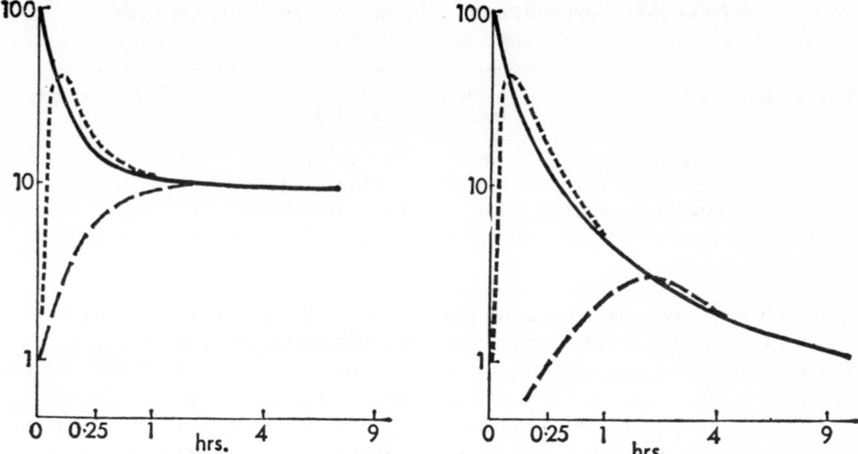

Fig. 2.1. Distribution of a drug after intravenous injection. The drug in the left-hand panel is equally soluble in oil and water and is not protein bound. That in the right-hand panel was about ten times as soluble in oil as in water.

——— Concentration in the plasma.
------ Concentration in rapidly perfused organs, i.e. brain, heart, liver, kidneys.
– – – – Concentration in slowly perfused organs, i.e. muscle, bone.

creased in proportion to the oil/water distribution coefficient and with which equilibration occurs with a half-time equivalent to the tissue mass × oil/water distribution coefficient divided by the blood flow. The right-hand part of Fig. 2.1 illustrates the effects produced. Notice that the fall in plasma concentration is not affected by high lipid solubility in the first 10–15 minutes after administration; it is in the later phases that the blood concentration continues to fall. This effect is important in determining the relative brevity of action of the barbiturate thiopentone (o/w 2) and the inhalational anaesthetic halothane (o/w 60). However, the reservoir effect also means that the concentration of drug in the adipose tissue takes a long time to be dissipated; with halothane the time for half removal may be as much as a week. The highly lipid-soluble insecticide dicophane (DDT) may remain in the body fat for many months after administration.

Protein binding of drugs

Many drugs are strongly bound to plasma proteins (mainly to plasma albumin). Apart from the effect on the distribution of the drug mentioned earlier, this also has some important effects. First, if the site of action of the drug is not within the circulation, the equilibrium concentration of the drug in the extravascular space will be that of the *unbound* fraction in the plasma. Plasma binding thus has the effect of reducing the effectiveness of the drug. Secondly, the excretion of the drug will normally be reduced so that its biological half time may be very long. Thirdly, because drugs may compete for binding sites on plasma albumin, the administration of a second drug may displace bound drug and so unexpectedly raise the level of free, pharmacologically active drug. For instance, the binding of the anticoagulant drug warfarin (p. 159) to plasma protein is decreased by barbiturates and by indomethacin, and their administration can therefore increase the amount of anticoagulation produced.

Drug penetration into the brain and cerebrospinal fluid

Drug penetration into the brain is governed by the unusual properties of the capillaries in this organ that are more complex and less permeable than capillaries elsewhere and are more like epithelia. Apart from a few substances that are transported through the capillaries by specific transport processes, penetration depends very much upon the lipid solubility of the drug. The behaviour of the choroid plexuses which secrete the cerebrospinal fluid is very similar. On the other hand, the outflow of cerebrospinal fluid into the venous sinuses is a wholly passive process of bulk flow which does not discriminate against any drugs. Because of this unidirectional flow of cerebrospinal fluid, substances present in the blood will never come into equilibrium with the cerebrospinal fluid unless lipid solubility is exceptionally high. For this reason the concentration of a drug of low lipid solubility such as penicillin in the cerebrospinal fluid will be very low and may be below the effective chemotherapeutic level. In some instances this low rate of penetration may provide a useful basis for selective drug action. For instance, the lipid-insoluble decarboxylase inhibitors carbidopa and benzerazide can be used to inhibit the metabolism of laevodopa in peripheral tissues without depressing its conversion into dopamine in the brain (p. 30).

As mentioned earlier, the brain has a high blood flow; however, the flow is not uniform but is highest in the cellular (grey) areas where it averages about 1 l/kg min. The half time of equilibration into these areas for a substance of high lipid-solubility will therefore be less than 1 minute. The general anaesthetics halothane and thiopentone come near to this value. On the other hand the half time of equilibration of barbitone, a hypnotic of much lower lipid solubility (heptane/water 0·002) is as long as half an hour.

Passage of drugs across the placenta

The foetal blood in the placental capillaries is separated from the maternal blood sinusoids by the trophoplastic epithelium, which offers a similar barrier to passage of drugs to that found in the brain. Once again it is lipid solubility which is the prime determinant of the rate at which equilibration between the two circulations occur. However, because there is no equivalent of the lymphatic system, or cerebrospinal fluid in this case, equilibration will eventually occur *even for lipid-insoluble drugs if they are administered for a long enough period.* The rule therefore is that if the drug is lipid insoluble and is administered only acutely there will be little penetration into the placenta; if it is administered repeatedly the plasma level in the foetus will eventually equal that in the mother.

ABSORPTION OF DRUGS WHEN INJECTED INTO THE TISSUES

When drugs are injected into a muscle in dissolved form the absorption into the local capillaries will depend essentially on the same factors discussed previously. At best the rate will be blood-flow limited—hence will depend on the local blood flow. This is especially the case since muscle capillaries are relatively permeable and will retard the absorption only of macromolecules.

The local blood flow may be affected by muscle work which increases muscle blood flow. The situation in the dermis is rather similar except that the blood flow is particularly involved in thermoregulation and is reduced when the environment is cold and is greatly increased when the environment becomes warmer. This can be of clinical importance. For instance, a dose of morphine injected subcutaneously into a cold shocked patient may be poorly absorbed and ineffective—when the patient is warmed up and the shock reversed in an ambulance or in hospital delayed absorption may occur with unforeseen consequences.

The absorption of drugs from injections into the tissues may also be modified by local pharmacological effects of the drug or constituents of the solution on the vessels. For instance, adrenaline is a powerful constrictor of skin vessels and consequently a subcutaneous injection is very slowly absorbed; however, it is a dilator of muscle vessels and so is well absorbed from an intramuscular injection. The use of injections of drugs into tissues is also influenced by whether they produce pain or tissue damage. In general the absorption of drugs by these two routes is rapid and is essentially complete within about 15 minutes. It is however sufficiently slow to greatly minimize the peak concentrations that occur in rapidly perfused organs after intravenous injection.

Macromolecules injected into the tissues may be too large to penetrate readily through the capillary wall. The absorption of these substances occurs mainly into the local lymphatics and the rate of absorption will depend on the rate of lymphatic flow, which may be fairly slow, and the half-time of absorption may be several hours.

Depot preparations

It is often convenient to slow the absorption of a drug from subcutaneous or intramuscular injection so as to produce a prolonged effect. The most common way of doing this is to use a preparation that is relatively insoluble in water and which is injected as a suspension of crystals or amorphous material. The absorption of the small fraction of drug that is in solution will occur as usual and this will be replaced by *dissolution* of the drug particles. It is easy to see that even if the dissolution process is not rate limiting, if say 90 per cent of the drug is injected as particles and only 10 per cent in solution, that the rate of absorption will be reduced by a factor of ten compared to wholly dissolved drug. Obviously the more insoluble the drug the greater the prolongation. In practice, the rate of dissolution is often rate limiting. We are all familiar with substances, like salt, that dissolve rapidly when put into water, and others like magnesium sulphate that need a great deal of stirring before they dissolve. When the rate of dissolution is slow it will depend critically on the physical state of the solid. Large crystals dissolve slowly, but if they are powdered they dissolve more rapidly and the more finely they are powdered the more rapidly they dissolve. These principles have been put to an important use in the various preparations of insulin (p. 170). The extreme of this principle is the implantation of a fused pellet of a drug which dissolves only over the period of many months. This method has been used for administering certain steroids.

Another approach to delaying absorption is to administer the drug as a solution or suspension in oil. The absorption is slow because it is only the drug partitioned into the tissue fluid surrounding the oil that is absorbed. If the drug is more soluble in the oil than in the tissue fluid this concentration will be low. This principle has been especially valuable in preparations of antipsychotic drugs, for instance fluophenazine decanoate need be injected only every few weeks.

ADMINISTRATION BY MOUTH

Most drugs are absorbed when taken by mouth unless they are broken down in the alimentary canal (e.g. insulin). The rapidity of absorption and the site of absorption depend on chemical and physical properties of the drug.

The barrier to absorption is the cell wall of the epithelial cells lining the gastro-intestinal tract and the ease with which a substance can penetrate through these cells depends on its partition coefficient between the aqueous phase in the gut lumen and cell cytoplasm and the 'lipid' phase in the cell membrane. Substances that are highly hydrophilic, for instance quaternary ammonium ganglion blockers (e.g. hexamethonium), are very poorly absorbed, whereas the more lipophilic ethanol is absorbed very rapidly. A great many drugs are weak cations, i.e. in acid solution they are cations and in alkali they are uncharged. At the pH corresponding to pK there are equal amounts of cation and uncharged form. The two forms differ in their partition coefficients, the cation being hydrophilic and thus poorly absorbed whereas the uncharged form is more lipophilic and thus more readily absorbed. The over-all rate of absorption will thus depend on the proportion of uncharged form present and this will be determined by the pH. Such a drug will be almost wholly cationic in the stomach and hence not appreciably absorbed there, but in the more neutral pH of the intestinal contents enough uncharged form is present to ensure good absorption. Needless to say, as the uncharged form is absorbed it is replenished from the cationic form by reequilibration.

In the case of anionic drugs (e.g. salicylates, barbiturates) the anion is poorly absorbed. Here the uncharged form predominates in the stomach so that absorption from the stomach may be quite significant although the major part of absorption is still in the small intestine.

As pointed out in connexion with absorption from the subcutaneous tissues, it is dissolved drug which is absorbed, so that insoluble drugs are slowly absorbed and the rate at which they are absorbed will be determined primarily by the rate of dissolution. It is therefore important that tablets of insoluble drugs should be composed of particles of the order of a few micrometres in diameter.

It is sometimes an advantage to coat tablets of drugs with protective coatings either to prevent dissolution in the stomach if they are liable to cause gastric irritation, or to prolong the period of absorption to give a longer effect. A typical 'enteric' coating is cellulose acetate phthalate which is insoluble in acid but dissolves quite rapidly in intestinal juice. In general, absorption of drugs taken by mouth begins in 15–60 minutes and reaches a peak in an hour or two so that oral administration produces less fluctuation in blood level than parenteral administration; a further difference is that since absorption from the intestine occurs into the portal venous system the drug must pass through the liver before reaching the general circulation. Since most of the drug metabolizing systems are concentrated in the liver, a higher proportion of the drug is metabolized when given by the oral route so that quite apart from the efficiency of absorption, less of the original drug reaches the general circulation and this means that doses must usually be higher to attain the same result when the drug is given by mouth.

A way round this for the tablet of the drug to be sucked rather than swallowed. Dissolution occurs in the mouth and adsorption occurs through the buccal mucosa directly into the systemic circulation. This is a useful method of getting rapid absorption of readily metabolized drugs and is used in the case of glyceryl trinitrate in the treatment of angina and of isoprenaline in asthma. The main limitation to this method is the objectionable taste of most drugs and the high proportion of drugs that are surface anaesthetics.

ADMINISTRATION BY INHALATION

For volatile drugs administration by inhalation may have particular advantages, notably the ease with which the concentration in the plasma and tissues may be controlled, and this is exploited in inhalational anaesthetics (Chapter 3).

However, non-volatile drugs may also be administered by this route as fine mists or dusts; these are frequently used in the treatment of asthma (e.g. isoprenaline and cromoglycate). The purported objective here is to produce a local action and for this the particles must be fine enough to penetrate into the smaller bronchioles. There is considerable doubt whether the local action is the dominant one and the effectiveness of the drug given by this route rests more on rapid and efficient absorption from the large absorbing area made available.

There may be cases where it is impracticable to administer the drug systemically because of poor oral absorption and rapid excretion. An example of this is the anti-allergic drug chromoglycate.

BIOAVAILABILITY

This term is used to describe the effectiveness of various methods of administration in delivering the drug to its site of action. This is a matter of considerable concern, particularly in the oral drugs in which different preparations of the same drug may show different absorbability. This has been identified as a considerable problem in the case of digoxin but is also known to be important in other drugs.

The absolute absorption of drugs can be determined by comparing the blood levels

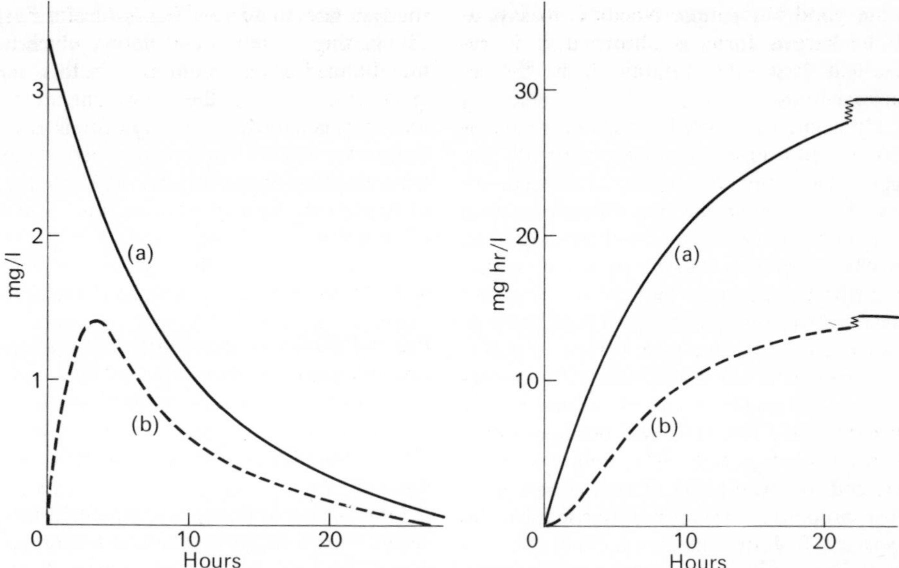

Fig. 2.2. A dose of 0·5 mg tetracycline/kg was given by two routes (a) intravenous and (b) by mouth. The curves in the left panel show the resulting levels of drug in the plasma. The cumulative (integral) blood levels are shown in the right-hand panel. It can be seen that the cumulative level after oral dosing is only about one half of the intravenous level, showing that only about half the dose has been absorbed by the gut.

obtained after oral dosing with those obtained after intravenous injection (Fig. 2.2). If the area under the oral curve is expressed as a fraction of that under the intravenous curve, this gives the fraction of the drug that has been absorbed. In the study of the absorption of tetracycline shown in Fig. 2.2 the area under the i.v. curve was 29·5 mg h/l and that under the oral curve was 14·4 mg h/l, showing that $(14{\cdot}4/29{\cdot}5)\times 100 = 49$ per cent of the drug was absorbed. This method can be used to arrive at suitable oral doses as well as comparing the behaviour of different preparations.

EXCRETION OF DRUGS

Most drugs are extensively metabolized, so that excretion of the unchanged drug is not usually the rate-limiting step in the disappearance of the drug from the body. The main groups of drugs in which urinary excretion is the major route of disposal are the chemotherapeutics (sulphonamides, penicillin, streptomycin, tetracycline, etc.) and the ganglion and neuromuscular blocking agents (tubocurarine, gallamine, mecamylamine, hexamethonium, etc.) Excretion by the kidneys depends first on glomerular filtration; the glomerulus does not filter proteins appreciably so only free unbound drug is filtered; the rate is such as to clear 28 per cent of the plasma free drug each minute. If the drug is extensively bound to plasma proteins, the total clearance rate will be much less. In the tubules the filtered drug is concentrated by the reabsorption of water and will tend to back diffuse along the concentration gradient into the peritubular blood. How far it will be able to do so will depend once more on its lipid solubility. As in the intestine, drugs that undergo protonation changes will tend to be lipid soluble in their uncharged form and much less lipid soluble as cations or anions. The clearance of the drug will therefore depend on the position of the ionic equilibrium which is dependent on the pK of the drug and the pH of the urine. If the urine is alkaline a higher proportion of a weak base will be in the uncharged form than if the urine is acid, more will diffuse back, and the excretion rate will be less. Conversely a weakly acidic drug will have a lower rate of excretion in acid urine. In the case of such drugs the pH of the urine may have an important effect on the blood levels of drug and the duration of drug action. For instance, this has been shown to be of some importance with amphetamine, mecamylamine, and salicylates.

Some drugs are also excreted by the tubular cells into the urine and may have a clearance rate greater than the glomerular filtration rate—this applies to acidic drugs such as penicillin, 4-aminohippurate, and cromoglycate, and to bases such as methoniums.

The presence of renal disease can make an important difference to the handling of drugs and if allowance is not made for this toxic effects can result. For instance, in severe chronic renal disease the glomerular filtration rate may be only 5–10 ml/min compared with the normal rate of 125 ml/min and rapid accumulation of streptomycin or gentamycin may occur. The dose of these drugs must therefore be adjusted in renal failure, and it is useful to use the plasma creatinine level for calculating the appropriate dose.

DRUG METABOLISM

A knowledge of how drugs are metabolized is very important. First, it relates to the duration of action of drugs as well as the possible route of administration, but the metabolites themselves may be biologically active and lead to unexpected effects, side effects or toxicity. In general it is lipid-soluble drugs that are most extensively metabolized and are converted to more polar derivatives that are more readily excreted.

The simplest metabolic reaction is hydrolysis and this occurs, for instance, with local anaesthetics like procaine (by cholinesterase) and is responsible for the safety of these substances. The same enzyme hydrolyses suxamethonium, a muscle relaxant. In about 1 in 3000 individuals the effects of suxamethonium are prolonged and this is due to the fact that these individuals have an atypical cholinesterase in their plasma which has a low affinity for suxamethonium and is inefficient in destroying the drug. The defect is due to a genetic variant. Hydrolysis is especially important for protein and peptide drugs whose actions are terminated by the action of proteases; this applies to vasopressin and oxytocin, angiotensin, insulin, etc.

Drugs may also be modified by conjugation with glycuronic acid, sulphate, acetic acid, or cysteine. Glycuronide formation occurs in the liver through the operation of a transferase which transfers glycuronic acid from uridine diphosphate-glycuronic acid. Glycuronide formation occurs especially with phenols, alcohols, and aromatic amines. It is worth bearing in mind that the enzyme responsible for glycuronide formation is not fully developed at birth, so that newborn infants and especially premature infants are deficient in this respect. It is well known that the failure to convert endogenous bilirubin to bilirubin glycuronide is responsible for the jaundice found at birth. Chloramphenicol is an example of a drug that is detoxified mainly by glycuronidation and before this was appreciated serious toxic effects were found when this drug was used in the newborn.

Conjugation with sulphate is confined to phenols, but is an important pathway for catecholamines, phenolic steroids, etc. Acetylation affects mainly aromatic amines and was first discovered when it was noted that *N*-acetylsulphonamides were the major excretion products of sulphonamides. Acetylation is also the major inactivation process for isonazid (isonicotinic hydrazide and in this case the acetylation enzyme is genetically determined by a recessive gene which determines whether individuals are slow or rapid (homozygous) or intermediate (heterozygous) acetylators.

Drug oxidation

The most versatile metabolic pathway for drugs is through oxidation in the liver by a system in the microsomes which is called a *mixed-function oxidase.* This enzyme system is able to utilize O_2 which is used to oxidize the drug and simultaneously to oxidize NADPH to NADP. This dual action is the basis of the name 'mixed function'. The oxidase system is complex and depends on a special group of cytochromes called **cytochrome P-450,** the number referring to their absorption maximum at 450 nm when reacted with carbon monoxide.

A characteristic oxidation is that of the side chain of barbiturates with aliphatic or alicyclic side chains (Fig. 2.3). Oxidative demethylation can occur as with aromatic ethers—for instance, phenacetin is converted into paracetamol and codeine can be demethylated to morphine. Incidentally these are two examples where metabolism produces active drugs!

Hydroxylation of aromatic compounds also occurs, a simple example being the conversion of acetanilide to 4-hydroxacetanilide. The evidence available suggests that aromatic hydroxylation proceeds through the intermediate formation of a 1,2-epoxide. This has special importance since the epoxide is capable of reacting with proteins to form covalent compounds without the intervention of an enzyme. Such a covalent compound may be of importance in three ways. First, it may act as a full antigen, and induce the formation of antibodies to the drug and hence is one way in which drug hypersensitivity can be produced. Secondly, it may react with liver constituents and cause liver necrosis; there is evidence for this mechanism with bromobenzene and with 3,4-benzpyrene. Thirdly, it may react with nucleic acid and be mutagenic. There is evidence that carcinogenic hydrocarbons need to be activated in this way in order to produce mutagenesis and malignancy.

The mixed-function oxidase can be induced (i.e. synthesis increased) by administration of suitable drugs. For instance, the activity in oxidizing pentobarbitone is greatly increased if phenobarbitone (a non-metabolized barbiturate) is administered to the animal some 24 hours earlier. This is due to synthesis of extra amounts of two components of the mixed-function oxidase, cytochrome P-450 and NADPH-cytochrome c reductase. This synthesis is prevented if the animal simultaneously receives an inhibitor of protein synthesis such as cycloheximide.

The pharmacological effects of this induction are readily demonstrated. If a rabbit was given a dose of 30 mg/kg pentobarbital the animal lost consciousness and the time before it was able to stand up again was just over an hour, but after the same dose had been given for three days the duration of unconsciousness was less than half this. When blood levels were examined it was found that the blood level of the anaesthetic at which consciousness returned was unaltered; however, the time taken for the blood level to fall to this critical value was accelerated in the animals that had had previous dosage.

A similar increase in rate of metabolism of pentobarbitone could be produced by quite unrelated drugs that also had this ability to

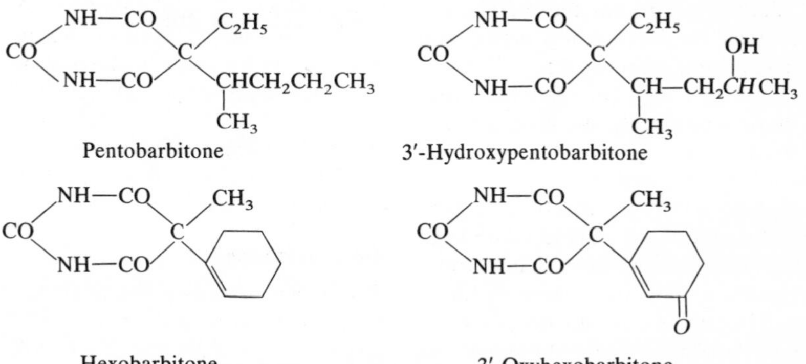

Pentobarbitone

3′-Hydroxypentobarbitone

Hexobarbitone

3′-Oxyhexobarbitone

Fig. 2.3.

induce the metabolizing enzyme system. We have the situation then, that repeated administration of a drug may change its characteristics so that the clinical effects are less then those of a single dose and that there may be interactions between drugs mediated by alterations in metabolism. This can have very important therapeutic consequences. For instance, the metabolism of the anticoagulant dicoumarol is also dependent on the microsomal system, and this activity is induced simultaneously with the barbiturate metabolism system. This means that if a patient who has been stabilized on dicoumarol to give an acceptable prothrombin time complains of insomnia and is put on a barbiturate, the rate of metabolism of dicoumarol may be increased, its mean blood level reduced, and the effect on prothrombin reduced to a level that is no longer therapeutically acceptable. Stimulation of the microsomal system is relatively long lasting and after the stimulating drug is withdrawn the system returns to its previous level slowly over many days (Fig. 2.4).

Drug metabolism by the microsomal system may be inhibited by certain drugs such as SKF 525A, but these compounds have not found a practical use in drug therapy, nor is a competitive interaction between drugs of much significance in the microsomal system although this may be of significance in other metabolic processes. An excellent example is the liver enzyme alcohol dehydrogenase which oxidizes ethanol through acetaldehyde to acetic acid, a harmless metabolic substrate for the citric acid cycle. This enzyme also oxidizes methanol to the highly toxic formaldehyde and to formic acid which produces a metabolic acidosis. Ethanol has a higher affinity for the enzyme than methanol and can therefore be used therapeutically in methanol poisoning to limit cell damage and acidosis. This enzyme also illustrates two other principles. **Pyrazole** is a simple substance of low toxicity (p. 252) which is a highly effective inhibitor of this enzyme and which therefore greatly prolongs the intoxicating effect of alcohol. Another drug **disulphuram** inhibits the conversion of acetaldehyde to acetic acid, so that after taking ethanol, acetyldehyde accumulates in the blood and produces unpleasant toxic symptoms. Disulphuram is sometimes used in the treatment of alcoholism.

Because the drug-metabolizing systems are concentrated in the liver, it does not come as a surprise that in degenerative liver disease, drug metabolism is grossly depressed and the doses of drugs may therefore need to be carefully adjusted to avoid excessive and prolonged blood levels.

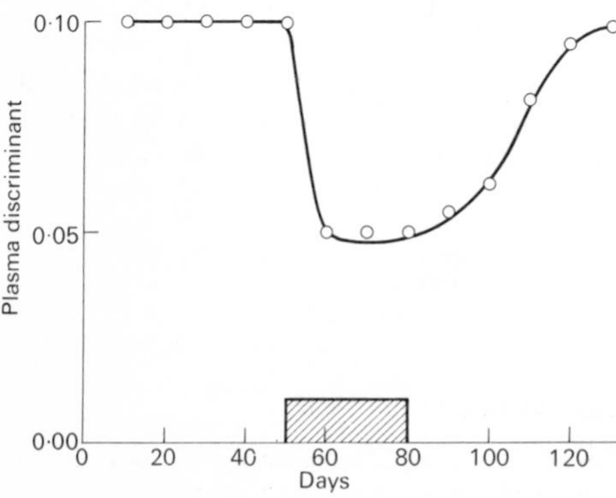

Fig. 2.4. Blood levels of dicoumarol given daily over a long period. From day 50 to day 80 the subject also received 65 mg phenobarbitone daily. The phenobarbitone induced a higher level of the enzyme system metabolizing dicoumarol, and the blood level fell to about one half. After discontinuing the phenobarbitone, the blood level climbs back to the earlier level quite slowly.

Accumulation of drugs

When drugs are administered for more than one dose, the aim is usually to produce as constant a pharmacological effect as possible. Excessively high levels are undesirable as they either produce a larger effect than desired or increase the risk of toxicity, whereas if the level falls too low the drug effect is insufficient. The spacing and amount of drug dosage should therefore be designed to reach a steady blood level in a predetermined time and to maintain it with minimum variation. Fig. 2.5 shows that dosage three times a day by injection if the biological half-life of the drug is 4 hours gives a very great fluctuation

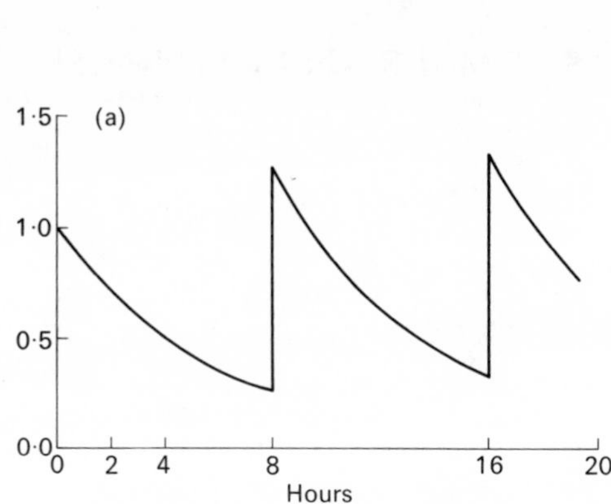

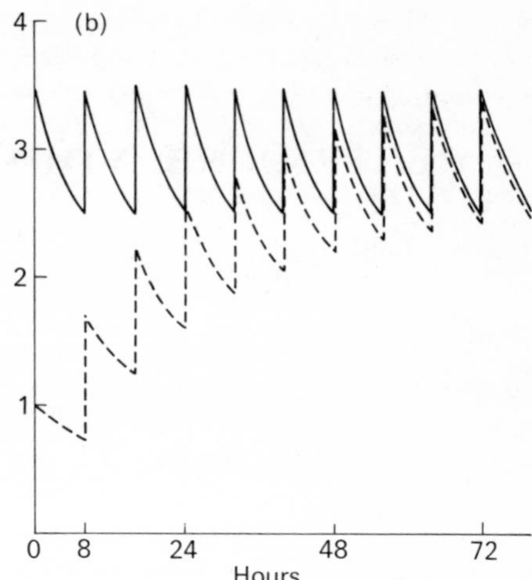

Fig. 2.5. Plasma levels of drugs after repeated dosage. (a) Plasma half-life 4 h. Note that with dosage three times a day the range of concentration is nearly 4 : 1 but there is little cumulation. (b) Plasma half-life 24 h. Note that with equal doses the plasma level cumulates to about 3·5 × the initial level (---). If the first (loading) dose is 3·5 × the subsequent doses, there is no cumulation (——). The ratio of maximum to minimum blood levels is only 1·4 : 1.

in blood level—this is the kind of blood level fluctuation seen with intramuscular penicillin. However, there is practically no cumulation, i.e. the peaks and troughs of concentration remain at very nearly similar levels. On the other hand if the half-life of the drug is 12 hours the ratio between the concentrations at the beginning and end of the run is much smaller, actually about 2 : 1, but the peaks and troughs continue to rise into the second day. This is even more obvious if the half-life is 24 hours. The drug is then said to *cumulate*. The problem of cumulation can be diminished by giving a larger initial dose—in Fig. 2.5 this was 3·5 times the repeated doses—with the consequence that the mean blood level becomes much more constant. When drugs are given by mouth the curve of blood level is smoothed out by the delay in absorption and it is easier to maintain a constant level (provided absorption remains constant).

Table 2.3. Biological half-lives of drugs

Suxamethonium	3·5 min
Benzylpenicillin	40 min
Paracetamol	2 h
Isoniazid	2·5 h
Tolbutamide	3·5 h
Dexamphetamine	7 h
Tetracycline	9 h
Sulphadiazine	17 h
Dicoumarol	32 h
Chlorpropamide	35 h
Digoxin	45 h
Phenylbutazone	72 h
Phenobarbitone	84 h

FURTHER READING

Binns, T. B. (1964). *Absorption and distribution of drugs*, Baltimore.

Gillette, J. R., Davis, D. C., and Sasame, H. A. (1972). *Cytochrome P-450 and its role in drug metabolism. Ann. Rev. Pharmacol.* **12.**

Goldstein, A., Aronow, L, and Kalman, S. M. (1974). *Principles of drug action*, New York.

Heffter, A. (1975). Handbook of experimental pharmacology, vol. XXVIII. *Concepts in biochemical pharmacology*.

Kalow, W. (1962) *Pharmacogenetics: heredity and the response to drugs*, Philadelphia.

La Du, B. N., Mandel, H. G., and Way, E. L. (1971) *Fundamentals of drug metabolism and drug disposition*, Baltimore.

Shanker, L. S. (1964). Physiological transport of drugs, *Adv. drug Res.* **1.**

Wagner J. G. (1975). *Fundamentals of clinical pharmacokinetics*, Hamilton.

3

CENTRAL NERVOUS SYSTEM TRANSMITTERS

EVERY function of the body is directly or indirectly controlled by the central nervous system and that in turn relies for normal operation on its chemical neurotransmitters. These chemicals have a fundamental and crucial role and yet their actions are vulnerable to natural malfunction and to modification by circulating chemicals and drugs. Malfunction or modification of their normal actions may result only in trivial observable effects but it can result in dramatic, prolonged, or fatal consequences. Whatever the consequence, the study of central transmitters, and the action that drugs have upon them, is of prime importance.

EXPERIMENTAL METHODS FOR THE STUDY OF CENTRALLY ACTING DRUGS ON TRANSMITTER MECHANISMS

An extremely wide range of techniques is now available for the study of centrally acting drugs. These techniques may be methods based simply on the observation of the whole organism or may involve sophisticated experiments which allow the effect of drugs on single nerve cells to be analysed.

The gross effects of drugs can be studied by direct observation of the movements of animals. No special skill or apparatus is needed to determine when an animal is anaesthetized or is convulsing but additional tests such as the recording of reflexes or the measurement of electrical activity in the brain usually provide valuable additional information.

Visual observation may be supplemented by automatic records of total activity by recording movements of a cage, or the floor of a cage, which is freely suspended and moves when the animal moves. A more satisfactory way of doing this is to arrange for movements of the animal to interrupt beams of light or infra-red rays and so signal movements. Drugs which alter behaviour, perhaps by reducing anxiety or stimulating exploratory activity, may be studied on animals placed in simple mazes.

The effects of drugs on reflexes can quickly be tested on frogs, by comparing reactions before and after the drug and by measuring the latent period and the duration of the effect. After strychnine, for instance, frogs give exaggerated responses to mild stimuli such as touching the skin.

More satisfactory ways for measuring the effect of drugs on reflex activity involve electrical and mechanical recording techniques. Early experiments made use of an automatic patellar tendon hammer and a myograph device for recording muscle shortening when the knee jerk reflex was evoked. Drugs were injected systemically and their effect on the characteristics of the reflex recorded. This type of experiment is rarely performed nowadays because the site of action of the drug cannot be properly localized. It is now much more convenient and informative to stimulate afferent nerves directly and to record the reflex responses evoked in nerves leaving the spinal cord. Drugs may be applied topically to the spinal cord or be given by close arterial injection and their effect on individual reflex pathways recorded. There are many variations of this basic type of experiment, the most recent being the introduction of methods for recording from single cells in the spinal cord and for applying drugs microelectrophoretically to these cells. Records are usually obtained from single cells by preparing glass micropipettes with tip diameters of a few micrometres. These pipettes are filled with a strong electrolyte solution, NaCl for extracellular recording, and are then coupled through a cathode follower to suitable amplifiers and display equipment. By moving the tip of the electrode through the tissue with a micromanipulator, the action potentials of individual cells are picked up, and displayed (Fig. 3.1).

To apply drugs to single cells, micropipettes are again used but they are filled with a strong solution of the drug to be tested. This drug must be at a pH which allows good ionization of the compound and the polarity of the charged ions must be known. If this pipette is now placed very near a nerve cell membrane and if a voltage, of the same polarity as the ionized drug, is applied to the drug solution, a current (measured in nA) will flow from the tip of the pipette and a small amount of the charged drug will be ejected. Numerous precautions have to be taken with this technique, a small 'braking' current must always be applied to the pipette to prevent the leakage of the drug by diffusion and controls must be performed to ensure that the electrophoretic current itself has no effect on the cells, It is usual for these micro-electrophoresis pipettes to be fused to at least one other micropipette so that electrical recordings may be made, and other drugs applied simultaneously, to the cell being studied. With this type of apparatus many detailed and valuable studies of the effect of drugs on reflex and nerve cell activity in the spinal cord and other parts of the central nervous system have been made.

Drug effects in the brain may also be studied by using electrodes which record the activity of whole populations of nerve cells. These electrodes, which need not be of very small dimensions, can be chronically implanted in the brain so that records are obtained from the conscious, free-moving animal.

The site of action of a drug may be determined by recording its effect before and after central lesions have been made. If the effect survives complete destruction of the nervous system it must, of course, be peripheral. If it does not survive then spinal, brain stem, and cerebral lesions can be produced in order to locate the approximate site of action. The central action of drugs can sometimes be determined, and their site of action located, by applying them locally. In this case the experiment is only convincing if very small doses are effective, since drugs which are given in this way may be absorbed by the blood stream and carried to a distant site of action. Drugs may be applied to the surface of the brain, to deep structures by microinjection, or injected into cerebral blood vessels or the ventricles.

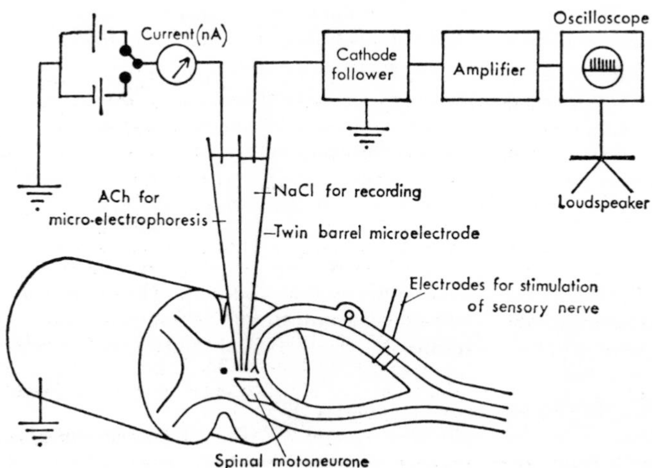

Fig. 3.1. Apparatus for recording from single nerve cells and for applying drugs by micro-electrophoresis.

If a drug can be made radioactive it is often possible to determine its distribution and predict its site of action, by making autoradiographs of brain sections after administration of the drug.

THE NEUROTRANSMITTERS

Although the action of drugs on the central nervous system has occupied the attention of pharmacologists for may centuries and spectacular advances have occurred, particularly in recent years, we still have scant knowledge of how most centrally active drugs really exert their effects. We do, however, have many drugs with powerful and useful actions on the nervous system but a majority of these have arisen more by good fortune than by design and in few cases can we define their mechanism of action.

In considering centrally active drugs it is helpful first to specify the sites at which these drugs can act and the mechanisms which they can affect. It is widely considered that most centrally acting drugs, apart from those which have generalized and non-specific excitatory or depressant effects, exert their actions at synaptic junctions in nervous pathways. These synaptic sites are not only highly vulnerable to drug action but they appear to be the sites at which malfunction, which may lead to mental disorders, tends to occur as opposed to the less vulnerable axons, supporting tissues, and cell bodies. The fact that there are about 300 000 million vulnerable synapses in one gram of cortical tissue emphasizes the possibility of disorders occurring and draws attention to the scope of drug treatment. At the synapse a prime target for any active drug will be the chemical neurotransmitter and its associated mechanisms for synthesis, release, efficacy of action, and termination of effect.

An applied drug may act pre-synaptically to affect neurotransmitter synthesis, storage, release, or reuptake. Alternatively, it may act post-synaptically to affect transmitter destruction or reuptake. It may have a direct agonist or antagonist action on the post-synaptic membrane or it may compete, or otherwise interfere, with the activity of the natural transmitter. Any of these actions will affect normal transmission at that synapse and thereby produce alterations in nervous function.

Before these drug actions are described it is appropriate to consider the identity, location, and role of the endogenous neurotransmitters. Although there is only reasonable certainty about the identity of two or three of these transmitters in the spinal cord and brain, there is suggestive evidence about many others. In order to be satisfied that a compound is acting as a central transmitter it should fulfil certain criteria, which, although useful, should never be regarded as inflexible, particularly as new classes of transmitter and transmitter actions are doubtless still to be discovered.

The most important criterion to be satisfied is that the suspected transmitter should occur naturally in the nervous system, usually in association with the enzymes and precursors required for its synthesis. It might be expected that the transmitter would occur in nerve terminals, often in vesicles or granules, but the synthesizing enzymes may be found in a remote part of the neurone from which the transmitter may be transported to the nerve terminal. Another criterion is that there should be a demonstrable mechanism for the termination of transmitter action. This may be by diffusion but is more usually affected by enzymic destruction or by reuptake of the transmitter into nervous or non-nervous tissue. An important but technically difficult criterion to satisfy is that a suspected transmitter should be shown to be released from nerve terminals following physiological stimulation of the pre-synaptic element. This is hard to demonstrate if the mechanism for terminating the action of the transmitter cannot be blocked.

Finally, the application of the suspected chemical transmitter from an external source, often a micropipette, to a receptive neurone must, in every respect, mimic the action of the naturally released endogenous transmitter. If release of the natural transmitter produces depolarization of the neurone then, if the exogenous chemical is identical, it should have exactly the same effect and these effects of the natural transmitter and exogenous transmitter must be affected in identical ways by the application of antagonists, uptake blockers, and other experimental procedures.

It has been impossible to satisfy completely all these criteria for any transmitter in the central nervous system but the evidence for ACh as an excitatory transmitter in the spinal cord and brain, and for γ-amino-butyric acid and glycine as inhibitory transmitters in the brain and spinal cord respectively is now almost complete. Evidence for other transmitters is less good but is being steadily amassed and is shown in Table 3.1 and in descriptions of the likely central neurotransmitters.

Acetylcholine (see also Chapter 7)

Transmission at Renshaw cells in the spinal cord is mediated by acetylcholine where its actions are excitatory and are effected mainly through nicotinic receptors to give characteristically fast on/off responses (see p. 86). Its actions are mimicked by nicotine, tetramethylammonium, and carbachol and are antagonized by hexamethonium, dihydro-β-erythroidine, tetraethylammonium, and, weakly, by curare. A second type of receptor with muscarinic characteristics is now known to be present on Renshaw cells and this is excited by muscarine and blocked by atropine.

In the brain there is good evidence for acetylcholine as a predominantly excitatory transmitter at receptors which have muscarinic-like characteristics. The main cholinergic pathways appear to be ascending and associated with the older parts of the brain and with the maintenance of arousal and consciousness (see Chapter 7).

γ-Amino butyric acid (GABA)

GABA hyperpolarizes most central neurones but it produces presynaptic inhibition in the spinal cord by depolarizing excitatory nerve terminals, an action which is antagonized by the convulsant picrotoxin.

In the brain, GABA appears to be an important inhibitory transmitter and it is found in nerve terminals in association with glutamic acid decarboxylase, its synthesizing enzyme. GABA is released from central nerve terminals by inhibitory physiological stimuli and its action is terminated by a powerful sodium-dependent uptake system into nervous tissue and into glial cells. Apart from an inhibitory GABA pathway running from Purkinje cells in the cerebellar cortex to various cerebellar nuclei, no other distinct GABA pathways have been mapped but much indirect evidence suggests their existence. The action of GABA is selectively antagonized by the convulsant bicucilline and GABA uptake can be blocked, at least to some extent, by mercurial compounds. This information, and a knowledge of the action of GABA agonists, has aroused interest in the possibility of developing drugs which will penetrate into the brain and mimic or potentiate the actions of GABA, therefore producing a possibly selective increase in inhibition which might be useful in the treatment of epilepsy or other central disorders where there is excess neuronal activity.

It has been recently been found that GABA and glutamic acid dehydrogenase are greatly reduced in *post mortem* samples of basal ganglia tissue obtained from patients who have suffered from Huntington's chorea. This disease involves neurological and psychiatric symptoms including choreic movements and it may be that a deficiency in the GABA transmitting systems underlies this disease.

Glycine

If the spinal cord is subjected to selective anoxia it is found that inhibitory spinal reflexes are quickly lost; so too are the spinal interneurones associated with these reflexes and glycine levels in the grey matter of cord drops simultaneously. This, together with histochemical and electrophysiological evidence,

Table 3.1. Possible transmitters in the central nervous system

	Acetylcholine	GABA	Dopamine	Noradrenaline	Glycine	5-HT	Substance P	Enkephalin	Glutamic Acid
Predominant action (E, Excitatory I, Inhibitory)	E	I	I	I	I	I	E	I	E
Evidence for transmitter role	Good	Good	Fair	Fair	Good	Fair	Fair	Poor at present	Poor
Antagonists	Nicotinic in cord. Mainly muscarinic elsewhere	Picrotoxin (cord). Bicuculline (brain).	Chlorpromazine. Haloperidol	β-blockers	Strychnine	LSD	?	?	HA966
Possible role (abbreviated)	Arousal, attention. Motor function	Presynaptic Inhibition in cord. Inhibition in CNS.	Mood regulation. Extra-pyramidal regulation	Mood regulation	Postsynaptic inhibition in sp. cord	Behaviour	Sensory signalling	Pain pathway signalling	Sensory pathways?
Termination of action	Hydrolysis by cholinesterase	Reuptake	Reuptake	Reuptake	Reuptake	Reuptake	Reuptake?	Enzymic degradation?	Reuptake

strongly suggests that glycine is a postsynaptic inhibitory transmitter at spinal motoneurones. This inhibitory action of glycine is selectively blocked by strychnine, which accounts for the convulsant properties of this compound (see p. 62).

DOPAMINE AND NORADRENALINE

There is now suggestive evidence that dopamine and noradrenaline are central transmitters and their roles seem particularly linked with the control of certain types of behaviour and mood. Fluorescent histochemical techniques have allowed the visualization of the amine pathways in the brain and this technique, together with the use of 6-hydroxydopamine (see Chapter 8) which selectively destroys noradrenergic and dopaminergic neurones, has allowed precise maps to be prepared. Noradrenergic terminals in the forebrain originate from cell bodies in the pons and medulla while others arise in the locus coeruleus and pass to the cerebellar cortex and the hippocampus. Descending fibres to the spinal cord originate in the pons and medulla.

The dopamine systems are mainly confined to the midbrain, anterior to the majority of noradrenergic neurones. Dopamine neurones are located in the substantia nigra and their fibres project into the medial forebrain forming the nigro-striatal pathway, terminating in the corpus striatum and globus pallidus. Other dopaminergic fibres arise medially to the substantia nigra and descend to innervate the nucleus accumbens, amygdala, the olfactory tubercle, and some parts of the cerebral cortex.

Unlike in the periphery, it is not possible to distinguish α and β receptors for noradrenaline in the central nervous system, but the usual response of neurones is inhibition although a few neurones may be excited under certain conditions. The inhibitory responses are blocked by β-receptor antagonists and, as in the periphery, the responses to noradrenaline involve stimulation of adenyl cyclase leading to the formation of cyclic AMP. The inhibitory effect of noradrenaline applied to Purkinje cells in the cerebellum can be mimicked by the application of cyclic AMP and this response, and that to noradrenaline itself, can be potentiated by theophylline and papaverine which inhibit phosphodiesterase that normally breaks down cyclic AMP.

The pharmacology of dopamine receptors is not well understood as they do not exist outside the central nervous system, but important experiments have shown that they can be stimulated by apomorphine and selectively antagonized by the neuroleptic drugs chlorpromazine, haloperidol, and related butyrophenones, and that a dopamine sensitive adenyl cyclase exists.

It appears that noradrenaline (like 5-hydroxytryptamine, see later) may be involved in regulating mood and that malfunction of noradrenergic mechanisms may lead to behavioural disorders associated with mood. This suggestion is supported by the fact that tricyclic antidepressants are potent inhibitors of noradrenaline uptake and therefore raise the levels of this transmitter. A similar increase in catecholamine level will occur in the presence of monoamine oxidase inhibitor antidepressants, so depressive disorders may be related to a reduced availability of noradrenaline and associated catecholamines.

Considerable evidence indicates that neuroleptic drugs, particularly those which are used to control schizophrenia, such as chlorpromazine and haloperidol, block dopamine receptor sites and therefore antagonize the inhibitory action of dopamine. It is interesting that the neuroleptic drugs are potent inhibitors of dopamine-sensitive adenyl cyclase and it may be that the neuroleptics block dopamine action, which requires the production of cyclic AMP, in this way. All this evidence suggests that the level of activity in dopaminergic pathways may determine normal behaviour patterns and that abnormal activity in these pathways may be relieved by blockade of dopamine inhibition.

A spectacular advance in our understanding

of a central disorder and its treatment has arisen in the case of Parkinson's disease. This disease is a neurological condition involving muscular rigidity, reduced voluntary movements (akinesia), and tremor. It is a progressive and serious illness which has long been known to be related to malfunction within the basal ganglia.

A variety of treatments have been used including surgical lesions in thalamic nuclei and the use of anticholinergic drugs such as atropine, benzhexol, and benztropine. It gradually became clear that the basal ganglia receive a strong dopaminergic innervation and that the dopamine levels in samples of caudate nucleus, taken *post mortem* from Parkinson's patients, were abnormally low and that this was associated with a loss of cells in the substantia nigra.

Since the disease appeared to be associated with a loss of dopamine in the brain it seemed logical to attempt to replace this chemical. Dopamine itself could not be used since it does not penetrate the blood–brain barrier but L-dopa, a precursor of dopamine, does so and produces dramatic improvements in the rigidity and akinesic symptoms of the disease. Since degeneration of dopaminergic fibres has occurred in the disease it is not possible to effect a cure with L-dopa, but its use has proved a major therapeutic advance. L-dopa is normally taken by mouth and, although it enters the brain freely, much will be converted to dopamine outside the brain and may cause unwanted side effects. In order to reduce these side effects, and to reduce the amount of L-dopa ingested, it is often given in conjunction with carbidopa which inhibits the conversion of L-dopa to dopamine outside the brain since it does not itself cross the blood–brain barrier.

It is interesting that the synthesis of dopamine in the nigro-striatal pathway is partly controlled by the influence of a cholinergic pathway, and the fact that anticholinergic drugs have some success in treating parkinsonism, suggests the existence of a cholinergic and dopaminergic balance in the basal ganglia involved in the control of motor function.

5-HYDROXYTRYPTAMINE (5-HT, SEROTONIN)

5-HT neurones can be visualized separately from noradrenaline and dopamine neurones using fluorescent histochemical methods, and they are located in the raphe system in the brain stem. Fibres from these neurones extend to the medulla and down to the spinal cord. Other neurones are located in the ventral part of the medial forebrain bundle. 5-HT axons innervate numerous structures including parts of the reticular formation, hypothalamus, lateral geniculate nucleus, and cerebal cortex.

The receptors for 5-HT have not been well defined but the application of 5-HT iontophoretically to central neurones usually produces an inhibition which may be blocked by lysergic acid.

The synthesis of 5-HT in the central nervous system can be effectively blocked by L-*p*-chlorophenylalanine (PLPA) and this has been used in studying the central role of 5-HT. As with the other catecholamines, there is a powerful uptake mechanism for 5-HT which probably is the major way in which its central action is terminated. This uptake system can be inhibited by analogues of 5-HT such as tryptamine and α-methyl tryptamine. Uptake of 5-HT, like that of noradrenaline, is also inhibited by the tricyclic antidepressant drugs.

Like noradrenaline, it appears that 5-HT systems may be involved in the maintenance of normal behaviour and there are strong suggestions that depression is associated with a deficiency of 5-HT in the brain. These suggestions arise partly from the observation that both the tricyclic and the monoamine inhibitor antidepressant drugs have powerful effects on 5-HT metabolism and uptake.

SUBSTANCE P

This substance was first extracted from the gut by von Euler and Gaddum in 1931 and in recent years has been identified as an undecapeptide (see Chapter 9) and synthesized in a pure form.

It is found in high concentration in the substantia nigra and is also present in the dorsal horn and roots of the spinal cord and has been shown to have powerful excitatory actions on mammalian spinal cord motoneurones and, on central neurones, it also has excitatory, though much slower and long lasting actions. Recent advances using immunocytochemical methods suggest that Substance P is much more widely distributed in the nervous system than had been thought, and particularly at sites where a sensory transmitter might be expected to be located.

THE ENKEPHALINS AND ENDORPHINS

Although the central effects of morphine and opiate-like drugs have been known for many centuries, it is only very recently that we have begun to understand how these drugs might act in the brain or the significance of receptors for opiates on central neurones. In 1975 two naturally occurring pentapeptides were discovered in brain and were named met- and leu-enkephalin; they were shown to mimic the properties of morphine. It soon became apparent that other larger, naturally occurring peptides have similar properties and these are now known as the endorphins and derive from the pituitary peptide β-lipotropin. One of these corresponds to the CO_2H-terminal portion of β-lipotropin (residues 61–91, β-endorphin) and has morphine like properties. Other fragments such as γ-endorphin (residues 61–87) and α-endorphin (residues 61–76) have similar properties. Met-enkephalin (residues 61–65) and all the other peptides share a common amino acid sequence at their NH_2-terminal region (Fig. 3.2).

It has been suggested that some, or all, of these peptides are naturally occurring morphine-like compounds which act as neurotransmitters at opiate receptor sites in the brain, but it has also been suggested that enkephalin is simply a breakdown product with no transmitter function of its own. Against this last suggestion is the evidence that enkephalins are rapidly destroyed by peptidases in the brain and have powerful actions, usually inhibitory and short lasting, on neurones in pain pathways. The enkephalins closely mimic morphine at a cellular level, stimulating cyclic GMP formation in rat striatal slices and in inhibiting cyclic AMP formation in other preparations. It has also been shown that the regional distribution of enkephalin in brain is very similar to that of the opiate receptor with high levels in the hypothalamus and low levels in the cerebellum. The calcium-sensitive release of enkephalin from brain nerve terminal preparations has also reported. At the present time, all this information adds up to an intriguing but confusing situation, but it does appear that opiate-like pentapeptides will shortly find their place amongst the most important neurotransmitters known to us. The significance of such discoveries will be widespread, allowing fresh approaches to the study of the transmission of noxious stimuli, tolerance, addiction and the development of powerful new analgesics.

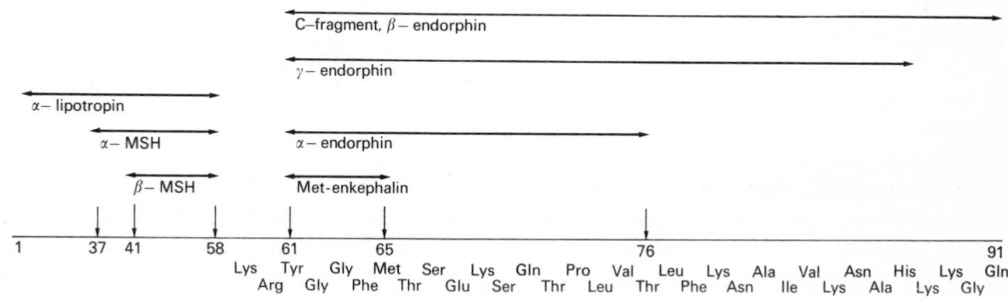

Fig. 3.2. Constituents of bovine β-lipotropin.

OTHER POSSIBLE CENTRAL TRANSMITTERS

There is some evidence that prostaglandins and histamine may act as transmitters, or at least modulators of nervous activity, in the brain and spinal cord but this evidence is based largely on the distribution and application of the substances, which alone is not convincing.

A number of amino acids, notably glutamic acid and aspartic acid (excitatory) and taurine (inhibitory) have been suggested as central transmitters at a variety of sites, but the evidence for this by no means complete and for each, is controversial. Despite this, it may well be only a matter of further investigation before a transmitter role for these compounds emerges since there is no doubt that the chemicals which we now recognize as transmitters function at only a very small proportion of the total synapses in the central nervous system. We undoubtedly have yet to learn of far more transmitters than those we have already recognized.

FURTHER READING

Bradley, P. B. (1975). *Methods in brain research.* Wiley, London.

Hall, Z. W., Hildebrand, J. G., and Kravitz, E. A. (eds.) (1974). *Chemistry of synaptic transmission.* Chiron Press, U.S.A.

Iversen, L. L. and Iversen, S. D. (1975). *Behavioural pharmacology.* Clarendon Press, Oxford.

Krnjevic, K. K. (1974). Chemical nature of transmission in vertebrates. *Physiol. Rev.* **54,** 418–540.

McLennan, H. (1970). *Synaptic transmission*, 2nd ed. Saunders, London.

4

CENTRAL NERVOUS SYSTEM DEPRESSANTS

ANAESTHETICS

THE drugs described in this section are probably the most important known to man. They include the general anaesthetics without which none but the most rudimentary surgery would be practicable. Although the mechanism and site of action of these compounds are still poorly understood, there have been notable advances in this field which now allow prolonged and complex surgery to be undertaken with excellent control of anaesthesia and its after effects.

Various drugs such as alcohol, opium, and hashish were amongst the first compounds used to reduce the pain of operations but effective general anaesthesia was only introduced in the nineteenth century. Although ether was known in the thirteenth century, it was only in the sixteenth century that its potential for relieving pain was suggested. This suggestion was forgotten and ignored until Sir Michael Faraday used ether for its anaesthetic power 200 years later. At about the same time, Sir Humphry Davy discovered the anaesthetic powers of nitrous oxide, but these discoveries were not immediately exploited. Only in 1846 when William Morton, an American dentist, used ether, first on dogs and then on man, for extracting teeth, did general anaesthesia begin to find wide acceptance. In 1847 Dr. James Simpson used chloroform to relieve labour pains and, despite opposition from many quarters, he persevered and then in 1853 the use of these agents gained a new respectability when Queen Victoria was given chloroform during the birth of her seventh child.

With early anaesthetics and anaesthetic techniques, the procedure of anaesthesia was both unpleasant and hazardous for the patient but advances in premedication and in the nature and purity of the anaesthetic compounds have now completely altered this picture. In addition, it is now possible to use much smaller doses of anaesthetic than before becasue separate drugs can now be used to secure the muscle relaxation required for surgery. Previously this was obtained by taking general anaesthesia to a very deep level. There is now a wide choice of anaesthetic compounds available and these include both volatile and non-volatile agents. Each type of agent tends to be particularly useful in a special situation and these are described under the appropriate headings for the individual anaesthetic agents.

THEORIES OF ANAESTHESIA

The mode of action of anaesthetics is still a matter for debate and, despite the advances made during the past decade in our knowledge of the functioning of nervous tissue, it is still impossible to decide the way in which anaesthetics act.

There is little doubt that anaesthesia is the result of a wide-spread depression of the CNS which is likely to arise from an action of the anaesthetic agent on either nerve axons, transmitter release from nerve terminals, or the excitability of postsynaptic membranes. It is difficult to obtain information about these possible sites of action by observing the action of anaesthetics on a complex structure like the brain, but experiments on peripheral tissues have shed some light on the problem.

Without doubt, all anaesthetics affect conduction in peripheral nerve axons but the concentrations of drug required to do this are much higher than those encountered in the brain during anaesthesia and, invariably, any associated synaptic junctions are much more vulnerable to the action of the anaesthetic. It has been convincingly demonstrated that anaesthetics block transmission through autonomic ganglia but the mechanism remains obscure although it is known that ether and chloroform, which block transmission, have no effect on the oxygen consumption of the tissue. Experiments on cells in the spinal cord have shown that ether diminishes reflex activity by reducing the evoked postsynaptic response to afferent nerve stimulation and by increasing the excitable threshold of the cell.

An effect of anaesthetics on transmitter release from nerve endings in the CNS is hard to measure directly but, on the guinea-pig intestine, volatile anaesthetics can block 80 per cent of the transmitter output. If these experiments are considered in conjunction with experiments that show an increase in acetylcholine content in the brain during anaesthesia coupled with a fall in acetylcholine release from the cortex, it seems possible that anaesthetics may act by reducing transmitter release in the brain. Anaesthetics also reduce the sensitivity of the neuromuscular end-plate to applied acetylcholine and so anaesthetic action at peripheral synapses suggests two possible mechanisms for their action in the brain: (1) a reduction of transmitter release from nerve endings: and (2) a reduction in the sensitivity of postsynaptic membranes.

Various theories have been proposed which, if confirmed experimentally, might suggest how these changes at a synaptic level could be brought about by anaesthetic drugs.

The theories fall into two main groups, biochemical and physical. The first group suggests that volatile anaesthetics depress enzyme systems, and the second that they interact with cell membranes.

Anaesthetics do interfere with brain enzyme systems but high concentrations of drug are required and it is not possible to be sure that these effects actually cause anaesthesia. High concentrations of anaesthetics lower brain tissue oxygen consumption and it has been suggested that barbiturates, chloral hydrate, and urethane interfere with the citric acid cycle. However, this is not accompanied by the decrease in the production of energy-rich phosphate compounds that would be expected. It is also possible that these changes occur as a result of reduced neuronal activity, and are therefore not concerned with the initiation of anaesthesia.

A suggestion by McIlwain briges biochemical and physical hypotheses. He suggests that depressant agents reduce ion movements across cells by an effect on the membrane and that this reduced activity allows a fall in tissue oxygen consumption and a rise, which can be observed, in phosphate energy stores. An action of some types of anaesthetics on the sodium carrier mechanism, which is activated during the generation of a an action potential, has been observed and, provided that the ionic movements affected by anaesthetics are concerned in the regulation of transmitter release or postsynaptic excitability, the hypothesis seems quite reasonable.

The first important physical theory of anaesthetic action was suggested by the early work of Meyer and Overton who proposed that the depression of activity caused by an anaesthetic was directly related to its lipid solubility. Certainly the correlation of anaesthetic potency with lipid solubility is striking and it is now known that highly fat-soluble anaesthetics, such as chloroform and ether, do stabilize the cell membrane and so reduce its sensitivity to electrical and other types of stimulation.

Other theories go further than explaining a correlation, they attempt to describe a mechanism of action at the cell membrane. Mullins suggests that anaesthesia occurs when 'pores' in the cell membranes are blocked by anaesthetic molecules so preventing the movement of ions. The portion of the membrane containing the 'pores' is considered to be of a lipid nature and so the relationship between anaesthetic potency and lipid solubility might be explained.

An intriguing suggestion by Pauling is that anaesthetics are able to form microcrystals of ice (clathrates) within the central nervous system. The microcrystals might interfere with synaptic tranmission or with the excitability of neuronal membranes. At body temperatures these microcrystals are not stable and Pauling suggests that they are stabilized by the charged side chains of proteins and solutes. There are modifications to this theory but all are proving difficult to test experimentally.

In 1939 Ferguson suggested that structurally non-specific drugs like general anaesthetics might have their potency determined by their thermodynamic activity. The thermodynamic activity is a measure of the number of molecules which are free to react with biologically important sites. The thermodynamic activity of a drug is not therefore necessarily determined by its concentration. A volatile anaesthetic given with oxygen has thermodynamic activity proportional to the partial pressure of the drug divided by the saturated vapour pressure of the anaesthetic alone at the same temperature. The theory predicts that structurally non-specific drugs will have similar biological activity if their thermodynamic activities are arranged to be the same. This imples that the potency of a structurally non-specific drug is inversely proportional to its solubility in water. The hypothesis complements that of Overton-Meyer since high lipid solubility is not the only property which is associated with low solubility in water.

None of the theories of anaesthesia which have been described is completely satisfactory and they are now under close examination using the sophisticated physical techniques which are now available. These studies have been directed at the interaction of anaesthetic molecules with membranes, particularly the red blood cell membrane. At this site all anaesthetics produce qualitatively similar results—at low concentrations the cells become more resistant to haemolysis but at high concentrations they tend to lyse.

It seems likely that the anaesthetic molecules enter the membrane and the increased molecular packing produces membrane stabilization. If too many molecules enter then the structure becomes unstable and is labilized and it is found that anaesthetic potency of a compound correlates well with this instability, anaesthetic concentration causing half maximal stabilization. In order to determine just what alters in the membrane when an anaesthetic penetrates it, the membrane behaviour is being studied by spectroscopic techniques (nuclear magnetic resonance and electron spin resonance) which allow the behaviour of molecules within the membrane to be studied.

Recent studies using electron spin resonance techniques—applied in analysing the action of anaesthetics on artificial phospholipid/cholesterol bilayer membranes have provided strong evidence that barbiturates and volatile anaesthetics act in a similar manner. With both types of anaesthetic the basic molecular mechanism of narcosis appears to result from an expansion and fluidization of the lipid phase of the nerve cell membrane.

Although the cause of anaesthesia is likely to involve both the protein and lipid components of a membrane, advances in this subject are only likely to follow further advances in our knowledge of membrane structure itself.

Neurophysiological approaches to the problem of the mechanism of action of anaesthetics have contributed evidence for the site of action of these compounds but little towards their mode of action, although they have resulted in the formation of many tentative theories of anaesthetic action. The most important piece of information to emerge has been that many anaesthetics exert their effect on the reticular formation, the brain stem network whose association with consciousness has been well demonstrated.

It is usually assumed that the reticular formation is particularly susceptible to the action of anaesthetics because of the abundance of synaptic connexions which are especially vulnerable to drug action, but evidence for this view is weak—the anesthetics could also be acting directly on reticular cell bodies.

In whatever manner anaesthetics may act on the reticular formation, the final result seems to be a non-specific inhibition of ascending reticular influences to higher centres and it is this effect which is thought to produce unconsciousness and anaesthesia.

Studies of the effect of anaesthetics on cell membranes, the electrical activity and the metabolism of single cells in the CNS may soon begin to provide important evidence on the mode of action of anaesthetics, a subject upon which, at present, one can do little more than speculate.

THE SIGNS OF ANAESTHESIA

Four stages of anaesthesia can be observed when induction is slow. With rapidly acting intravenous anaesthetics the earlier stages are passed so quickly that they are not normally encountered.

1. Stage of analgesia. The patient is conscious and can talk and obey commands. Awareness of pain is reduced towards the end of this stage.

2. Stage of excitement. This stage begins with loss of consciousness and extends to a level where surgery is possible. The patient can no longer exert control over himself, the pupils dilate and the pulse is rapid and strong. Muscular tone and movement may increase. This stage of anaesthesia is maintained for as short a period as possible.

3. Stage of surgical anaesthesia. Excitement disappears, respiration becomes regular, the pulse slows, and reflexes disappear. Reflexes are not all lost simultaneously, the reflexes controlling voluntary muscles go first. The conjunctival and eyelid reflexes are abolished and the cough and vomiting centres in the medulla become paralysed. The third stage of anaesthesia is sometimes subdivided in four planes.

4. Stage of respiratory paralysis. At this stage the medulla becomes severely depressed and the result is shallow, irregular respiration, a rapid pulse, a fall in blood pressure, and pupil dilation. Death is due to a stoppage of respiration as the respiratory centres in the brain stem become paralysed.

THE ELECTROENCEPHALOGRAM AND ANAESTHESIA

Spontaneous electrical rhythms can be recorded from the brain of all living mammals. In a relaxed human subject with eyes closed, the dominant frequency in the electrical waves is about 10 cycles per second but the administration of an anaesthetic causes marked, but reversible, changes in this rhythm and in the amplitude of the recorded waves.

During induction with most anaesthetics the pattern of the dominant rhythm (the high-voltage α rhythm) becomes desynchronized and a high-frequency, low-voltage pattern emerges. This usually coincides with the stage of delirium in the subject.

STAGE		I CONSCIOUS	II EXCITED	III SURGICAL ANAESTHESIA				IV DEAD
PLANE				1	2	3	4	
RESPIRATION	DIAPHRAGM							
	INTER-COSTAL							
EYE MOVEMENTS		VOLUNTARY	+ + + + +	+ + + + + + + + + + +	FIXED			
MUSCLE TONE								
PUPIL DIAMETER		N	+	−	−	N	+	+
SWALLOWING VOMITING								
E.E.G. αWAVES	VOLTS	0	+++	++	+	+	+	0
	RATE	0	3 PER SEC. DECREASING TO 0·1					0

Fig. 4.1. Effects of anaesthesia.

As anaesthesia develops, the electroencephalogram again becomes synchronized and the voltage of the waves increases, with a well-defined rhythm which gradually becomes more complex as slow frequency waves are super-imposed.

Further deepening of anaesthesia results in diminution of the voltage and in the eventual disappearance of all electrical activity.

Although different anaesthetic agents may produce their own series of characteristic changes in the electroencephalogram it has been possible to correlate the concentration of a given anaesthetic in the arterial blood with the pattern of the electrical rhythm. The clinical signs of anaesthesia may lag behind the changes in the electroencephalogram, especially during induction and termination of anaesthesia, but nevertheless, the use of this technique has become a valuable aid in the control of anaesthetic depth especially when neuromuscular blocking drugs are employed which may mask some of the clinical manifestations of anaesthesia.

Several methods have been described whereby the electroencephalogram from the patient can be used to control, automatically, the amount of anaesthetic delivered so as to maintain a constant and predetermined depth.

PREMEDICATION

Before giving a general anaesthetic it is usually desirable to reduce anxiety and pain if these are present and also to produce sedation in the patient to allow a smooth induction of the anaesthetic. It is also an advantage to reduce bronchial and salivary secretion in order to prevent choking when the swallowing reflex becomes paralysed. The sedative drugs commonly used are morphine, papaveretum, and pethidine, the latter compound has no sedative action but relieves anxiety and produces a feeling of well-being.

Barbiturates are also used, but less frequently now than in the past, because their effect is somewhat unpredictable when given orally. Phenothiazine derivatives may also be employed and their anti-emetic properties may be of especial value in some patients.

Excessive salivary and bronchial secretions may be stopped by the use of an anticholinergic drug such as atropine, which blocks muscarinic receptors. The use of atropine-like drugs has the additional advantage of reducing reflex bradycardia mediated by the vagus. Vagal bradycardia is especially liable to occur with halothane and cyclopropane anaesthesia and this may lead to cardiac arrest. This effect may be abolished by the use of atropine-like compounds, although the release of catecholamines which occurs during cyclopropane anaesthesia may produce cardiac arrhythmias more readily when vagal tone to the heart is reduced. Hyoscine is often preferred to atropine because it is more effective in reducing secretions and has marked sedative properties of its own, although it is less effective in preventing vagal slowing of the heart.

Atropine-like compounds are usually given intravenously shortly before induction of anaesthesia, this has the advantage of ensuring that the patient is adequately atropinized during surgery and removes the discomfort to the patient of long periods of waiting with a dry mouth before the operation.

VOLATILE AND GASEOUS ANAESTHETICS

Volatile anaesthetic are absorbed from the lungs and largely excreted again unchanged. The passage of an anaesthetic like chloroform from the lungs to the blood is very rapid but many hours of absorption may be required before the body becomes saturated. This delay occurs because the gas passes slowly from the blood into other tissues and particularly into tissues rich in fat. In the early stages of administration the concentration of the anaesthetic in the venous blood is much less than in the arterial blood but both these concentrations increase and the difference between them becomes less. As the concentration in the blood rises the rate of absorption by the tissues gradually decreases until the blood is in equilibrium with the concentration of the anaesthetic which is used. Excretion is rapid at first, so that when administration ceases the blood concentration falls to about half its original value in 5 minutes.

The solubility of an inhalation anaesthetic in blood is important because it largely determines the rate of induction and recovery from anaesthesia. With gases of low solubility the tension rises quickly in the blood and therefore acts rapidly on the brain.

Table 4.1. Partition coefficients of some gases at body temperature

	Blood/gas	Tissue/blood	
		Brain	Fat
Nitrogen	0·1	1·1	5·2
Cyclopropane	0·46	..	20·0
Nitrous oxide	0·47	1·0	3·0
Halothane	2·3	2·6	60·0
Chloroform	7·3	1·0	68·5
Trichlorethylene	9·0	..	107
Diethyl ether	15	1·14	3·3

THE VOLATILE AND GASEOUS ANAESTHETIC AGENTS

Halothane ($CHBrCl.CF_3$)

Halothane is a colourless liquid with a sweet, non-irritant odour. It is non-flammable and not explosive alone or in mixture with air or oxygen. It is now used in about 70 per cent of all operations requiring general anaesthesia.

The stage of excitement during induction is brief and recovery from full anaesthesia is rapid and not unpleasant.

Halothane tends to lower blood pressure, probably by a combination of effects including the block of sympathetic ganglia, increase in vagal tone, direct myocardial depression, central vasomoter depression, and an increase in afferent discharge from the baroreceptors.

The most common arrhythmias associated with halothane anaesthesia are nodal rhythm and ventricular extrasystoles. Catecholamines should not be injected during anaesthesia because halothane is known to sensistize the myocardium to these compounds.

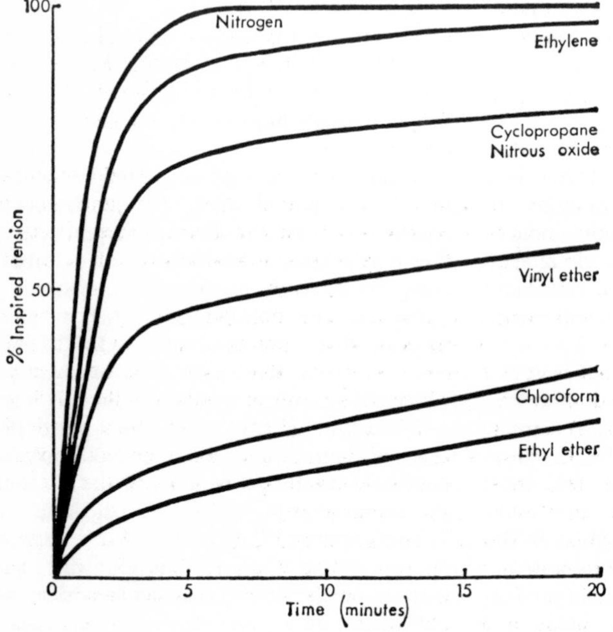

Fig. 4.2. The effect of the blood solubility of anaesthetic gases on their alveolar or arterial uptake curves. The rate of induction and recovery with these anaesthetics is largely a function of their solubility in blood.

Halothane potentiates the action of curare-like drugs but antagonizes the effect of suxamethonium. There have been some reports of liver damage following the use of halothane but the incidence of the complication is extremely low and is often referable to a previous history of liver disease.

Methoxyflurane

Methoxyflurane is a non-flammable gas which is not explosive when mixed with oxygen and is stable in contact with soda lime. Because it has a low vapour pressure, induction is slow but when used with thiopentone this disadvantage is overcome. Methoxyflurane produces good muscular relaxation. Although the use of this anaesthetic is contra-indicated in the presence of liver disease and, like halothane, it may occasionally produce a fall in blood pressure and respiratory depression, it is regarded as a safe anaesthetic and is in wide use.

Fluoroxene

Fluoroxene is a volatile anaesthetic which is flammable and explosive. It must be used in a closed-circuit system and is suitable for the induction of light anaesthesia.

Diethyl ether (anaesthetic ether $(CH_3CH_2)_2O$)

Apart from nitrous oxide, ether is the oldest volatile anaesthetic still in use. Ether is a volatile (boiling point 35° C), colourless liquid, with a pungent smell. It decomposes in air and in the presence of light and heat. Mixtures of ether with air, oxygen, or nitrous oxide are dangerously flammable and explosive.

An unexpected property of ether is that it has a neuromuscular blocking action and reduces the contraction of skeletal muscle evoked by nerve stimulation or by the close-arterial injection of acetylcholine. This effect is similar to that obtained by curare-like compounds whose action it potentiates. Before the introduction of neuromuscular blocking drugs, this effect of ether in producing a reduction of muscle tone made it a popular anaesthetic but its use has diminished in recent years.

Ether is a safe and versatile anaesthetic and, although it is not now used alone in major surgery, it is still used for short operations after anaesthesia has been induced by some other agent.

Ethyl chloride (C_2H_5Cl)

The boiling point of ethyl chloride is 12·5° C so that this substance is a gas at ordinary temperatures and pressures but a liquid if kept under slight pressure. It is slightly soluble in water and is flammable and forms explosive mixtures with air and with oxygen.

Ethyl chloride has been used as a general anaesthetic since the beginning of the century and for local analgesia by virtue of its cooling effect when applied locally.

It is still used as the sole anaesthetic for short operations on children and for the induction of anaesthesia prior to the use of another anaesthetic but it is being increasingly replaced by safer compounds.

Nitrous oxide (N_2O)

Nitrous oxide was the first general anaesthetic to be used. It is a colourless gas, heavier than air, with a faint sweet smell. It is not flammable but, like oxygen, it supports combustion.

Nitrous oxide is a weak anaesthetic and is therefore commonly used in conjunction with analgesics or for the maintenance of anaesthesia after the administration of a rapidly acting barbiturate.

The gas can only be given in concentrations up to 80 per cent with oxygen; higher concentrations than this produce hypoxia which may result in damage to the CNS.

When used without other drugs, an 80 per cent mixture of nitrous oxide with oxygen does not usually produce more than second stage anaesthesia.

The gas may be used alone for very brief operations and it is used, in a 35–50 per cent mixture with oxygen, as an analgesic in obstetrics.

There is little difference in the analgesic action of nitrous oxide when mixed with air instead of oxygen and this suggests that hypoxia is not responsible for the analgesic effect of nitrous oxide inhalation.

Cyclopropane

Cyclopropane is a colourless gas which is heavier than air, explosive, and flammable. It is a potent but expensive anaesthetic gas and was extensively used until the advent of balanced anaesthetic techniques.

Cyclopropane is usually given from a closed-circuit anaesthetic machine and it acts rapidly after a not unpleasant induction.

The gas is safe but, because it is potent and rapidly absorbed, it is easy to give an overdose. Recovery from the anaesthetic is rapid but may be followed by restlessness due to a lack of analgesic activity during the recovery phase.

Apart from the risk of explosion it is a useful anaesthetic especially as it allows good oxygenation and has no serious toxic actions.

ANAESTHETIC SOLUTIONS

Various attempts have been made to produce anaesthetics that could be given in solution either intravenously or rectally. It is not usually considered safe to produce full and prolonged anaesthesia by a single dose in this way because the appropriate dose varies in an unpredictable way for different individuals. A dose which is large enough to produce surgical anaesthesia in a reasonable proportion of people would be fatal for some, and once the anaesthetic has been administered, it is impossible to recall it. On the other hand, some barbiturates are quickly taken up by body fat or are very rapidly destroyed in the body, so that it is possible to inject them more or less continuously throughout the operation and to control the depth of anaesthesia by controlling the rate of infusion.

Thiopentone sodium (sodium thiopental)

This is the most widely used intravenous anaesthetic. It acts rapidly and is used to induce anaesthesia. Because thiopentone acts so rapidly the classical stages of anesthesia are rarely seen and the first signs of an overdose may be apnoea.

Thiopentone is not an analgesic and it cannot therefore be used by itself for painful operations. The drug is highly fat soluble and this means that it will have a rapid onset of action. It also means that, despite the fact that it is only metabolized slowly in the liver and other body tissues, there will be a rapid recovery from its effects because it will be taken up in body fat. This explains why rapid recovery from the anaesthetic may follow several repeated injections of the drug up to a point when no more can be stored in the fat. A further dose then gives prolonged anaesthesia and recovery only occurs as the drug is destroyed.

Propanidid

Propanidid is a phenoxy-acetic acid derivative which is given intravenously and produces short-acting anaesthesia (4–5 minutes) which makes it useful for minor dental and surgical procedures.

Ketamine

This is known as a dissociative anaesthetic because it produces a state of dissociation from the environment with analgesia, amnesia, and light sleep. The action of the drug appears to be mainly on the higher centres in the brain with little effect on medullary centres. Muscle relaxation is poor but anaesthesia can be produced rapidly when the drug is given intravenously and lasts for 5–10 minutes. Recovery from ketamine anaesthesia may be slow and accompanied by 'nightmares'.

STEROID ANAESTHETICS

The anaesthetic properties of steroids have been known for over 30 years following the first observations published by Selye in 1941. Steroid anaesthetic have two major advantages over barbiturates but one major barrier to their widespread use in clinical medicine. Their advantages are, first their greater therapeutic ratio and their large safety margin, and secondly, their progressive elimination from blood by the liver so that the recovery from an anaesthetic dose does not rely solely on the redistribution of the drug. The drawback to the use of these compounds in clinical medicine was that they are hard to dissolve and insoluble in water and therefore could not be given intravenously.

Early work showed that steroid anaesthesia was not associated with any one particular hormone or property but it was shown that an oxygen atom had to be present at either end of the steroid molecule and that increasing the double bonds in the A or B ring decreased anaesthetic potency.

In 1955 hydroxydione was introduced; this compound is similar to pregnanedione except that the Na succinate group was replaced by a hydrogen atom in the 21-carbon position. There were problems associated with this drug, particularly involving post-anaesthetic thrombophlebitis, pain at the site of injection, and slow induction of anaesthesia which made it unsuitable for clinical use (Fig. 4.3).

Many related compounds were then developed and tested by intravenous injection into mice and the most potent was found to be 3α-hydroxy-5α-pregnane-11, 20-dione (alphaxalone) which is insoluble in water but very potent and with a high safety margin and rapid induction. This compound was soluble in polyoxyethylated castor oil (Cremophor EL) with the addition of a small amount of a related steroid called alphadolone acetate. This mixture was known as Althesin. Althesin given intravenously rapidly induces a dose-dependent anaesthesia of moderate duration. It has a high therapeutic index, is non-cumulative, and is only slightly potentiated in patients with acute liver damage. There is no vascular irritation and it can be used with all the common pre- and post-anaesthetic medicaments, with inhalational anaesthetics, and with muscle relaxants.

Both steroids enter the brain and are concentrated in the liver and kidney and are not redistributed into the body fat. They are excreted as metabolic products in the faeces or urine within 5 days of injection. The way in which they produce anaesthesia is at present completely unknown. They compare favourably in clinical usefulness with thiopentone, and methohexitone as an intravenous anaesthetic for major and minor surgery.

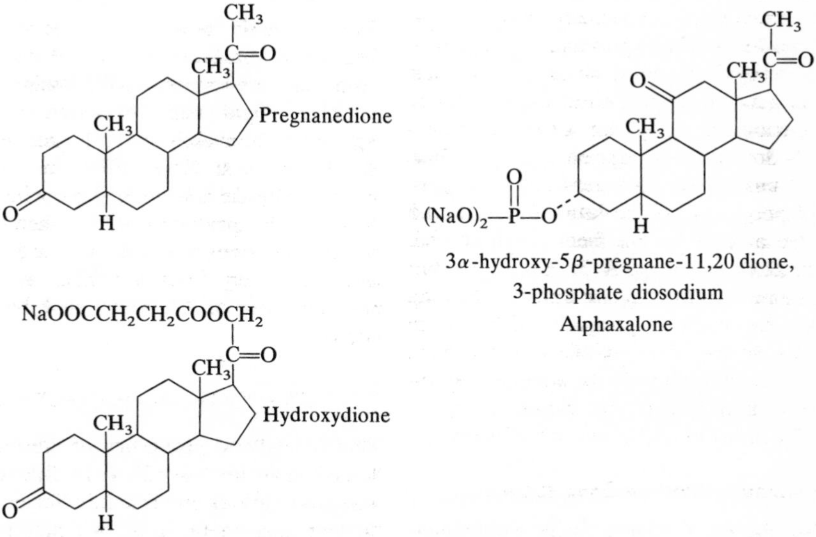

Pregnanedione

3α-hydroxy-5β-pregnane-11,20 dione,
3-phosphate diosodium
Alphaxalone

$NaOOCCH_2CH_2COOCH_2$

Hydroxydione

Fig. 4.3. The structures of some steriod anaesthetics.

HYPNOTICS AND SEDATIVES

The drugs described in this section all have important and often strong depressant actions on the CNS. In sufficiently large doses, most of them will produce anaesthesia by a non-specific depression of the nervous system, but their main usefulness is found in a specific depression of certain central functions obtained with lower, and sometimes very small, doses.

Like other compounds which act directly on the nervous system, our knowledge of their mode of action is meagre.

Sleep is as necessary as food, and lack of it is a serious complication of disease. A hypnotic is a drug which produces sleep, and a very large number of hypnotics are available. However, none of them should be used if the patient can be made to sleep by more simple means because dependence upon a hypnotic may become a habit which is difficult to break.

The difference between a hypnotic effect and general anaesthesia is largely a matter of degree. Any hypnotic given in a large dose causes general anaesthesia, but few drugs are used for both purposes because few drugs have the necessary combination of properties.

Many drugs have some degree of hypnotic activity but their predominant effect may be another type of CNS inhibition and this determines their classification. One can then talk of the hypnotic effects of such a drug but not of the drugs themselves as hypnotics.

Sedatives are agents used to relieve tension and anxiety and make sleep more possible, and they should not, as hypnotics do, actually make the patient sleepy. They act by causing a mild degree of cortical depression. Sedative drugs are usually the common hypnotic agents given in small does throughout the day.

BARBITURATES

The formulae of a number of barbiturates are shown in Table 4.2. They are derivatives of barbituric acid in which all the substituted groups are H. Barbituric acid may be regarded as a derivative of malonic acid ($COOH \, . \, CH_2 \, . \, COOH$) and urea and it is therefore sometimes called malonylurea. Barbituric acid is not itself a hypnotic but substitution of various organic radicals for the hydrogen atoms on C_5 gives compounds with hypnotic actions, the barbiturates.

Replacement of the oxygen atom on C_2 by a sulphur atom gives thiobarbituric acid, the basis of the thiobarbiturates.

Barbiturates are almost insoluble in water but possess weak acidic properties because they exist as an equilibrium mixture of keto (—CO—NH—) and enol (—C(OH):N) forms. The hydrogen of the enol form can be substituted by sodium or other metals to form soluble salts.

Certain features of the structure of the barbiturates allow some generalization of their actions to be made. If the alkyl groups on C_5 are increased in length the potency increases but the duration of action is reduced. A similar change in effect occurs if the alkyl groups on C_5 are substituted by alicyclic, branched or unsaturated side chains and by the attachment of an alkyl group to one of the nitrogen atoms of the ureide. Anticonvulsant properties appear in the barbiturates when a phenyl group is present on C_5 and are more marked in straight-chained alkyl derivatives than in those with branched chains.

Most barbiturates, except hexobarbitone and thiopentone, are absorbed when given orally and most of them may also be given intravenously. They are excreted in the urine partly unchanged, although most of them are also metabolized in the liver.

It has been usual to classify barbiturates according to their duration of action but this arbitrary division is not based on measurement in man and cannot be regarded as satisfactory. It is now known that hypnotic barbiturates fall only into the longer and shorter acting groups and even this classification may not be valid because there is evidence that the incidence of hangover with phenobarbitone is no greater than with quinalbarbitone.

Table 4.2. Derivatives of barbituric acid

```
           (6)
  R1       CO—NH
    \     /     \
     C         CO
    /(5)  \     / (2)
  R2       CO—N
           (4)  |
                R3
```

Duration of action	Trade name	R_1	R_2	R_3	Main use
'Long' Acting (longer than 8 hours)					
Barbitone	Veronal	Ethyl	Ethyl	H	Hypnotic
Phenobarbitone (Phenobarbital)	Luminal	Ethyl	Phenyl	H	Hypnotic, sedative, anticonvulsive
'Short' Acting (up to 8 hours)					
Amylobarbitone (Amobarbital)	Amytal	Ethyl	Isoamyl	H	Sedative, hypnotic, premedicant
Allobarbitone	Dial	Ethyl	Allyl	H	Sedative, hypnotic
Butobarbitone	Soneryl	Ethyl	*n*-butyl	H	Sedative, hypnotic
Cyclobarbitone	Phanodorm	Ethyl	Cyclohexenyl	H	Sedative, hypnotic
Pentobarbitone (Pentobarbital)	Nembutal	Ethyl	1-methylbutyl	H	Sedative, hypnotic, premedicant
Quinalbarbitone (Secobarbital)	Seconal	Allyl	1-methylbutyl	H	Hypnotic, pre-medicant
'Very Short' Acting (I.V. Injection)					
Hexobarbitone	Evipan	Methyl	Cyclohexenyl	1-methyl	Anaesthetic
Methohexitone	Brevital	Allyl	1-methyl-pentynyl	H, S replaces O on C_2	Anaesthetic, hypnotic
Thiopentone Sodium (Thiopental)	Pentothal	Ethyl	1-methylbutyl	H, S replaces O on C_2	Anaesthetic
Thialbarbitone	Kemithal	Allyl	Cyclohexenyl	H, S replaces O on C_2	Anaesthetic

Except for barbitone and phenobarbitone, equilibrium between the brain and the plasma is quickly attained. The fat depots of the body are important repositories for some barbiturates, particularly short acting ones like thiopentone.

The classical barbiturates are broken down by oxidation of their alkyl side chains and produce hypnotically inactive compounds. *N*-methyl derivatives, such as hexobarbitones, are demethylated to give hypnotically active barbiturates and these quickly appear in the urine.

Thiobarbiturates undergo desulphuration to give barbiturates with activity similar to that of the parent compound and these can be found in plasma and must therefore play a part in the anaesthetic and post-anaesthetic action of thiobarbiturates.

Barbiturates are used as sedatives, hypnotics, basal narcotics, anaesthetics, and anticonvulsants, the appropriate compound being chosen on the basis of its duration of action (see Table 4.2). With the exception of the very short-acting compounds, most of the derivatives can be used as hypnotics but those in most common use are phenobarbitone, amylobarbitone, pentobarbitone, and quinalbarbitone.

Those who take barbiturates reqularly are liable to become physically dependent on them and withdrawal symptoms may be observed following prolonged use of the drugs. The first dose may weaken the memory so that the patient forgets he has taken a dose and takes more. Overdosage may cause incoordination and prolonged sleep or profound anaesthesia with paralysis of the respiration. Barbiturate poisoning produces cyanosis and markedly depressed respiration which may result in respiratory failure followed by cardiovascular collapse and death. The most important way to treat barbiturate poisoning is by instituting artificial respiration and clearing the stomach contents if the drug has only recently been taken. If the drug has been absorbed, it may be advisable to produce forced diuresis.

When the barbiturate overdosage is not too great the depression of respiration may of barbiturates on the medullary respiratory centres. The slow-acting barbiturates like barbitone and phenobarbitone have a cumulative action when taken every day. Barbiturates should be used with caution in severe liver and kidney disease as metabolism and excretion will be delayed.

Tolerance to barbiturates develops when they are taken repeatedly due to the activation of liver enzyme systems which metabolize the drug so reducing the effect of a given dose.

NON-BARBITURATE HYPNOTICS AND SEDATIVES

Various halogen derivatives are used as anaesthetics, basal narcotics, and hypnotics. They are all liable to cause toxic effects and should be avoided in patients who are liable to ketosis or who have damaged livers.

Chloral hydrate ($CCl_3CH(OH)_2$)

This was the first hypnotic, having been introduced in 1868 by Liebreich, who knew that alkaline solutions liberated chloroform, and hoped that the same change would occur in the body. It is now known that chloral hydrate is reduced in the body to trichlorethylalcohol ($CCl_3 . CH_2OH$), and that it is this substance which is active in the body. It combines in the liver with glycuronic acid to form urochloralic (chloraluric) acid ($CCl_3 . CH_2O \ (CHOH)_5 . COOH$). Urine containing urochloralic acid acquires the power of reducing Fehling's solution. Chloral hydrate is widely used, especially in the elderly and in children, as a hypnotic which is taken by mouth and causes sleep in about half an hour, and lasts 6–8 hours. It is especially valuable in manic states and to treat delirium tremens. Chloral hydrate should be well diluted before administration because it irritates the gastric mucosa and may cause nausea and vomiting.

Dichloralphenazone is a combination of chloral with phenazone that is also used as a hypnotic.

Nitrazepam

Nitrazepam is a benzodiazepine with more pronounced hypnotic properties than other compounds in this group. It is proving a useful alternative to barbiturates as an hypnotic since it is considerably safer when taken as an overdose. Prolonged use may lead to physical dependence but again, this appears to be less of a problem than with barbiturates. Drowsiness and lightheadedness have been reported to follow an hypnotic dose of nitrazepam.

Glutethimide

Glutethimide is a piperidinedione derivative with actions rather similar to the barbiturates. It is a CNS depressant with strong hypnotic activity and was introduced in the hope that it would prove less addictive than the barbiturates, but several cases of withdrawal symptoms, following discontinuance of the drug, have been reported and it must be considered a drug of addiction. It resembles phenobarbitone structurally and quinalbarbitone in its onset and duration of action. It is well tolerated and relatively non-toxic. It forms a useful alternative to barbiturates as a hypnotic.

Methyprylone

Methyprylone is used as a sedative and mild hypnotic, it acts within an hour and its effects last about 6 hours. Little is known about its side-effects but in normal dosage they appear to be absent.

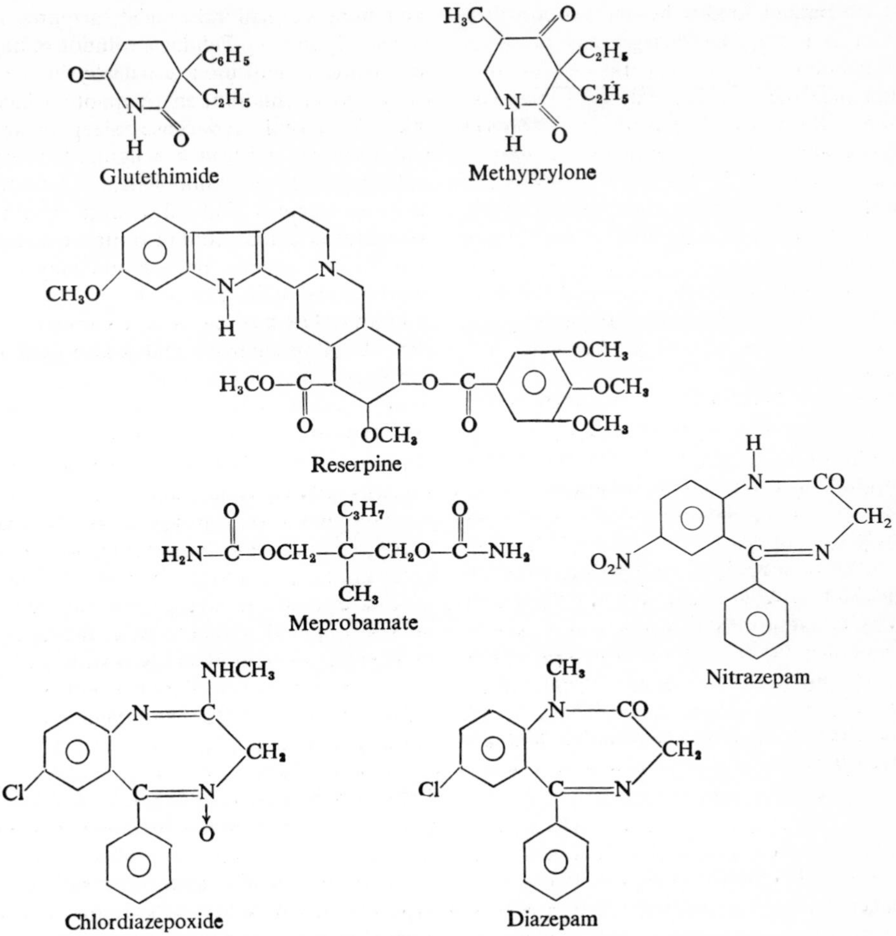

Glutethimide

Methyprylone

Reserpine

Meprobamate

Nitrazepam

Chlordiazepoxide

Diazepam

Fig. 4.4. The structures of some hypnotic and tranquillizing drugs.

Bromides

The bromides have a general depressant effect on the central nervous system with specific anticonvulsant activity. Their hypnotic and analgesic effects are weak in normal doses.

They are readily absorbed from the small intestine and are only excreted slowly in the urine. Complete elimination of the drug may not take place for 6 weeks or more and therefore their action is cumulative.

Bromides are not normally preferred to barbiturates and are no longer used except in some proprietary preparations.

ANTICONVULSANTS

The term 'epilepsy' describes a variety of disorders which may involve loss of consciousness, convulsions, and changes in the electroencephalogram.

The three major types of epilepsy are: (1) grand mal, in which major convulsions occur; (2) petit mal, in which there may be loss of consciousness with only mild convulsion and

Table 4.3. Drugs used to treat epilepsy

Grand mal	Phenobarbitone Phenytoin Carbamazepine Sulthiame
Petit mal	Troxidone Ethosuximide
Psychomotor	Diazepam Nitrazepam Phenacemide Phenytoin

autonomic disturbance; and (3) psychomotor epilepsy in which there may be various types of confused behaviour.

The anticonvulsant drugs used to treat these different types of epilepsy are shown in Table 4.3.

The initiation of epileptic seizures appears to be due to a suppression of central inhibition and the development of abnormal nerve impulse activity in small feed-back loops, possibly as a result of enhanced post-tetanic potentiation (P.T.P.) effects in these circuits.

It seems that the most important action of anticonvulsants is to lower the excitability of certain central neurones and so diminish the excessive firing which would otherwise result in a seizure.

Most anticonvulsants are related to phenobarbitone, which is itself the oldest and best-tried anticonvulsant. Considerable efforts have been made to produce more potent anticonvulsants, without the disadvantages of barbiturates, by making small changes in the basic barbiturate molecule.

Most of the anticonvulsants contain a common basic ring structure and in all drugs except a few which are used for petit mal epilepsy only, the addition of a phenyl ring to the nucleus is essential for activity. The effect of structural changes on the central actions of these compounds can be followed in Table 4.3 and Fig. 4.5.

None of the anticonvulsant drugs at present in use is ideal because of their side-effects and because their action is not always predictable. These difficulties would be largely overcome if a drug were developed which could specifically potentiate central inhibitory processes. It is now known that γ-amino butyric acid is an inhibitory transmitter in parts of the brain including the cerebral cortex (see Chapter 3) and drugs which pass the blood–brain barrier and then mimic or potentiate its action may be highly effective anticonvulsants. It is already known that if γ-amino butyric acid itself, which does not pass the blood–brain barrier, is injected in very small amounts directly into the cerebral ventricle in man, it has a dramatic effect in alleviating the symptoms of epilepsy and produces no side-effects.

Phenobarbitone (phenobarbital)

This was the first effective anticonvulsant known and is still in wide use. The upper dose limit is set by the appearance of sedation but this can be offset by combining the drug with a central stimulant like amphetamaine.

Phenytoin (diphenylhydantoin)

Phenytoin was developed in 1938 as a result of a planned search for a drug to diminish convulsions during electro-shock therapy. The drug is important because it is not a sedative and is particularly effective in suppressing electrically evoked convulsions in sub-hypnotic doses.

The mode of action of phenytoin appears to be to limit the spread of an epileptic focus rather than to increase the seizure threshold. It is known that the drug is able to reduce P.T.P. in the spinal cord and a similar stabilizing action in higher centres could prevent the spread of epileptiform seizures. In petit mal attacks, where P.T.P. is thought not to be involved, this drug is ineffective. Phenytoin is well absorbed from the intestine and mostly destroyed in the body. Toxic effects are common and some may be serious. The less serious effects include dizziness, nausea, and skin rashes. The more serious complications are megaloblastic anaemia, morbilliform rash with fever, exfoliative dermatitis, and gingival hypertrophy.

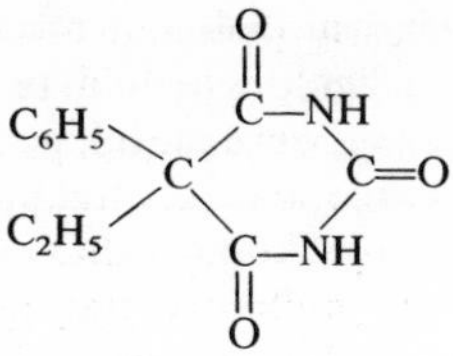

Phenobarbitone.

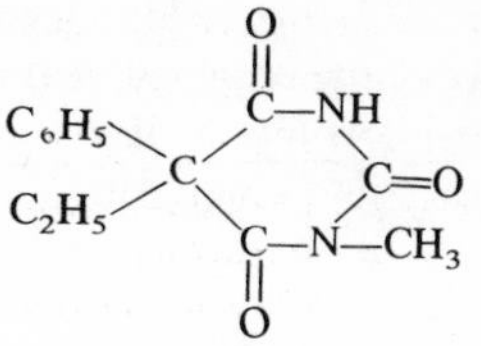

n-Methylphenobarbitone.

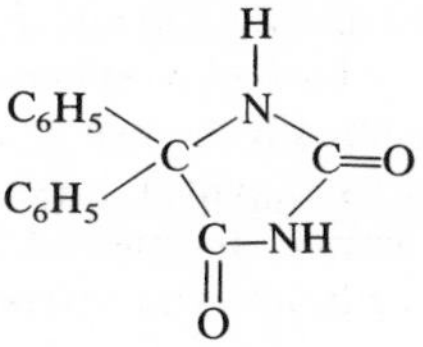

Phenytoin.

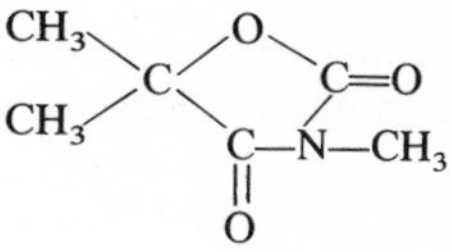

Troxidone.

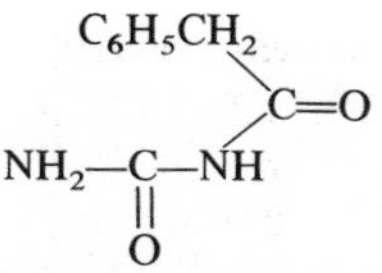

Phenacemide.

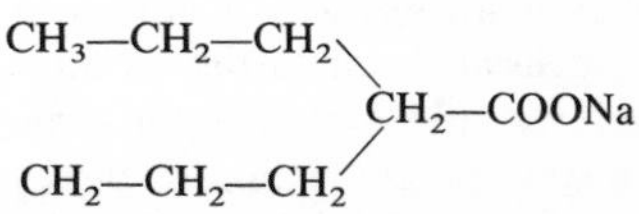

Sodium valporate

Fig. 4.5. The structures of some anticonvulsants.

Troxidone (trimethadione)

The alkyl substituents in this compound confer a selective action on petit mal epilepsy and, unlike phenytoin, it has a marked effect on the electroencephalogram. Troxidone is a toxic drug and may cause rashes, photophobia, and, occasionally, agranulcytosis and aplastic anaemias.

Phenacemide

Phenacemide is used in the treatment of psychomotor epilepsy but only if other treatment fails because it is potentially toxic to the liver and bone marrow.

Carbamazepine

This compound is related to the tricyclic antidepressant drugs, but it is useful in treating grand mal epilepsy. Some psychotropic effects have been reported but these do not seem serious.

Ethosuximide

Ethosuximide is commonly used, largely replacing troxidone, to treat petit mal conditions and it can be combined with those anticonvulsants used to treat major epilepsy when both these conditions exist. Toxic effects may include nausea and vomiting, dizziness, and leucopenia.

Sulthiame

This has been widely used in treating grand mal conditions and, although it appears to have weak anticonvulsant activity of its own, it seems to inhibit the metabolism of other anticonvulsants given concurrently.

Sodium valporate

Sodium valporate is unlike other anticonvulsant drugs in chemical structure but appears to be effective in controlling grand mal epilepsy.

Diazepam

Diazepam, given intravenously, is the drug of choice for the interruption of status epilepticus but its use for chronic oral therapy of epilepsy is not clearly defined. Chronic oral administration in does which may control seizures can give rise to sedation, ataxia, and incoordination.

TRANQUILLIZING DRUGS

Tranquillizing drugs have been called the drugs of civilization and as modern society proceeds so the demand for these compounds rises.

Although their increasing and often indiscriminate use may be deplored, there is no doubt that they have revolutionized the treatment of the mentally ill and transformed the lives of many people who would otherwise have been condemned to institutions.

These drugs are used to treat conditions of fear, anxiety, and violence and have a particular use in the alleviation of the symptoms of schizophrenia and allied disorders. They do not have significant hypnotic or anaesthetic actions.

The development of effective tranquillizing drugs has progressed in a somewhat haphazard and arbitrary manner and some of the earlist tranquillizers arose from the observation that an antihistaminic compound, promethezine, calmed excited emotional states. This led to the production of analogues of promethezine and so produced the phenothiazine class of tranquillizers. One reason for this unsatisfactory manner of progress has been the difficulty of testing and evaluating the effect of centrally acting drugs and in understanding their mechanisms of action in the brain.

Mental disorders cannot be produced in experimental animals and so tests for psychotropic drug action are necessarily empirical. These tests usually involve the comparison of the effect of a new drug with that of a drug of proved therapeutic value on the behaviour of animals. The actual tests involved are varied and large in number and the use of various combinations of them may provide a useful profile of a potential psychoactive drug, but screening procedures of this kind are unlikely to produce entirely new classes of useful drugs.

The tests usually employed often begin with a preliminary screening test by observing the effects of a drug on the general behaviour of animals. Following initial screening there may be tests on the spontaneous motor activity, exploratory activity, motor coordination, and muscle tone. More elaborate experiments assess the action of drugs on conditioned avoidance responses and on operant conditioning where the effect of a drug on an animal trained to perform tasks by reward and punishment can be studied. Aggressive and neurotic behaviour can be induced in rats and mice by means of brain lesions or by applying repeated electric shocks, and experimental neuroses can be produced by frustrating conditioned responses in animals. The action of drugs can be tested on all these experimental models but the interpretation of results has to proceed with great caution as extrapolation from animal models to man can produce grossly misleading results.

It only begins to be possible to be confident about the potential therapeutic value of a centrally acting drug after it has been tested in man under well-controlled conditions. The development of entirely new classes of centrally acting drugs depends largely on developing an understanding of the basic mechanism underlying a particular mental disorder and then attempting to affect this mechanism in a logical manner, usually by employing basic experimental techniques in the first instance.

The tranquillizing compounds may be classified into two main groups, the major and the minor tranquillizers.

1. Major tranquillizers.

   Rauwolfia derivatives, i.e. reserpine.

Phenothiazine derivatives, i.e. chlorpromazine, promazine, triflupromazine.

2. Minor tranquillizers.
   Propanediol derivatives, i.e. meprobamate.
   Benzodiazepine derivatives, i.e. chlordiazepoxide, diazepam.

MAJOR TRANQUILLIZERS

Rauwolfia deriatives

Reserpine is the most important of the many alkaloids found in extracts of the climbing shrub known as *Rauwolfia serpentina* which has long been used in India for treating snake bites, hypertension, insommia, insanity, and noisy children.

In recent times reserpine was used to relieve hypertension but the calming effect of this drug led to it being used as an effective tranquillizer. It is absorbed from the intestine and is commonly given by the mouth. Its action develops slowly during 2–4 hours and may last several days, even when the drug is injected intravenously, but the highest concentration in the brain is found comparatively soon, before any obvious effects on the whole animal are seen. It is hydrolysed in the body to methyl reserpate which appears in the urine.

It is generally agreed that the tranquillizing action of reserpine is quite different from the sedative action of barbiturates. Its mode of action is not known but what is known is that it depletes the brain of 5-hydroxytryptamine and noradrenaline, the latter about 10 per cent of its original level within 4 hours and for about 8 hours, but it is unlikely that these effects alone are responsible for the tranquillizing action of reserpine.

Reserpine has a prolonged sedative action without narcosis and is not an anticonvulsant. It inhibits the activity of sympathetic but not parasympathetic centres and as result there is a fall of body temperature, constriction of the pupil, a fall in blood pressure, loss of pressor reflexes, and diarrhoea. The central side-effects of reserpine include fatigue, nervousness, insomnia, nightmares; tolerance and addiction do not occur. There is now little doubt that reserpine may also produce suicidal tendencies in some patients and for this reason it is not now in wide use.

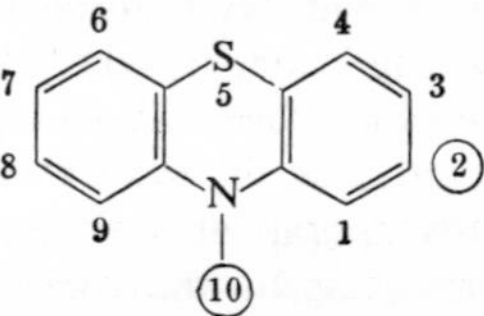

Fig. 4.6. The phenothiazine nucleus.

Phenothiazine derivatives

This group forms the largest and most important group of major tranquillizers. They are all based on the phenothiazine nucleus, differing only in their substituents at positions 2 and 10. These compounds share the same general properties but differ quantitatively in their tranquillizing potency and side-effects.

There are many phenothiazine derivatives in addition to those shown in Table 4.4 but the most important changes that may be made to the phenothiazine nucleus are illustrated by these examples. The most potent tranquillizers have a three-carbon chain attached at position 10 and the addition of a fluorine radical or a piperazine ring as in trifluoperazine raises their potency still further.

Table 4.4. Phenothiazine derivatives

	10	2	Tranquillizing potency
Chlorpromazine	$(CH_2)_3—N(CH_3)_2$	Cl	1·0
Promazine	$(CH_2)_3—N(CH_3)_2$	H	0·5
Triflupromazine	$(CH_2)_3—N(CH_3)_2$	CF_3	4
Trifluoperazine	$(CH_2)_3—N\langle\ \rangle NCH_3$ (piperazine ring)	CF_3	10

Chlorpromazine was first used in Paris in 1951 by Laborit and Huguenard to lower the body temperature and so cause 'artificial hibernation' during operations.

The most important effect of chlorpromazine is to cause tranquillization and in normal dosage it does not affect higher mental function.

It is widely used in mental hospitals to treat seriously disturbed patients and is often so effective they can return home. Like reserpine it increases the action of hypnotics, but unlike reserpine it does not reduce the amounts of 5-hydroxytryptamine and noradrenaline in the brain. It is known that chlorpromapine blocks dopamine receptors in the central nervous system and this action may underlay its therapeutic effects. It has an anti-emetic action on the vomiting centre in the medulla and it antagonizes the actions of various drugs on this centre. It has little or no action on motion sickness.

Its main peripheral action is to antagonize the α-receptor actions of catecholamines (Chapter 8). It has local anaesthetic action and has an effect like that of quinidine on the heart. It does not block autonomic ganglia and in spite of its chemical similarity to promethazine, it has practically no atropine-like or antihistamine-like action.

Its effect on the circulation may be largely due to depression of the central and peripheral sympathetic nervous system. Under its action the blood pressure is low, the skin warm and dry, and the pulse rapid. It causes a marked reduction in temperature, partly due to cutaneous vasodilatation and partly due to the inhibition of shivering. The fall in temperature causes a fall in the metabolism of the tissues and this may protect them from harm when their circulation is depressed during operations, and in some other conditions where shock may occur. Some the sedative effects may be secondary to the fall of temperature.

A single large dose may cause postural hypertension. Repeated doses may cause excessive sedation, Parkinson-like tremor, various allergic effects, leucopenia, and obstructive jaundice, the latter effect being the result of hypersensitivity in a few people to the drug.

Minor side-effects include a dry mouth, constipation, and urinary frequency.

Promazine and trifluoperazine have similar actions to chlorpromazine.

MINOR TRANQUILLIZERS

Propanediol derivatives

These compounds are used for the treatment of anxiety states; they are not effective in the treatment of psychoses.

Meprobamate blocks neuronal conduction in the hypothalamus and spinal cord and it produces mild tranquillization without drowsiness. It is used in the treatment of neuroses, alcoholism, and anxiety states but it does carry a serious addiction risk. It also reduces tolerance to ingested alcohol.

Mephenesin is a muscle relaxant and an interneuronal blocker. It is now a very effective tranquillizer but it has few side-effects. Mephenesin carbamate is more widely used than mephenesin because it is more slowly absorbed from the gastro-intestinal tract and has a longer duration of action.

Benzodiazepines

Chlordiazepoxide and Diazepam form a new chemical class of tranquillizer. Chlordiazepoxide was the first to be used and diazepam, a more potent compound, was then introduced. These drugs are widely used for a variety of conditions, particularly anxiety states, to secure muscle relaxation, and in the rehabilitation of alcoholics. The tranquillizing effect of these chemicals was first used to tame tigers but they are now more extensively used on man.

They block electroencephalogram arousal patterns following stimulation of the reticular formation and reduce after-discharges in higher centres but, like all tranquillizers, their precise mode of action is unknown.

A great advantage of these drugs is that, although they are rapidly absorbed from the gut, their action is prolonged, the plasma half-peak concentration occurring after about 24 hours.

Unpleasant side-effects are only seen in very high doses when drowsiness and ataxia may be apparent. There appears to be little, development of tolerance or addiction and the drugs are safe, 2·25 g having been taken over 24 hours without death.

ALCOHOL (C_2H_5OH)

Alcohol is an anaesthetic, a disinfectant, a protein precipitant, a local irritant and, in discreet doses, it may also be regarded as a valuable minor tranquillizer.

Alcohol is rapidly absorbed from the stomach and if any reaches the intestines it is rapidly absorbed from there. It can also be absorbed as a vapour through the lungs. Once absorbed, alcohol is quickly distributed throughout the body water.

Up to 98 per cent of the alcohol that enters the body is completely oxidized; the rate at which this oxidation takes place is related more to body weight than to the concentration of alcohol present. About 10 ml of alcohol can be oxidized by a normal adult per hour.

Primary oxidation of alcohol by alcohol dehydrogenase occurs in the liver where acetaldehyde is formed which is then converted to acetyl CoA. This is then further oxidized through the citric acid cycle or utilized in the synthesis of tissue constituents. The rate of conversion of alcohol is maximal when the dehydrogenase system is saturated and this occurs at blood levels of about 0·1 per cent alcohol.

Alcohol which is not oxidized in the body is excreted almost entirely through the kidney and lungs. As the amount of alcohol removed from the body in this way comprises only a small part of that ingested the use of diuretics does little to remove the signs of intoxication.

Action of alcohol

The effect of alcohol on the CNS tends to overshadow the numerous actions of this drug on other tissues.

Contrary to popular opinion, the action of alcohol on the CNS is mainly inhibitory and the apparent excitatory action of this drug results from the depression of inhibitory systems in the higher centres of the brain. These higher centres normally exert an inhibitory influence enabling the organism to behave sensibly. When these centres are suppressed the cruder instincts appear to be released and behaviour becomes more spontaneous, more childlike, and less critical.

Human alcohol intoxication is commonly divided into four stages:

1. In the first stage there is a slight loss of efficiency, a dulled critical ability, and spinal reflexes are slower and weaker but the subject feels pleased with himself.
2. In the second stage, the novice drinker loses all self-control, the hardened drinker speaks and moves with exaggerated care.
3. In the third stage the subject is unconscious with a flushed face, active sweat glands, red eyes, and dilated pupils.
4. In the fourth stage there is danger of death from paralysis of the respiratory and vasomoter centres in the medulla.

Alcohol affects the electroencephalogram, causing a slowing of the dominant rhythm and this has been used as a guide to the state of intoxication.

The mechanism of action of alcohol on cells in the CNS is obscure. It does seem to have a non-specific depressant action on the excitability of all neurones and this may be through a local anaesthetic action.

Serious additive effects are known to occur when alcohol is taken in addition to various psychotropic drugs. Chlorpromazine, for instance, greatly increases the expected impairment of judgement and co-ordination following alcohol ingestion.

Very small amounts of alcohol are sufficient to reduce skilled performance and blood alcohol levels of 50 mg/100 ml of blood produces significant slowing of reaction time in most people. Sensible legislation in most European countries now sets maximum blood alcohol levels for driving cars which varies from zero in some countries to 80 mg/100 ml blood in Great Britain.

Alcohol causes an increase in blood flow through the skin, probably by direct inhibition of the vasomotor centre. This leads to a feeling of warmth and a fall in body temperature. In reasonable doses, alcohol does not appear to have any direct effect on cardiac output, coronary or cerebral blood flow.

The increase in peripheral blood flow following alcohol ingestion causes a fall in body temperature and this may be aggravated by the occurrence of sweating. As with general anaesthetics, large doses of alcohol may inhibit the central temperature regulating mechanisms and so cause a pronounced fall in body temperature.

Alcohol produces diuresis partly because of the extra fluid that is ingested and also by a direct action inhibiting the release of antidiuretic hormone from the posterior pituitary. The diuretic effect is proportional to the level of circulating alcohol in the blood and is usually only seen as the alcohol level rises.

Chronic alcohol poisoning

The constant drinking of alcohol injures the CNS so that the drinker becomes careless, untidy, forgetful, and irritable. At the same time he acquires a certain amount of tolerance so that large quantities of alcohol have no apparent effect on him. This is mainly due to a real insensitivity of the nervous system, and to the fact that the persistent drinker has much practice in concealing the effects of drink. As time goes on the drinker becomes more irritable and more anxious and may eventually develop delirium tremens. In this condition he is very restless and may suffer a variety of hallucinations. This condition may eventually lead to permanent mental disturbance or to death.

Chronic alcoholism has many ill effects, some of which are due to associated factors such as vitamin deficiency. The stomach shows chronic gastritis; the kidneys show fatty changes and hypertrophy of connective tissue, and cirrhosis of the liver may occur. One of the most important effects is neuritis involving both sensory and motor nerves and causing loss of sensation in the skin and loss of power in the muscles. This neuritis is due to a deficiency of aneurine and can be cured by the injection of this substance. The diet of chronic alcoholics is usually deficient in this vitamin and absorption is poor.

Tetraethylthiuram disulphide (disulfiram, *Antabuse*) is a drug now used to treat cases of chronic alcoholism. This substance was originally tested as an anthelmintic but when first tested on man it was noticed that it produced disturbing and unpleasant symptoms when alcohol was ingested. Given by itself disulfiram is relatively non-toxic but it greatly alters the intermediate metabolism of alcohol by inhibiting the oxidation of acetaldehyde in the liver thus allowing the concentration of this substance in the body to rise. The symptoms of acetaldehyde poisoning include excessive flushing, headaches, palpitations, giddiness, and nausea and are so unpleasant that alcohol will be avoided as long as disulfiram is present.

ANALGESICS

Pain saves many lives, since it compels those who can, to avoid harm and to seek treatment when harm has been done. The relief of pain is always desirable, but the use of drugs for this purpose is dangerous if it makes diagnosis more difficult, or if it is allowed to take the place of more fundamental treatment.

Pain can be relieved by general anaesthetics, local anaesthetics, counter-irritants, or by various drugs which act centrally without producing general anaesthesia. The best known of these are morphine and its derivatives, but various synthetic drugs are equally effective, and the antipyretics (Chapter 12) have a weak action of the same kind.

Painful stimuli cause a number of reactions, such as a sudden intake of breath, withdrawal from the source of pain, vocalization, a fall of blood pressure, and the psychogalvanic reflex, which consists of changes in the electrical resistance of the skin. It is difficult to compare the relative potency and effectiveness of different analgesics because it is not easy to assess pain quantitatively. Weakly painful stimuli can be applied by a measured prick with a needle, heat, cold, or electric shocks which produce some unconditioned responses, such as the sudden intake of breath, without enough pain to disturb the animal. Analgesics such as morphine diminish these effects and their action can be measured in this way.

Another method of studying analgesics involves experiments on man. The pain may be due to disease or produced artificially. Painful agents used include ischaemia, pressure, and electrical currents and the effect may be judged by the man's response or description of his sensations. Such experiments are said to be subjective and are notoriously difficult, since the result may be affected by a multitude of factors.

OPIUM

Opium consists of dark resinous lumps, made by drying the milky juice that exudes when an incision is made in unripe seed capsules of the Oriental poppy (*Papaver somniferum*). It contains about twenty-five different alkaloids, the most important of which are morphine (3–20 per cent), codeine (methylmorphine) (0·3–0·4 per cent), narcotine (2–8 per cent), and thebane (0·2–0·5 per cent). The other alkaloids, including narceine and papaverine, constitute just over 1 per cent of the drug.

MORPHINE

Morphine (Table 4.5) is the most important alkaloid in opium; it is readily absorbed when eaten, smoked, or injected. Its effects are seen in about half an hour and begin to pass away after 3–5 hours but may last for at least 12 hours. It is mostly oxidized, mainly in the liver, and a certain amount is excreted into the stomach and probably into other parts of the alimentary canal.

Morphine exerts its most important effects on the CNS where it causes depression and excitation of certain centres. It depresses the cerebral cortex and reduces the powers of

Table 4.5. The structure of some morphine-like compounds and their antagonists

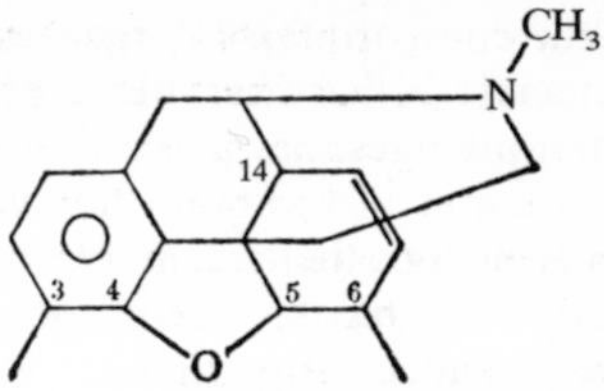

The morphine skeleton

	Substituents on morphine skeleton			
	3	4–5	6	N–
Morphine	HO	O	HO	CH_3
Codeine	CH_3O	O	HO	CH_3
Diamorphine	CH_3COO	O	CH_3COO	CH_3
Dihydromorphinone	HO	O	=O	CH_3
Levorphanol	HO	—	H	C_3H_5
Metopon	CH_3O	O	=O	CH_3
Nalorphine	HO	O	HO	C_3H_5
Levallorphan	HO	—	H	C_3H_5

concentration, fear, and anxiety. Pain particularly prolonged, as opposed to acute pain, is reduced and this produces a great feeling of contentment.

The effect on the cerebellum is mainly depressant and there may be motor incoordination. Various centres in the medulla are affected. The vomiting centre and the associated centres for salivation, sweat, and bronchial secretion are stimulated at first, though become depressed by large and subsequent doses. The sweating is associated with vasodilatation of the skin vessels, so that morphine increases heat loss and is a mild antipyretic.

The respiratory centre and the cough centre are depressed. The respiration is slow and deep and may be periodic. Large doses kill by stopping the respiration altogether. The parasympathetic portion of the oculomotor nucleus is stimulated and the pupils become constricted and, in morphine poisoning, may be of pinpoint size. Other effects mediated via the CNS include a feeling of heaviness in the limbs, a dry mouth, itching, and the reduction of hunger sensations.

Until recently little was known about how morphine exerts these effects on the CNS. It does inhibit the hydrolysis of acetylcholine and in low concentrations it reduces the release of acetylcholine from nerve endings in the guinea-pig intestine. If acetylcholine is a neurotransmitter in the brain this may have some bearing on the action of morphine. Morphine also blocks the action of 5-hydroxytryptamine at peripheral sites and although there are indications that this chemical may be concerned in central transmission, it is again not possible to say if morphine works by this kind of action.

With the recent discovery of discrete opiate receptors within the brain the mode of action of morphine has become easier to explain. It now appears that morphine may be mimicking the action of a chemical normally produced in the brain, an endogenous opiate which may be enkephalin or peptides from the endorphin series (see chapter 9).

The enkephalins and endorphins share many properties in common with morphine and will produce a naloxone-sensitive analgesia when injected into the brain; they also appear to produce tolerance and dependence like other opiates.

Of the more peripheral actions of morphine, constipation is one of the most important. The constipation produced is unaffected by denervation of the intestine or by atropine, and is largely due to an increase in the tone of the gut and sphincters and an inhibitory action on Auerbach's plexus. Other factors which probably increase this action of morphine are inhibition of the secretion of the intestinal glands and depression of the reflexes responsible for defaecation.

Morphine also causes retention of both urine and bile by closing the sphincters. It raises the pressure in the common bile-duct and may cause biliary colic. It should therefore not be used in the treatment of pain due to biliary colic.

Tolerance and dependence

Tolerance to morphine occurs and, over a period of time, the dose taken has to be increased to produce the same degree of effect. Tolerance in man usually takes 2–3 weeks to acquire on normal therapeutic doses and it applies only to the depressant action of the drug, the respiratory depression shows tolerance but the effect on the pupil and on the intestine continues unabated. People receiving morphine regularly are liable to become physically dependent on the drug. When this has occurred, withdrawal of the drug produces symptoms within 15–20 hours. In addicts, the morphine antagonist nalorphine can produce withdrawal symptoms within 30 minutes. The withdrawal symptoms commence with yawning, sweating, and running of the eyes and nose. There will then be restlessness for 18–24 hours. After this period there is mydriasis, 'goose flesh', cramp, nausea, insomnia, vomiting, and diarrhoea. Tolerance to morphine is rapidly lost during this period and the withdrawal symptoms may be terminated by a suitable dose of morphine.

Many theories have been advanced to explain the mechanism of tolerance and dependence but none has proved completely satisfactory. The discovery of opiate receptors and opiate-like peptides within the brain has, however, allowed more logical explanations to emerge. Dependence on opiate drugs is likely to be the result of some interaction between synthetic and endogenous analgesic chemicals and it has been reported that the development of morphine dependence in rats is paralleled by an increase in the levels of enkephalin in their brains. This seems to be paradoxical since morphine dependence is accompanied by a decrease in effectiveness of the drugs (tolerance) and it might be expected that an increase in enkephalin would enhance its effect. In fact, an increase in brain transmitter often means it is not being released (cf. acetylcholine) and therefore its effects are diminished at the receptor sites. This may be happening in the development of morphine dependence, morphine acts on the same receptors as enkephalin and, through a feedback mechanism, enkephalin release from nerve terminals is reduced. The brain then becomes dependent on morphine as a substitute for enkephalin.

Further research may well provide further modifications of our ideas about dependence but it does seem that many facets of the problem are now becoming unified into a convincing hypothesis.

MORPHINE-LIKE COMPOUNDS

Pethidine (meperidine)

Pethidine is a piperidine compound and has many properties in common with both morphine and atropine. This drug has a slightly higher analgesic potency than codeine. It causes euphoria and may lead to physical dependence. Its actions differ in many ways from those of drugs in the morphine group. It is not an effective sedative or hypnotic and its direct effect on smooth muscle is inhibitory; it does not constrict the pupil or cause constipation. On the other hand, like morphine, it closes the sphincter of Oddi and thus increases the pressure in the gall-bladder, so that it should not be used in the treatment of biliary colic. Tolerance is not as complete as with morphine and with the doses that some addicts take, convulsions may occur.

Pethidine is used for acute pain in pre- and post-operative stages and for chronic pain associated with cancer. It may be used as a premedicant, in the early stages of labour, for incomplete anaesthesia during minor surgical procedures, and to produce basal narcosis in conjunction with drugs like chlorpromazine and promethazine. It is particularly useful in pulmonary and cardiac surgery because it depresses cardiac and bronchial reflexes.

Codeine

The actions of codeine are much weaker than those of morphine and it is less likely to cause unpleasant side-effects and, even in large doses, it does not depress respiration. It is not as addictive as morphine and unlike morphine, is not destroyed in the body, but is mostly excreted in the urine. It is used to treat minor pain and as an antitussive agent.

Pholcodine

Pholcodine resembles codeine in suppressing cough and is particularly useful in the treatment of unproductive cough. It is less toxic than codeine, does not cause constipation, and is well tolerated by children.

Diamorphine (heroin)

Diamorphine is a slightly more powerful analgesic than morphine with fewer side-effects. Diamorphine is used nowadays only to relieve very severe pain, usually in a terminal illness.

Dihydromorphinone

Dihydromorphinone is a synthetic derivative of morphine with a similar but weaker analgesic activity. It may be used as a substitute for morphine and unpleasant side-effects are said to be less severe.

Levorphanol

Levorphanol acts like morphine but its effect is more prolonged. It has little hypnotic activity and anxiety is not relieved. Levorphanol is used for the relief of severe pain. Its lack of sedative action is an advantage in some patients.

Methadone

Methadone is a strong analgesic of similar potency to morphine but it has less sedative and euphoric action. Tolerance to the analgesic, sedative, and respiratory depressant effects has been observed. It is a drug of addiction. It is used to treat severe pain and in premedication. It is also used to treat morphine dependence because it may be withdrawn with few unpleasant consequences.

Phenazocine

Phenazocine is a synthetic analgesic with similar actions and uses to morphine but it is effective in smaller doses and has a more prolonged action. It was developed in the hope that it would be less addictive than morphine but this hope has not been fulfilled.

Etorphine

Etorphine is a new synthetic agent which is from one thousand to eight thousand times more potent than morphine. It has a powerful central depressant action which can be antagonized with nalorphine.

ANTAGONISTS OF MORPHINE ACTION

Naloxone

Unlike other antagonists of opiate action, naloxone is an almost pure antagonist at the opiate receptor. When given in high doses to man it does not produce drowsiness or the side effects associated with morphine and the less specific morphine antagonists. Naloxone prevents, or promptly reverses, the effects of opiates in man and in patients with respiratory depression there is relief within minutes. For this reason, naloxone is invaluable in treating opiate overdosage.

Nalorphine

This is a partial antagonist of morphine and is used as an antidote not only for morphine but also for synthetic substitutes such as pethidine and methadone. Structurally it only differs from morphine in the replacement of the methyl radical attached to the nitrogen atom with an allyl group.

The actions of nalorphine alone are similar to those of morphine. Respiration and blood pressure are depressed and it has a slight sedative, but little analgesic, action.

When respiratory depression is established with morphine the administration of nalorphine will stimulate breathing. This probably occurs because nalorphine competes successfully with morphine for receptor sites in the respiratory centre, and while alone it would depress respiration, it would do so less than morphine so the net result is a reduction in the morphine depression.

Nalorphine can be used to establish whether addiction to morphine-like drugs is present because withdrawal symptoms will quickly follow the injection of nalorphine to the addict.

Levallorphan

Levallorphan is a morphine-like compound having the same relationship to levorphanol as nalorphine has to morphine.

Like nalorphine this compound antagonizes respiratory depression due to morphine-like drugs and will prevent respiratory depression if given with them. It also reduces the analgesic action of these drugs so the agonist and antagonist are not normally given together.

ANTIPYRETIC–ANALGESICS

These are considered, with their role in lowering body temperature, in Chapter 12.

FURTHER READING

Bovet, D., Longo, V. G., and Silvestrini, B. (1957). Electrophysiological methods of research in the study of tranquillizers. Contribution to the study of the reticular formation, in *Psychotropic Drugs*, Amsterdam.

Brazier, M. A. B. (1961). Some effects of anaesthesia on the brain, *Brit. J. Anaesth.* **33,** 194.

Domino, E. F. (1962). Sites of action of some central nervous depressants, *Ann. Rev. Pharmacol.* **6,** 217.

Eger, E. I. (1962). Atropine, scopolamine and related compounds, *Anesthesiology*, **23,** 365.

Faulconer, A., and Bickford, R. G. (1960). *Electroencephalography in anesthesiology*, Springfield, Ill.

Fields, W. S. (1957), *Brain mechanisms and drug action*, Springfield, Ill.

Lasgna, L. (1954). A comparison of hypnotic agents, *J. Pharmacol. exp. Ther.* **111,** 9.

Millichap, J. P. (1965). Anticonvulsant drugs, in *Physiological pharmacology*, ed. Root, W. S., and Hofmann, F. G., Vol. 2, New York.

Mullins, L. J. (1954). Some physical mechanisms in narcosis, *Chem. Rev.* **54,** 289.

Papper, E. M. and Kitz, R. J. (1963). *Uptake and distribution of anaesthetic agents*, New York.

Paton, W. D. M. and Speden, R. N. (1965). Uptake of anaesthetics and their effect on the central nervous system, *Brit. med. Bull.* **21,** 44.

Shearer, W. M. (1961). The evolution of premedication, *Brit. J. Anaesth.* **33,** 219.

Spinks, A. (1963). Anticonvulsant drugs, *Progr. Med. Chem.*, **3,** 261.

Steinberg, H. (1964). *Animal behaviour and drug action*, London.

5

CENTRAL NERVOUS SYSTEM STIMULANTS

THE drugs described in this chapter excite both mental and motor activity but they often act in very different ways to achieve these ends.

Many of these compounds have more than one type of action on the nervous system but they are classified, and will be discussed here, under the heading of their most important action.

These compounds may act directly on the CNS by increasing the effectiveness of excitatory synaptic signalling or they may work by reducing central inhibition. There are numerous ways in which these changes may be effected by stimulant drugs and it is only in recent years that details of some of these actions are beginning to be understood. There are now plausible explanations for the actions of some convulsants and it is likely that this understanding will aid studies on the actions of other stimulant compounds.

ANTIDEPRESSANTS

Drugs in this class are used widely for patients who are socially maladjusted, apathetic, and depressed. They may be divided into four major classes: (1) the direct stimulants; (2) monoamine oxidase inhibitors; (3) dibenzazepine derivatives; and (4) xanthine derivatives.

DIRECT STIMULANTS

Amphetamine

Amphetamine increases the speed of mental arithmetic, delays fatigue, and produces a general feeling of well-being. It stimulates respiration and is used to treat poisoning by depressant drugs and as an adjuvant in the treatment of mild depressive neuroses. It helps to reduce obesity by reducing the appetite. Amphetamine has, like adrenaline, α and β peripheral actions and a powerful direct stimulant action on the CNS, particularly in the region of the reticular formation. This stimulant action occurs even when brain catecholamines have been depleted by reserpine and in the presence of monoamine oxidase inhibitors.

Amphetamine and amphetamine derivatives are now in wide use with and without medical supervision. This has led to considerable problems because of the addictive nature of these compounds. These drugs should only be taken for short periods and always under medical supervision. There is now good evidence that this class of compound may precipitate dangerous psychoses in some types of patient.

Dexamphetamine (dextro amphetamine)

This is the dextro-isomer of amphetamine and it is three to four times as potent as the L-isomer. It has similar pharmacological actions to amphetamine but its central effects, in relation to its peripheral actions, are stronger than those of amphetamine. The side-effects of this drug are as dangerous as those of amphetamine.

Dexamphetamine is often mixed with a CNS depressant, usually a barbiturate, and is officially used in this form to treat obesity. It is in this form that the drug is taken unofficially for its CNS stimulant activity. A common mixture is that of dexamphetamine with amylobarbitone (*Drinamyl*, *Dexytal*, 'Purple Hearts').

MONOAMINE OXIDASE INHIBITORS (Fig. 5.2)

The drugs in this section are all antidepressants and inhibit monoamine oxidase and

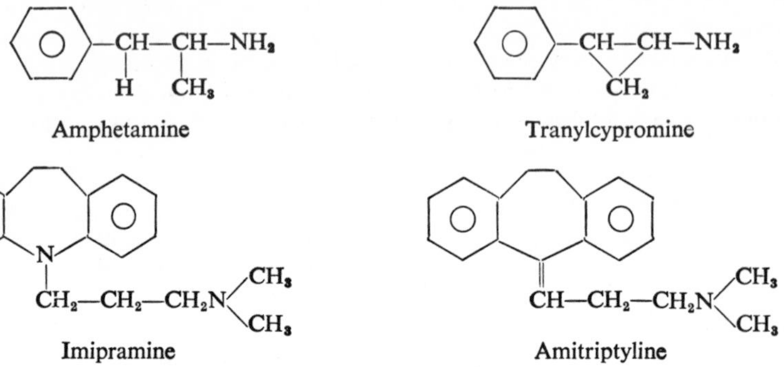

Amphetamine

Tranylcypromine

Imipramine

Amitriptyline

Fig. 5.1. The structures of some antidepressant compounds.

there is evidence to suggest a link between these two actions. It is possible, however, that these compounds have a central action quite distinct from their ability to block monoamine oxidase systems (see Chapter 2).

The early monoamine oxidase inhibitors were hydrazine derivatives and were highly toxic and are therefore no longer in use (iptoniazid, pheniprazine) but modifications to the structure of iproniazid have yielded less toxic hydrazines which are only slightly less effective as antidepressants (isocarboxazid, nialamide, phenelzine). Tranylcypromine, a monoamine oxidase inhibitor which is not a hydrazine derivative, has also been developed.

Iproniazid, pheniprazine, isocarboxazid, nialamide, phenelzine

These compounds are all derivatives of hydrazine and inhibit monoamine oxidase. Iproniazid was originally introduced as an antitubercular drug but its stimulating action on the CNS led it to be used for this action. This resulted in the development of related compounds with similar central actions but fewer toxic side-effects. The most serious side-effects encountered with iproniazid result from over-stimulation of the nervous system and include manic symptoms and insomnia. Liver damage and hypertension may also occur. Isocarboxacid has a more delayed onset

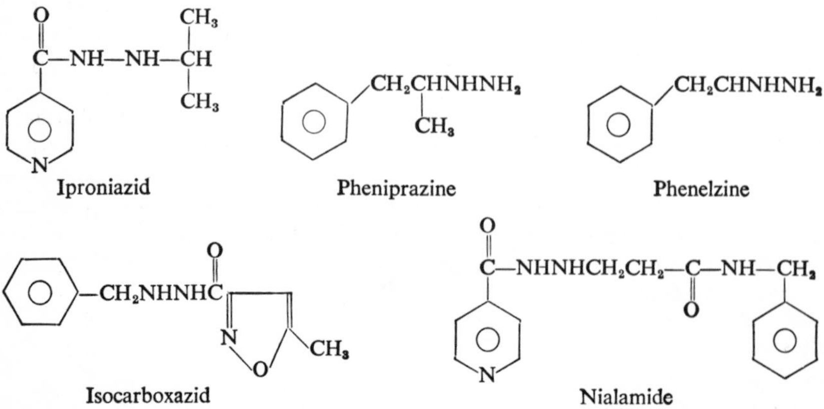

Iproniazid

Pheniprazine

Phenelzine

Isocarboxazid

Nialamide

Fig. 5.2. Hydrazine derivatives which are antidepressants.

of action but its side-effects are less serious than those of iproniazid. Phenelzine may cause hypertension as may pheniprazine but this latter drug is a more effective monoamine oxidase inhibitor than iproniazid and is quicker acting and less toxic.

Tranylcypromine

This compound is not a hydrazine derivative but inhibits monoamine oxidase. Caution has to be exercised in the use of all the compounds which inhibit monoamine oxidase because serious complication can ensue when patients under their influence eat certain foods containing large amounts of tyramine (see Chapter 8).

DIBENZAZEPINE DERIVATIVES

These drugs are now the most widely used ones for the treatment of mental depression. They were discovered in 1958 during clinical trials of phenothiazine tranquillizers. It was found that one compound, imipramine, had a low tranquillizing potency but that it helped certain types of depressed patients.

This is remarkable since imipramine only differs from promazine, a useful tranquillizer, by the replacement of the sulphur atom which links the benzene rings, by a CH_2—CH_2 chain.

Imipramine, desmethylimipramine

These compounds have only very weak monoamine oxidase inhibitory activity and, not surprisingly, they share many common properties with the phenothiazines, having some local anaesthetic action and mild atropine-like and antihistamine effects. The way in which they stimulate the nervous system is unknown but, unlike amphetamine, they are ineffective if brain catecholamines have been depleted by reserpine.

It has been demonstrated that imipramine has a cocaine-like effect on sympathetic nerve terminals and prevents the re-uptake of noradrenaline. This greatly reduces the inactivation of noradrenaline and therefore potentiates its action and this may account for the stimulant action of the drug on the CNS.

Amitriptyline

Amitriptyline is chemically and pharmacologically related to imipramine. It has atropine-like properties and the side-effects of its use include a dry mouth, tachycardia, blurred vision, and constipation.

Although imipramine, desmethylimipramine, and amitriptyline are all mild tranquillizers their clinical usefulness is found as antidepressants. It may be that the removal of anxiety from patients with some kinds of depression is sufficient to relieve the illness.

XANTHINE DERIVATIVES

Caffeine, theobromine, theophylline

The xanthine derivatives (Fig. 5.3) have many pharmacological properties in common. They stimulate the CNS, act on the kidney to produce diuresis, stimulate cardiac muscle, and relax smooth muscle (Chapter 10). Although they share these properties it is usual to find that they are not all equally effective for each type of action.

The effectiveness of the pharmacological actions of each compound are shown in Table 5.1.

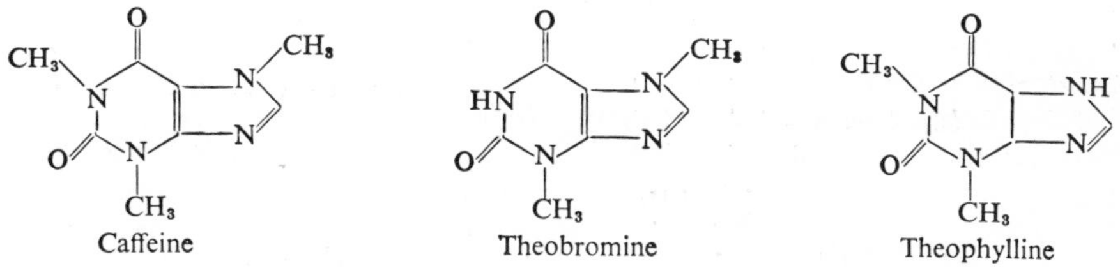

Caffeine | Theobromine | Theophylline

Fig. 5.3. The structures of some xanthine derivatives.

Table 5.1

	CNS and respiratory stimulation	Smooth muscle relaxant	Diuresis	Cardiac stimulation	Skeletal muscle stimulation
Caffeine	+++	+	+	+	+++
Theobromine	+	++	++	++	+
Theophylline	++	+++	+++	+++	++

Caffeine is completely absorbed from the small intestine and most of it is oxidized to urea and carbon dioxide. Some is excreted as methyl-uric acids and some as methylxanthines and a very small amount is excreted in the urine unchanged. None of the xanthines is completely demethylated so there is no increase in the excretion of uric acid.

Caffeine is a strong CNS stimulant, theophylline is less powerful, and theobromine has only a weak action. Caffeine excites the CNS at all levels but the cortex appears most vulnerable and the spinal cord least vulnerable. Its main effect is to produce clear thought and to reduce drowsiness and fatigue. It increases the motor effects of conditioned reflexes and improves the higher functions of the brain such as those involved in mental arithmetic. These effects may be obtained with about 100–250 mg of caffeine, the amount contained in one or two cups of coffee.

The xanthines also stimulate the respiratory, vagal, and vasomotor centres in the medulla. Caffeine is a particularly effective respiratory stimulant and it is used for this purpose. If very large doses are injected they cause strychnine-like convulsions by stimulating the spinal cord.

It has been known for some time that the methylxanthines have marked effects on cellular metabolism. Caffeine increases the oxygen consumption and lactic acid output of skeletal muscle and the twitch strength is increased. This may occur because methylxanthines, especially theophylline, are competitive inhibitors of phosphodiesterase, an enzyme that inactivates cyclic 3′, 5′-AMP. The concentration of cyclic AMP rises and tissue glycolysis therefore increases. In this way metabolic activity may be increased and may account, at least in part, for the stimulant action of these drugs on the nervous system.

These compounds are used therapeutically for their actions on the myocardium, smooth muscle, and CNS. Caffeine is mostly used only as a CNS stimulant while theobromine and theophylline are used most frequently for their effects on the myocardium.

CONVULSANTS AND ANALEPTICS [Fig. 5.4]

These drugs may produce stimulation of many regions of the CNS but their most important actions are often on the medulla.

Drugs which are used specifically to produce convulsions are called convulsants. Therapeutically they have limited applications although leptazol has been used in place of electro-convulsive therapy.

Drugs which overcome depression of the CNS due to overdoses of barbiturates, morphine, and similar compounds are known as analeptics. Their most important action is to stimulate centres in the medulla, but a sufficiently high dose of any of these drugs will produce generalized convulsions.

The mechanism of action of a few convulsants is now beginning to be understood. It appears that they have no important direct

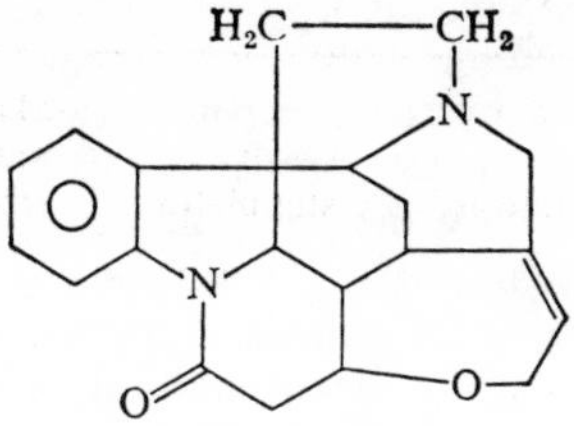

Strychnine

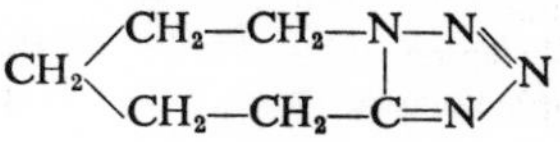

Leptazol

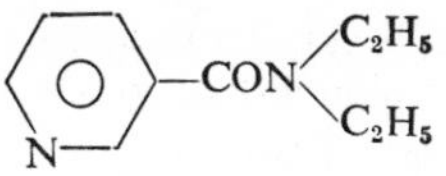

Nikethamide

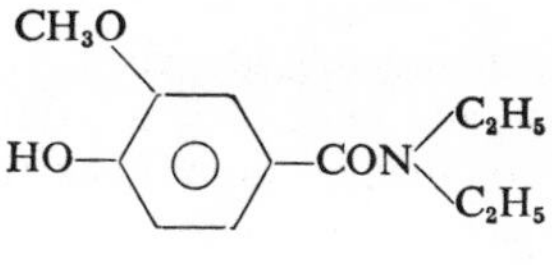

Ethamivan

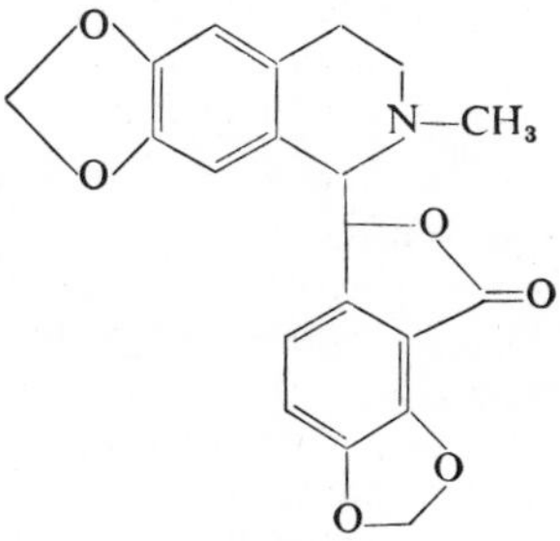

Bicuculline

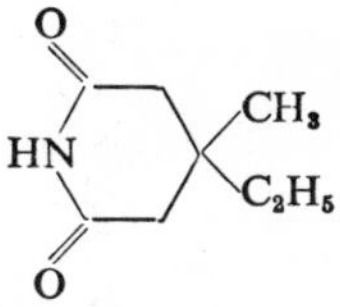

Bemegride

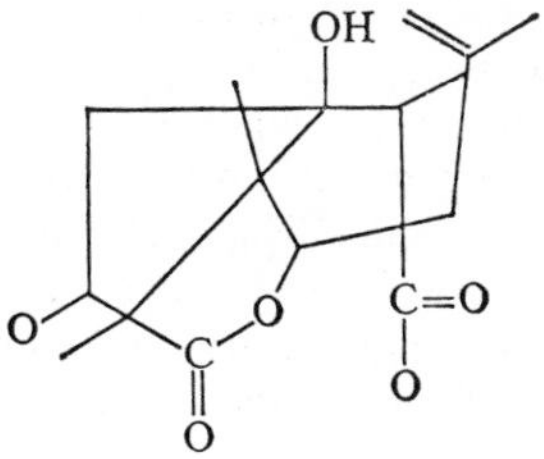

Picrotoxin

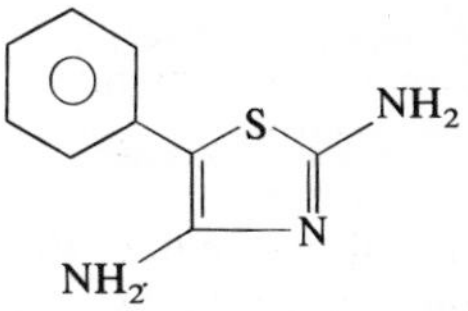

Amiphenazole

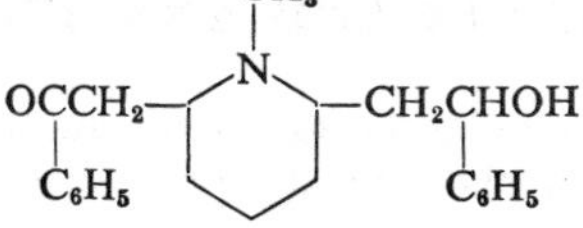

Lobeline

Fig. 5.4. The structures of some convulsants and analeptics.

stimulant action but that they work by antagonizing the action of natural inhibitory transmitters at central synapses. These effects are so clear for certain convulsants, e.g. strychnine, bicuculline, and picrotoxin, that central inhibition at various sites is now often described in terms of the convulsants that do or do not antagonize them.

Strychnine

Strychnine has no important therapeutic value but has proved useful in the investigation of the mode of action of convulsant drugs. Its mechanism of action on the CNS is better understood than that of any other stimulant compound.

Action. Strychnine's most striking effects are on the CNS and consist of the stimulation, followed by the depression of reflexes. After strychnine the motor effects of spinal reflexes are increased and the latent period is diminished. Reflexes become more generalized and, after large doses, small sensory disturbances will send all the voluntary muscles in the body into violent and painful convulsions.

The main site of action of strychnine is on the spinal cord and convulsions occur after removal of the rest of the nervous system. This action of strychnine has been analysed in considerable detail by Sir John Eccles and his co-workers, and it is known that strychnine does not excite directly but acts by inhibiting inhibition. This has been discovered by recording intra- and extracellularly from spinal motoneurones and stimulating inhibitory afferent nerves to these cells. Strychnine was given intravenously or by micro-electrophoretic application directly on to the motoneurones. It was found that strychnine did not alter membrane potentials, or the excitability of motoneurones, but that it did reduce the membrane hyperpolarization (inhibitory post-synaptic potential) generated by stimulation of the appropriate inhibitory afferent nerve.

This inhibitory postsynaptic potential can be exactly mimicked by glycine applied to the motoneurones by micro-electrophoresis. This evidence, together with recent information concerning the regional distribution of glycine, its uptake by nerve tissue, and its release, makes it very likely that it is an important postsynaptic inhibitory transmitter.

Strychnine does not affect presynaptic inhibition in the spinal cord and so it is unlikely that glycine mediates this effect.

In the brain strychnine does not antagonize postsynaptic inhibition and this suggests that the inhibitory transmitter is different to that in the spinal cord.

Strychnine has an excitatory action on the medulla, where it will stimulate the vasomotor and vagal centres. It has a remarkable effect in enhancing the sensations of

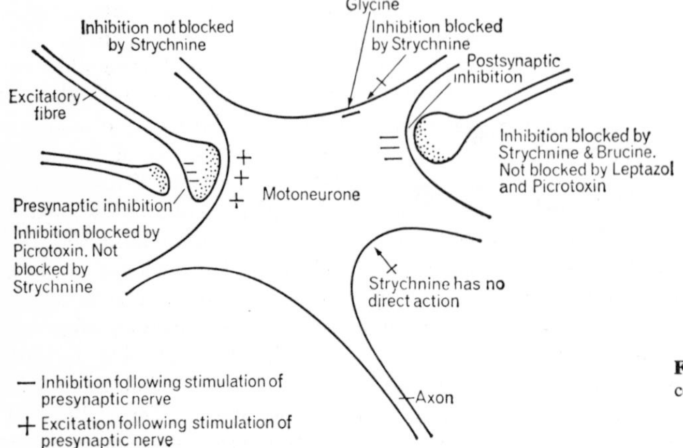

Fig. 5.5. The site of action of convulsants in the spinal cord.

touch, smell, hearing, and sight. After strychnine small differences of colour or illumination are more easily discriminated and the field of vision is increased.

Strychnine also acts on the alimentary canal. It has a bitter taste and therefore increases the appetite. It has a peripheral stimulant action on intestinal muscle, which is probably due to an action on Auerbach's plexus and the drug has been used in the treatment of constipation.

Strychnine poisoning

After a high dose the subject will become restless and small sensory stimuli will cause jerking of the limbs and this quickly leads to generalized convulsions. The trunk and limbs become rigidly extended and the face distorts. Each convulsion lasts a few minutes, is very painful, and is followed by a period of exhaustion. After five or six convulsions the respiration fails to return and he dies of asphyxia.

Strychnine is one of the very few poisons whose effects can be counteracted after absorption. It is important to stop the convulsions and to achieve this sensory stimuli must be reduced to a minimum and a general anaesthetic can be administered. Treatment with one of the barbiturates or with mephenesin is often an effective antidote.

Picrotoxin

The active principle in picrotoxin is picrotoxinin and it is a powerful stimulant which affects all parts of the nervous system to some extent. It is extremely effective in restoring respiration that has been depressed by barbiturates or by morphine. The stimulant action of picrotoxin potentiates the excitatory actions of morphine on the CNS.

The difference between a therapeutic and a toxic dose of picrotoxin is small and convulsions are easily produced so that it is rarely used today. Picrotoxin is known to act in the spinal cord by blocking the action of GABA-mediated presynaptic inhibition.

Leptazol (pentylenetetrazol)

Leptazol stimulates the brain and, to a lesser extent, the spinal cord. It is particularly effective in stimulating the medulla which has been depressed by drugs and it is therefore a useful analeptic but it is less effective than picrotoxin. The use of leptazol in place of insulin or electroconvulsive therapy has not proved successful. Leptazol is sometimes used in the diagnosis of epileptic conditions. It is injected intravenously in subconvulsive doses while the electroencephalogram is recorded and this will often reveal potential epileptic foci. It seems unlikely that leptazol blocks either pre- or postsynaptic inhibition, nor does it seem to excite motoneurones by causing depolarization.

Nikethamide

Nikethamide is a weak analeptic and, in high doses, produces convulsions similar to those obtained with leptazol. The myocardium may be depressed but stimulation of the vasomotor centre will cause vasoconstriction and a rise in blood pressure. Nikethamide is used as a stimulant when respiration is depressed by barbiturates. It has been used in the past as a cardiovascular stimulant but it is not now used for this purpose because of its action on the myocardium.

Bicuculline

Bicuculline is a phthalide-isoquinoline alkaloid isolated from corydalis species and is as potent a convulsant as strychnine. It is known to be a specific and reversible antagonist of the inhibitory action of GABA on some central neurones and its site of action is likely to be in those regions of the brain where GABA is a major transmitter. Considerable evidence has accumulated to make it very likely that GABA is an inhibitory transmitter in the brain. This evidence includes the identical nature of natural IPSP and a GABA-induced hyperpolarization, the regional and subcellular distribution of GABA, its uptake by nerve tissue, and its release during central inhibition. The action of GABA is not antagonized by strychnine or picrotoxin but the specific antagonism of bicuculline to GABA hyperpolarization and natural IPSPs confirms GABA as a transmitter in those regions of the brain so far studied, namely the cerebral cortex, Purkinje cell neurones, mitral and thalamic cells.

Bemegride

Bemegride resembles leptazol in its stimulant action on the CNS. It has been used as an antidote to barbiturate poisoning but it is rarely used for this purpose now. Like leptazol it may be used for the diagnosis of epilepsy.

Amiphenazole

Amiphenazole is a central stimulant which was originally thought to be a specific antagonist of certain depressant actions of morphine without affecting analgesia. It now seems that it is a straightforward analeptic. Large doses will produce convulsions.

It has been used as a respiratory stimulant during respiratory insufficiency but its effectiveness is in doubt.

Lobeline

Lobeline is a powerful alkaloid obtained from *Lobelia* and has general actions like nicotine. Its most marked action is to stimulate respiration via the carotid sinus receptors, and it has been used to revive patients who have had an overdose of a narcotic. It causes stimulation and then depression of autonomic ganglia, the adrenal medulla, and the neuromuscular junction.

It is not now normally used as a respiratory stimulant because its action is rather unpredictable and it may have unpleasant and dangerous side-effects.

Ethamivan

Ethamivan is a vanillic acid derivative with a structural resemblance to nikethamide. It is a respiratory stimulant and is usually preferred to nikethamide to treat cases of barbiturate poisoning. Ethamivan has proved particularly useful, when given by mouth, in the treatment of respiratory distress in the new-born.

HALLUCINOGENS

Compounds which act on the CNS to produce hallucinations can be loosely classified as stimulants although their mode of action is completely unknown and their effects are certainly not always of a stimulating nature.

Many hallucinogenic compounds are known and they have always proved attractive to those who hope to enrich and widen their perception and who seek novel experiences. Although these compounds have become rather widely used in some sectors of society, their use is like the use of any powerful and poorly understood drug and is fraught with danger.

The effects of these compounds are hard to predict from one individual to another and may cause permanent or semi-permanent psychological damage in some people. In addition to this danger there are reports of genetic effects associated with these compounds and the possibility of the development of serious dependence.

Because these drugs are subject to strict controls they can normally only be obtained from illegal sources and this always raises the possibility that they are contaminated by other more harmful compounds.

Animals appear to be remarkably resistant to LSD and although many species have been subjected to tests with the drug, only primates show any response in doses up to ten times those effective in man.

The effect of LSD in man has been claimed to resemble, in some aspects, the symptoms of schizophrenia and as little is known of the mechanism of action of the drug as is known of the causes of schizophrenia.

It is well known that LSD antagonizes the action of 5-HT *in vitro* and since 5-HT may be a control neurotransmitter it has been suggested that this may form the basis of action of LSD. This hypothesis became less tenable when it was found that powerful 5-HT antagonists, such as bromo-lysergic acid diethylamide, had no hallucinogenic activity. It is also now known that LSD and 5-HT act in a similar way at central synapses, for instance in the lateral geniculate nucleus, apparently to compete with action of the natural neuro-transmitter.

With high doses of LSD there are signs of sympathetic stimulation and an amphetamine-like desynchronization of the electroencephalogram occurs so the basis of action of LSD may be associated with central noradrenergic mechanisms.

Many of the effects of LSD can be relieved with chlorpromazine. Tolerance to the behavioural effects of LSD develops quickly and there is cross-tolerance between LSD and mescaline. LSD is used in psychotherapy but its usefulness in this field is not yet proven. On the other hand it has been widely used as a research tool in the study of central synaptic transmission and, because of its high potency and specificity, it is likely to continue to be used in the study of sensory transmission processes.

Cannabis (marihuana)

Hallucinations are only caused by large doses of cannabis but it is the most widely used drug of this type.

The drug is obtained from the hemp plant (*Cannabis sativa*) and has been in use longer than almost any other drug. It may be taken in the form of a cigarette ('joint') but can be taken orally.

The active principle is tetrahydrocannabinol and many synthetic derivatives of this compound have been produced and many are more potent than the parent compound.

In small amounts cannabis produces euphoria and elation and there is often a loss of appreciation of time and space.

The mode of action is unknown although it does appear that changes in the catecholamine content of the brain occur.

The dangers associated with the use of cannabis are still controversial but as research proceeds so these dangers become more apparent. There is evidence that prolonged use may produce liver enzyme induction and reports of permanent brain damage have appeared. Another complication seems to be that short-term recall memory is impaired and this may prove to the most serious side effect of the drug, particularly when it is used by young people. Another danger is that the drug may be adulterated with more habit-forming compounds or that the consumer will be persuaded or will desire to proceed to the use of more dangerous drugs.

Recent work suggests the possibility of an interesting therapeutic use for tetrahydrocannabinol. It appears that the compound greatly reduces the abstinence syndrome occurring after the withdrawal of a narcotic analgesic such as morphine. At present methadone is commonly used, but this itself produces physical dependence whereas physical dependence has not been associated with the use of cannabinoids in men. It is thought that tetrahydrocannibinol may be acting by reducing the release of acetylcholine in the central nervous system, which would be consistent with evidence that links cholinergic systems with physical dependence.

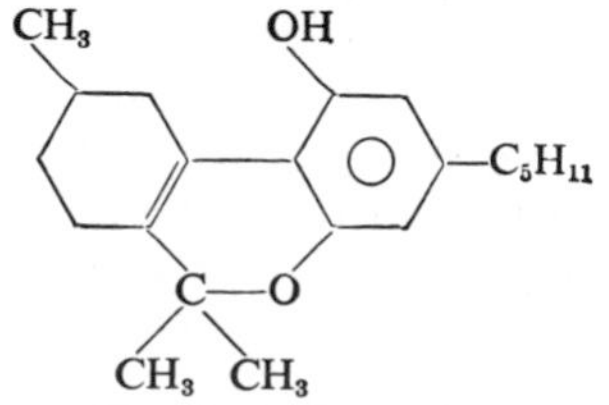

CH_3 OH C_5H_{11} C—O CH_3 CH_3

Tetrahydrocannabinol

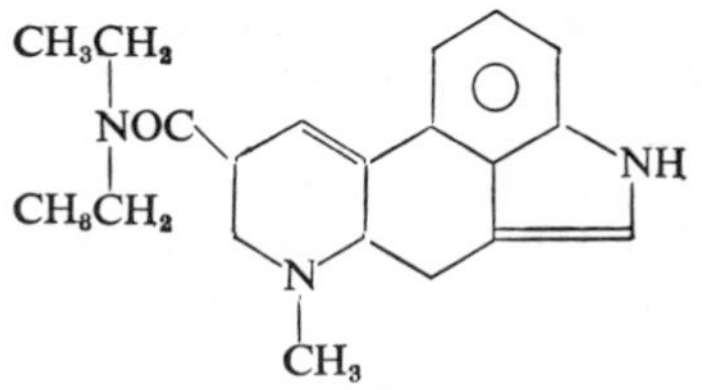

CH_3CH_2 NOC CH_3CH_2 NH N CH_3

Lysergic acid diethylamide

Fig. 5.6. The structures of hallucinogenic compounds.

Lysergic acid diethylamide (LSD)

Powerful hallucinogenic drugs such as mescaline, which were isolated in 1896 from the peyoti cactus, have been used for various reasons, often involving religious rites, from the early nineteenth century. In 1943 the phychological effects of a much more powerful synthetic hallucinogen, lysergic acid diethylamide, were discovered accidentally by Hofmann. This compound will produce hallucinations in man in doses as low as 20 μg taken orally but has few actions outside the CNS at this or at higher dose levels.

FURTHER READING

Curtis, D. R. (1963). The pharmacology of central inhibition, *Pharmacol. Rev.* **15,** 333.

Feldberg, W. (1963). *A pharmacological approach to the brain from its inner and outer surface*, London.

Hahn, F. (1960). Analeptics, *Pharmacol. Rev.* **12,** 447.

Holtz, P. and Westermann, E. (1965). Psychic energizers and antidepressant drugs, in *Physiological Pharmacology*, ed. Root, W. S., and Hofmann, F. G., Vol. 2, New York.

Krnjevic, K. (1967). Chemical transmission and cortical arousal, *Anesthesiology* **27,** 100.

6

LOCAL ANAESTHETICS

MECHANISM OF ACTION

Local anaesthetics prevent the generation and conduction of nerve impulses and, while this is a property of a great number of drugs, only those which have this as a predominant characteristic when in low concentrations are classed as local anaesthetic agents. Their site of action is the cell membrane and the block they produce is the result of interference with changes in membrane permeability to potassium and sodium ions. These permeability changes are responsible for the rising and falling phases of the action potential and they follow depolarization of the membrane. In the presence of a local anaesthetic the electrical excitability of the tissue gradually decreases until, eventually, complete block ensues.

How local anaesthetics affect the transient changes in ionic permeability is unknown but the potency of these compounds is matched by their ability to increase the surface pressure of monomolecular lipid films. It has been suggested that the anaesthetic 'squeezes' the lipid molecules closer together. In the lipid membrane layers of nerves this could have the effect of closing membrane 'pores' so reducing ionic permeability; this would have the effect of stabilizing the membrane and reducing its excitability.

DIFFERENTIAL SENSITIVITY OF NERVE FIBRES

Not all nerve fibres are equally vulnerable to the actions of local anaesthetics. As a general rule, small diameter fibres are more easily blocked than large one and if cocaine is applied to a mixed nerve trunk it is found that the small diameter γ fibres block first and the large α fibres last. The sensitivity of nerve fibres is not, however, entirely determined by their diameter, because some small myelinated fibres block more easily than even the small diameter C fibres.

It is now known that there is no difference in the vulnerability of motor and sensory fibres of the same diameter.

After administration of a local anaesthetic the various sensations are not lost simultaneously, probably because they are mediated by nerves of different diameters. The order of sensation loss is rather variable but usually pain is abolished first, followed by the sensations of cold, warmth, touch, and deep pressure in that order.

THE EFFECT OF pH

The most useful local anaesthetics are secondary or tertiary amines and they can exist as uncharged or positively charged molecules, depending on the pH of the solution and on the pK_a of the compound.

Procaine, for instance, is a weakly basic tertiary amine and in solution may exist as a mixture of the uncharged compound (B in Fig. 6.1) and the cationic form present in a given solution will depend on the pH of the solution according to the equation $\log [B]/[BH^+] = pH - pK$.

Since the pK_a of procaine at 20° C is 8·7 at pH 7, 2 per cent of the drug will be in the uncharged form and at pH 9, 67 per cent of the procaine will be in the uncharged form.

The penetration of a local anaesthetic to its site of action depends on its ability to cross lipid barriers and the uncharged form has a high oil/water distribution coefficient and can therefore penetrate into lipid layers with ease. The cationic form is hydrophilic and therefore penetrates lipid layers very slowly. It would be expected, therefore, that procaine would be more effective at the higher pH because of the much larger fraction of the uncharged form that is present in solution.

$$B + H_3^+O \leftrightharpoons BH^+ + H_2O$$

$$NH_2\text{—}Ph\text{—}COOCH_2CH_2N(C_2H_5)_2 \xrightarrow{H_3^+O} NH_2\text{—}Ph\text{—}COOCH_2CH_2N^+\begin{cases} C_2H_5 \\ H \\ C_2H_5 \end{cases}$$

Fig. 6.1. The ionization of procaine.

This is not, however, the whole story, because once the drug has penetrated the lipid barriers and reached its site of action it appears that the charged, rather than the uncharged, form is most effective in producing an anaesthetic effect. This suggestion has been confirmed by Ritchie and his co-workers who showed convincingly that alkaline anaesthetic solutions were more effective in nerves with their outer sheathing intact but that neutral solutions were more effective in desheathed nerves, the cation being the active form of the anaesthetic and the uncharged molecule being important only for penetration.

PHARMACOLOGICAL ACTIONS

In addition to their action in blocking conduction in nervous tissue, the local anaesthetics interfere with the function of all organs in which the transmission of electrical impulses occurs. The most important effects are on the CNS and heart.

Central nervous system

Most local anaesthetics stimulate the CNS and overdoses may lead to tremors, restlessness, and convulsions. Central depression may occur later and death may result from respiratory depression. The stimulant action may be the result of a block in vulnerable central inhibitory pathways. Although all local anaesthetics cause stimulation, cocaine is unique in having a powerful effect on the cerebral cortex and it may be this which makes cocaine addictive. Synthetic local anaesthetics have less stimulant actions on higher centres and do not cause addiction.

Cardiovascular system

If given systemically, local anaesthetics have a quinidine-like action on the myocardium and reduce its excitability and force of contraction; they also prolong the refractory period and slow conduction. These effects cannot easily be taken advantage of because the drugs are rapidly destroyed and their CNS effects usually predominate.

All local anaesthetics except lignocaine and cocaine produce vasodilatation by a direct action on arterioles.

FATE AND METABOLISM OF LOCAL ANAESTHETICS

All local anaesthetics are broken down in the liver to non-toxic products and procaine is also inactivated in the plasma by circulating cholinesterase.

CHEMISTRY OF LOCAL ANAESTHETICS

The very large number of local anaesthetics available have many actions in common and their chemical structures show many similarities. They are all water-soluble salts of lipid-soluble alkaloids and consist basically of three parts, an amino group, a connecting group which is an ester or amide, and an amino alcohol residue in which the amino group may be substituted by alkyl groups or form part of an alicyclic ring. Alterations in

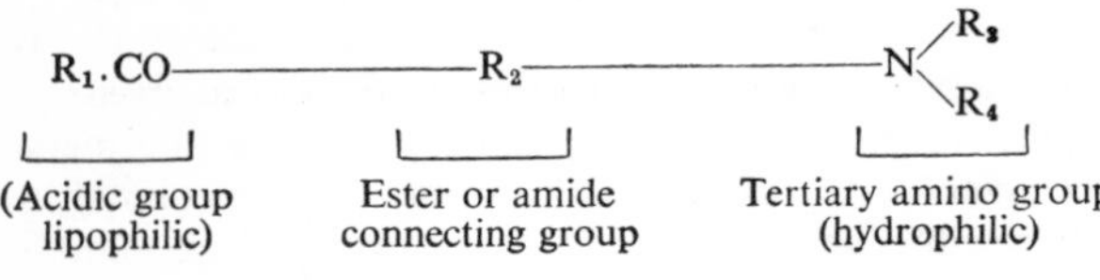

Fig. 6.2. The basic structure of local anaesthetics.

all three parts of the molecule give compounds of varying potency and toxicity. Local anaesthetics may be divided into three main groups; (1) cocaine, a naturally occurring alkaloid and the first local anaesthetic to be used; (2) para-aminobenzoic acid derivatives (procaine, amethocaine, etc.); (3) agents including lignocaine, cinchocaine, benzocaine, many of which chemically resemble the para-aminobenzoic acid drugs.

THE ADMINSTRATION OF LOCAL ANAESTHETICS

Local anaesthetics may be administered in a number of ways. (1) As a cream, ointment, spray, solution, or powder to mucous membranes or to damaged skin around wounds. (2) By infiltration. The drugs may be injected locally into subcutaneous tissue to block sensation for the performance of minor, superficial surgery. (3) By injection into the subarachnoid space of the spinal cord to procure block of motor and sensory roots and autonomic fibres. This is known as spinal anaesthesia and will block the sensation of pain from the regions of body innervated by the affected segments of the cord. (4) By injection near major nerve trunks to block sensation from the innervated region of the body, e.g. brachial plexus block.

Amethocaine (tetracaine)

This compound is suitable both for injection and application to mucous membranes. It is the most powerful local anaesthetic after cinchocaine and is used for infiltration anaesthesia, spinal and extradural block. It is often mixed with procaine or lignocaine to combine the rapid action of these compounds with its own more prolonged effect.

Like most other local anaesthetics, amethocaine is usually administered with adrenaline in order to constrict blood vessels and thus reduce absorption and thereby confine the area of anaesthetic effect and increase the duration of action.

Cinchocaine (dibucaine)

Cinchocaine is a powerful local anaesthetic with an onset of action slower than procaine

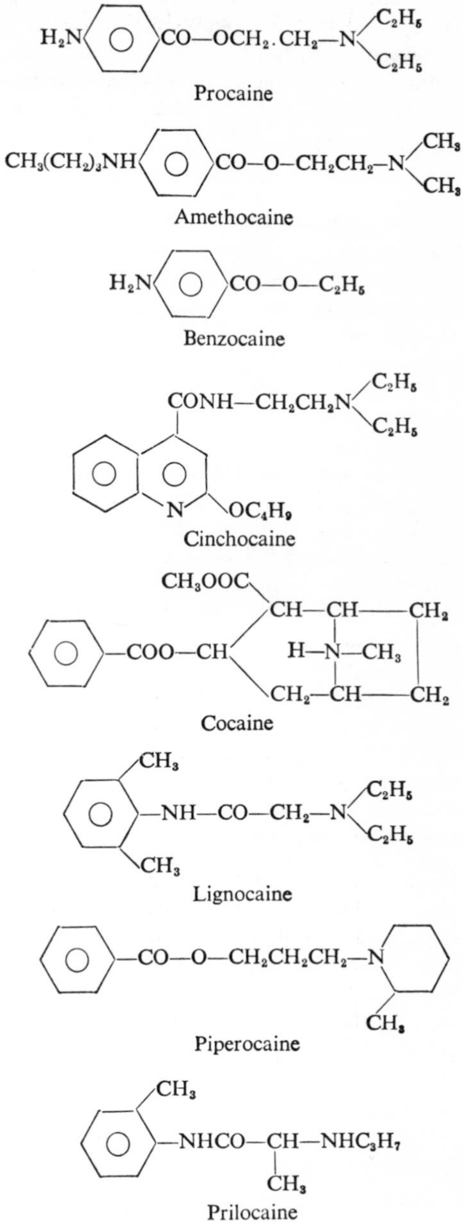

Fig. 6.3. The structures of some local anaesthetics.

but with a longer duration. It is absorbed from mucous membranes and is 2–5 times more toxic than cocaine but, because it is more active, it can be used in lower concentrations. It sometimes produces inflammation at the site of injection. It is still widely used for spinal anaesthesia.

Cocaine

Cocaine is obtained from the leaves of *Erythroxylon coca,* a tree found in South America.

It has pharmacological actions on the nervous and cardiovascular systems similar to those of other local anaesthetics.

In some respects it differs from other local anaesthetics because it has its own adrenergic action and blocks the uptake of catecholamines into adrenergic nerve terminals and so enhances the action of adrenaline, noradrenaline, and sympathetic nerve stimulation (Chapter 18).

It produces marked stimulation of the higher centres in the brain which results in restlessness and euphoria. This stimulation will give way to depression, paralysis of medullary centres, and death.

Cocaine potentiates the excitatory and inhibitory responses of sympathetically innervated tissues to the action of noradrenaline and adrenaline and to stimulation of sympathetic nerves. This effect is produced because cocaine prevents the reuptake of noradrenaline into nerve terminals and thus produces a buildup of the neurotransmitter. The increased concentration of neutrotransmitter at the receptors causes a type of supersensitivity to develop. Probably the most important result of this action is possible occurrence of ventricular fibrillation. It is a potent surface anaesthetic and produces intense vasoconstriction. Because of its toxic actions in the body its use is mainly limited to surface anaesthesia.

Cocaine is a drug of addiction and the results of its persistent adminstration are unpleasant and the victims, who become tolerant to the drug and therefore increase their intake, lose all self-control. They develop tremors, hallucinations, and eventually become melancholic and insane. Treatment for cocaine addiction consists in withdrawal of the drug, which does not cause serious symptoms like those following the withdrawal of morphine, but relapses are common.

Poisoning by cocaine. The early symptoms of poisoning are due to actions on the CNS. There is excitement, restlessness, and mental confusion with giddiness, fainting, and vomiting. Due to stimulation of the sympathetic nervous system the skin is pale, the pupils dilated, and the temperature raised. Large doses cause convulsions followed by central paralysis and death from failure of respiration.

Lignocaine (lidocaine)

Lignocaine acts rapidly and has a strong anaesthetic action on mucous membranes. It has no action on blood vessels and produces long-lasting general analgesia when given intravenously. It is used for local anaesthesia by infiltration, nerve, epidural, and caudal block. It is not used widely for spinal anaesthesia.

Lignocaine is also used to produce general analgesia and toxic side-effects are rare except when high doses are administered intravenously.

Prilocaine

Prilocaine closely resembles lignocaine in structure. It is as effective as lignocaine as an anaesthetic but it is less toxic and lasts longer. It is also active topically and on mucous membranes. There is not yet full clinical data on this local anaesthetic but it appears to be safe and free of serious side-effects.

Procaine

Procaine is a safe and effective local anaesthetic. It is used for infiltration anaesthesia and all types of regional, spinal, and extradural block. Its duration of action may be prolonged by combination with amethocaine. It is also used for the relief of post-operative pain by producing general analgesia, to prevent cardiac arrhythmias during cyclopropane and trichlorethylene anaesthesia, and as a supplement to nitrous oxide and oxygen anaesthesia.

Procaine has a vasodilator action so it is rapidly absorbed after local injection and this action is used to produce vasodilation in peripheral vascular disease, acute arterial spasm, and in venous spasm.

Procaine antagonizes the actions of sulphonamides and anticholinesterase drugs inhibit its hydrolysis and therefore its removal. It is normally rapidly hydrolysed by pseudocholinesterase in the plasma to give para-aminobenzoic acid and diethylaminoethanol, the former being excreted in the urine and the latter being largely metabolized in the liver.

FURTHER READING

Adriani, J. (1960). The clinical pharmacology of anaesthetics. *Clin. Pharmacol. Ther.* **1,** 645.

De Jong, R. H. and Wagman, I. H. (1963). Physiological mechanisms of peripheral nerve block by local anesthetics, *Anesthesiology* **24,** 684.

Douglas, W. W. and Ritchie, J. M. (1962). Mammalian non-myelinated nerve fibres, *Physiol. Rev.* **42,** 297.

Matthews, P. B. C. and Rushworth, G. (1957). The relative sensitivity of muscle nerve fibres to procaine, *J. Physiol.* (*Lond.*) **135,** 263.

Ritchie, J. M. and Greengard, P. (1966). On the mode of action of local anaesthetics, *Rev. Pharmacol.* **6,** 405.

Skou, J. C. (1961). The effect of drugs on cell membranes with special reference to local anaesthetics, *J. Pharm. Pharmacol.* **13,** 204.

Wiedling, S. (1963). Local anaesthetics, *Progr. Med. Chem.* **3,** 332.

7

CHOLINERGIC SYSTEM

THERE is now sufficient evidence to be sure that acetylcholine is liberated from motor nerve terminals and that it transmits the nerve impulse across a synaptic gap to the end-plate region on skeletal muscle cells. There is also good evidence that acetylcholine acts as a neurotransmitter at Renshaw cells in the spinal cord and at autonomic ganglia. It seems likely that a similar mechanism of transmission occurs at some motor terminals on smooth muscles and there is growing evidence that cholinergic synapses are present in the brain.

Since acetylcholine has important actions at so many sites in the body it is not surprising that its effects, and the effects of acetylcholine-like drugs and their antagonists, are varied and often complex.

A convenient division of the actions of cholinergic drugs exists because it has long been recognized that they act on two main types of membrane receptor. These receptors are called 'muscarinic' and 'nicotinic' receptors because muscarine and nicotine were found to stimulate them selectively before other, even more specific, drugs were discovered.

The effects of acetylcholine-like drugs on nicotinic receptors are blocked by curare and muscarinic actions are blocked by atropine.

Although it is now becoming clear that the differences between these two types of receptors may not be as clear-cut as was previously thought, they still form a useful way of classifying the action of acetylcholine.

This chapter is divided in the following way:

1. Methods of studying the cholinergic system.
2. Nicotinic receptors—drugs acting at the skeletal neuromuscular junction.
   Nicotinic receptors—drugs acting at the autonomic ganglion.
3. Muscarinic receptors—drugs acting at parasympathetic, postganglionic nerve junctions.
4. Mixed receptor sites—the spinal cord and brain.
5. Individual cholinergic drugs and their antagonists.

METHODS OF STUDYING THE CHOLINERGIC SYSTEM

DRUGS WHICH ACT AT NICOTINIC RECEPTORS

The action of drugs on nicotinic receptors can best be studied by their effect on neuromuscular transmission. This can be most easily investigated by recording muscle contractions evoked by the direct application of drugs or by maximal stimulation of the motor nerve in the presence of drugs. The drugs may be applied over the whole muscle or injected into the blood vessels entering the muscle. The latter method of drug application has been more widely used, the injection being made into an artery as near as possible to the insertion of the nerve. This is known as a close arterial injection and ensures a high concentration of drug at the neuromuscular junction. Acetylcholine delivered in this way will produce a twitch of voluntary muscle.

Maximal stimulation of the motor nerve produces contraction of the muscle and the effect of drugs on neuromuscular transmission may be tested by recording changes in the extent of the contraction.

Among the muscle preparations commonly used are the cat tibialis anterior, the frog gastrocnemius, and the rat diaphragm. The first preparation is used *in situ* but the other two are conveniently used as isolated preparations. They are illustrated in Fig. 7.1.

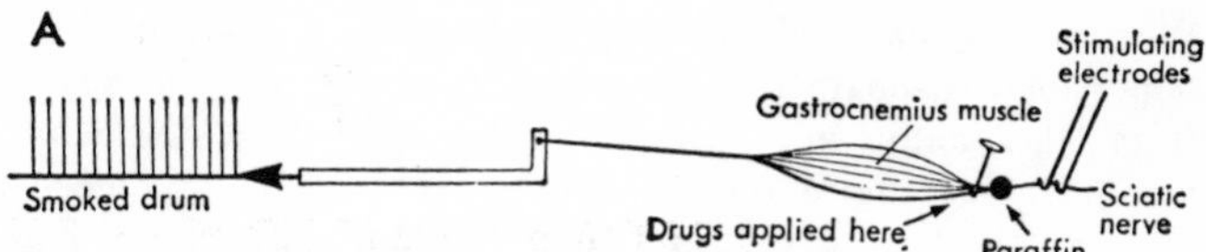

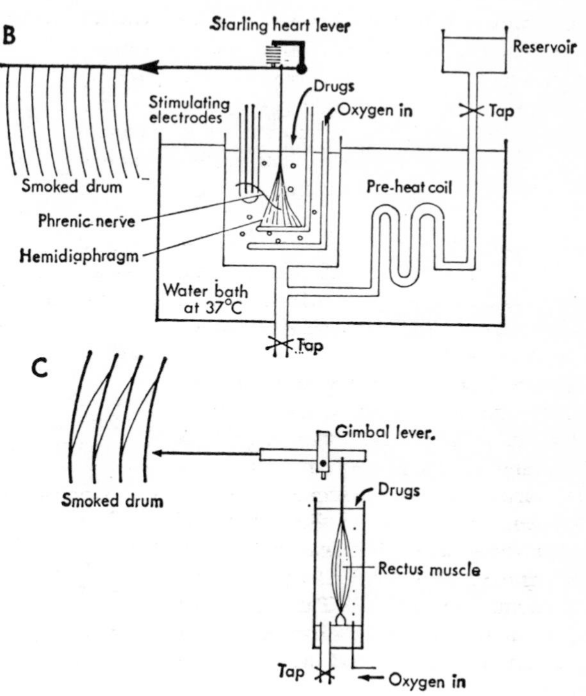

Fig. 7.1. Schematic illustrations of three simple, isolated preparations, which can be used to study the action of drugs on the neuromuscular junction.

A. The frog sciaticgastrocnemius preparation. Notice use of paraffin to prevent short-circuit of stimulating electrodes by drug solutions.

B. Isolated rat phrenic nerve-diaphragm preparation.

C. Frog rectus preparation.

Information about acetylcholine-like drugs may also be obtained from muscles containing multiply-innervated fibres. These fibres are especially sensitive to the action of acetylcholine-like compounds and respond with a prolonged, non-propagated contracture rather than a twitch. Examples of this type of preparation are the frog rectus and the dorsal muscle of the leech. Because of their sensitivity, these techniques are useful for assaying very small smounts of acetylcholine.

Since microelectrophoretic techniques were introduced, many advances have been made in understanding the mechanism of neuromuscular transmission, and the pharmacology of drugs which affect nicotinic receptors. The basic techniques for recording membrane potentials and applying drugs are described on p. 25. Variations of this technique are now used almost exclusively for the detailed study of pharmacological events at the neuromuscular junction, and other cholinergic receptor sites.

TESTS FOR MUSCARINIC ACTIVITY

The muscarinic activity of a drug may be conveniently tested on the isolated guinea-pig ileum preparation (Fig. 1.1). It should be remembered that when a drug like acetylcholine is being tested for its muscarinic activity it is essential to eliminate any interference due to its action on nicotinic receptors.

With the guinea-pig ileum preparation it is impossible to separate the muscle receptors from the autonomic ganglia which are nicotinic, but effects on the latter may be blocked by the use of a ganglion blocking drug such as hexamethonium.

The muscarinic activity of a drug may be estimated by its ability to lower blood pressure (Fig. 7.9) and it can be tested on the rate and force of contraction of the isolated perfused heart. If the drug is acting on muscarinic receptors its action should always be abolished by atropine.

Another convenient, but less quantitative test of muscarinic activity, is on the diameter of the pupil of the eye and on the blood vessels of the perfused rabbit ear or the perfused rat hind quarters.

THE BIOLOGICAL ASSAY OF ACETYLCHOLINE

One of the most sensitive assay preparations for acetylcholine is the dorsal muscle of the leech treated with an anticholinesterase. This tissue contracts in a concentration of about 1×10^{-9} g/ml of acetylcholine.

The frog rectus preparation, which is easier to use, is about ten times less sensitive than leech muscle. The heart of the clam (*Venus mercenaria*) is extremely sensitive but lacks the specificity to choline esters that is shown by the leech and frog rectus preparations. Other useful preparations are the cat blood pressure, the frog heart, and the rabbit auricle. All these methods involve a comparison of the activity of the unknown solution with a solution containing a known amount of acetylcholine. If two or more tests on different preparations agree quantitatively in terms of acetylcholine it is good evidence that the test solution contains acetylcholine or a very similar choline ester. The presence of acetylcholine in the test solution can only be confirmed by the used of further tests including: (1) the abolition of activity on the frog rectus and leech preparations by the addition of D-tubocurarine; (2) the blocking of a depressor response in blood pressure preparations by the addition of atropine-like compounds; (3) loss of activity in the test solution following alkali hydrolysis; (4) loss of activity in the test solution following incubation with acetylcholinesterase; and (5) chromatographic analysis of the active principle and a comparison of its Rf characteristics with those of acetylcholine and similar choline esters.

NICOTINIC RESPONSES

Peripheral nicotinic receptors are located on the postsynaptic membrane of the neuromuscular junction and on autonomic ganglion cells. A considerable amount is now known about the actions of agonist and antagonist drugs at these sites and they will be considered in the following section.

THE NEUROMUSCULAR JUNCTION

Detailed accounts of the histology and general properties of the neuromuscular junction and the electrical changes which occur during the transmission of an impulse may be found in most textbooks of physiology.

As shown in Fig. 7.2, the myelinated motor nerve fibre loses its myelin sheath near the tip and the axon spreads under the sarcolemma where it is separated by a cleft of about 300 Å from the folded structure of the muscle end-plate (the post-synaptic membrane).

Although the nerve terminal and the postsynaptic membrane lie close together there is no continuity between them and it is this gap which acetylcholine bridges to generate an electrical potential at the end-plate.

The sequence of events which results in a muscle contraction may be summarized as follows:

1. An action potential travels down the motor nerve fibre and invades the fine, unmyelineated terminal.

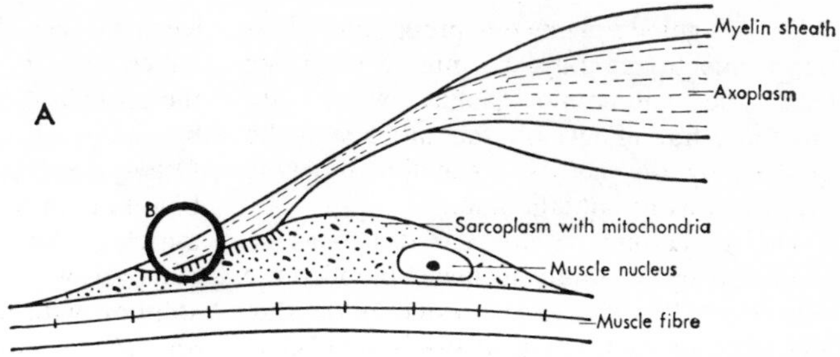

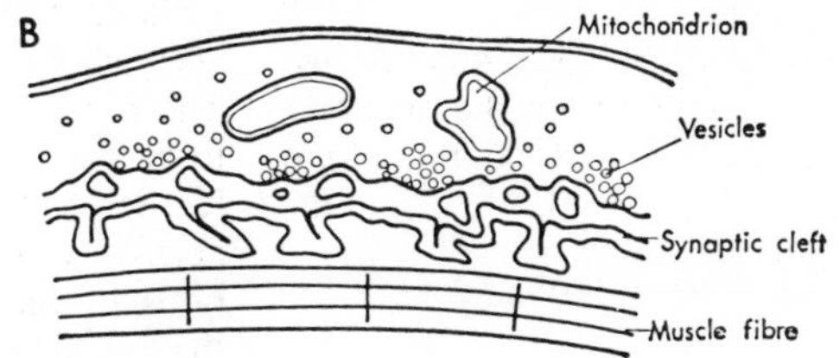

Fig. 7.2. A. Diagram of frog neuromuscular junction.
B. End-plate region of frog neuromuscular junction magnified × 19 000.

2. Depolarization of the terminal causes the release of about 100 'quanta' of acetylcholine each containing roughly 10^6 molecules. Each quantum is thought to be the contents of one synaptic vesicle. The vesicles are concentrated in the motor nerve terminal, close to the presynaptic membrane.
3. The liberated acetylcholine quickly diffuses across the synaptic gap and interacts with receptors on the end-plate of a muscle fibre. The receptors can be shown to be on the outer surface of the muscle fibre membrane, because when acetylcholine is injected intracellularly it is ineffective.
4. The action of acetylcholine on the receptor results in a massive increase in the ionic permeability of the end-plate region allowing Na^+ and K^+ ions to flow down their concentration gradients and so reduce the membrane potential from above −70 mV to near zero. The acetylcholine is then rapidly hydrolysed by cholinesterase.
5. If the evoked end-plate potential is sufficiently large, if will trigger off a further sequence of events resulting in the generation of a propagated muscle action potential which in turn activates the contractile processes of the muscle fibre. When no action potentials are passing down the motor nerve there is a continuous, spontaneous release of acetylcholine quanta from the nerve ending which produces miniature end-plate potentials (mepps). These potentials are not large enough by themselves to produce muscle spikes and are thought to be the result of the random bursting of single vesicles.

The synthesis of acetylcholine occurs in the motor nerve terminals and requires glucose, oxygen, sodium ions, choline, and the enzyme choline acetyltransferase, for its maintenance. If synthesis is blocked then transmission fails and this happens rapidly at high rates of stimulation of the motor nerve.

One way of stopping synthesis is by interfering with the uptake of choline by the nerve terminal. This can be achieved with **hemicholinium** (HC-3) which has some structural similarities to choline and appears to compete for a choline carrier in the nerve membrane. The transmission block which occurs can be overcome with excess choline. A striking demonstration that HC-3 reduces

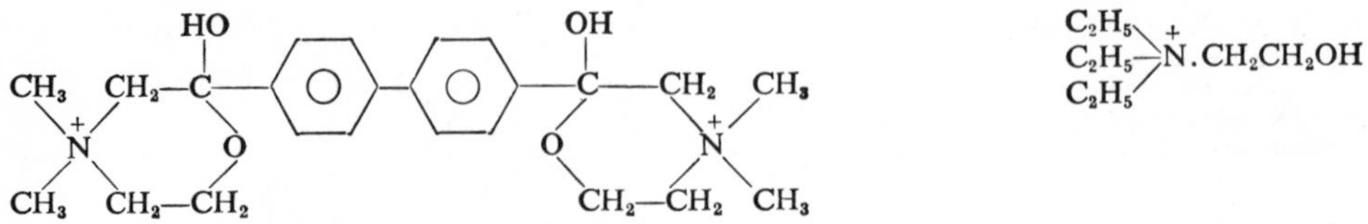

Hemicholinium (HC–3)

$(C_2H_5)_3\overset{+}{N}.CH_2CH_2OH$

Triethylcholine

Fig. 7.3. Drugs which interfere with the synthesis of acetylcholine.

acetylcholine synthesis and hence the content of each vesicle was provided by the demonstration that the size of mepps, but not the frequency, was reduced after the drug. A compound with an effect similar to that of HC-3 is **triethylcholine** (Fig. 7.3).

Myasthenia gravis, a disease characterized by muscular weakness, is likely to be due to a defect in acetylcholine synthesis because the amplitude of the mepps is reduced.

Little is known of the way in which acetylcholine is released from the motor nerve terminal but it is known that a reduction in extracellular calcium or an increase in magnesium reduces spontaneous acetylcholine release and that local anaesthetics, acting on the fine terminals of the nerve, stabilize the membrane and so block release.

Botulinum toxin causes muscular fatigue and paralysis due to the abolition of acetylcholine release. This is well illustrated by the reduced frequency but unimpaired amplitude of mepps which follows botulinum poisoning.

Black widow spider venom produces paralysis of skeletal muscle and it does so by causing the explosive release of all the acetylcholine stores in motor nerve terminals. The use of this venom experimentally has shown that the synaptic vesicles disappear from the motor nerve terminal when the acetylcholine is lost, thus adding support to the idea that they contain the transmitter.

There is some evidence that cholinergic receptors exist on the presynaptic motor nerve terminal and these may be affected by acetylcholine if anticholinesterase drugs are present. The result of this will be increased depolarization of the terminal and a consequent increase in acetylcholine release, leading to enhanced muscle activity.

Most drugs which affect neuromuscular transmission do so by an action at the postsynaptic membrane. Acetylcholine has important effects at this site and, although its action is too brief to make it of clinical importance, its mode of action is relevant to the action of many other drugs which are clinically useful.

The close arterial injection of acetylcholine to a skeletal muscle causes a twitch, and if an anticholinesterase is present to prevent enzymic destruction of acetylcholine, there may be prolonged fasciculations. The twitch and fasciculations are the result of the depolarizing action of acetylcholine on the end-plate region. If a large amount of acetylcholine is

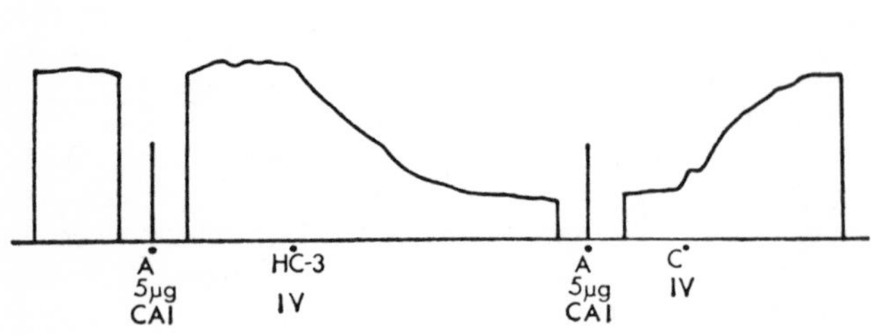

Fig. 7.4. The effect of HC-3 on neuromuscular transmission. Maximal twitches of the cat tibialis anterior muscle elicited by stimulating the motor nerve at a frequency of 1/s.

In this, and in all subsequent diagrams of the effect of drugs on muscle twitches, the individual records of twitches are not shown. Instead they are enclosed in a common envelope, the top edge of which indicates the height of the twitches.

A, acetylcholine; C, choline; CAI, close arterial injection.

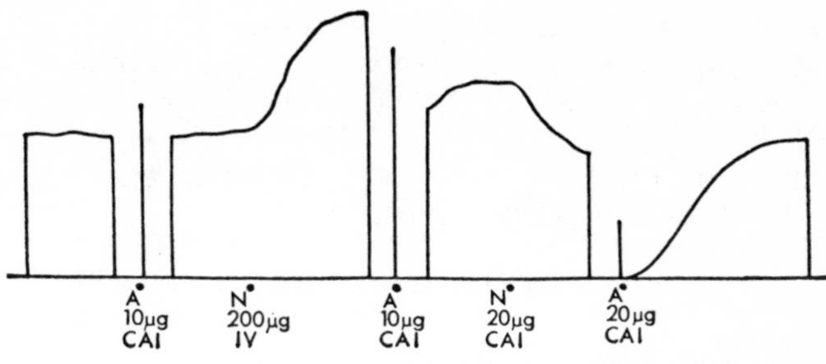

Fig. 7.5. A depolarizing block of neuromuscular transmission by acetylcholine. Cat tibialis anterior muscle. Stimulus frequency, 0·1/s. A, acetylcholine; N, neostigmine. Note the potentiating effect of intravenously injected neostigmine on the maximal twitches and on the effect of injected acetylcholine. When neostigmine is injected arterially it reaches the end-plates in a high concentration and a depolarizing block occurs as the acetylcholine accumulates. A further injection of acetylcholine makes the block worse.

injected, and if there is abundant antichlolinesterase present, the stage of excitation may develop into a stage of block known as a depolarizing block.

This depolarizing action of acetylcholine is an effect on nicotinic receptors and is antagonized by curare-like compounds which act as antagonists to acetylcholine by competing for the receptors and thereby preventing depolarization.

An acetylcholine block is made worse by tetanic stimulation of the motor nerve and by the addition of drugs which depolarize the membrane.

There are other important drugs, notably the methonium compounds, which depolarize the end-plate and thereby block neuromuscular transmission.

Suxamethonium, which resembles two molecules of acetylcholine laid end to end, has this property and so does **decamethonium.** The former drug is hydrolysed by pseudocholinesterase but has a sufficiently prolonged action to make it clinically useful. Decamethonium is not hydrolysed and so it has a longer action. Both these compounds may cause an initial facilitation of transmission in the period before a block develops.

It is interesting that both these compounds which activate the nicotinic receptor are long, slender molecules having a pair of charged groups separated by a carbon chain. It is known that the neuromuscular blocking activity in methonium compounds is greatest when the charged nitrogen groups are separated by ten to twelve carbon atoms. Any

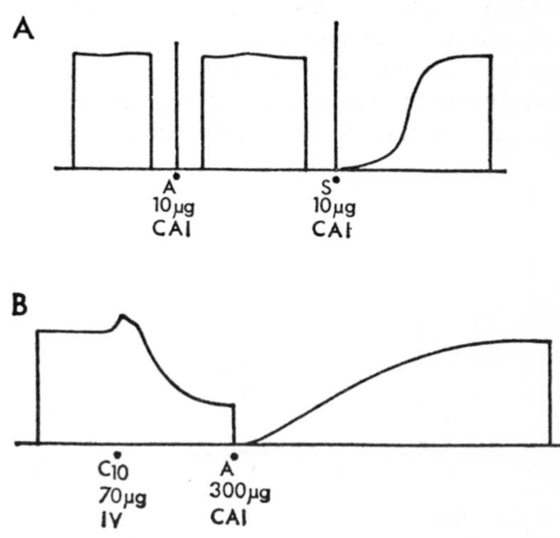

Fig. 7.6. The blocking action of suxamethonium decamethonium on the cat tibialis neuromuscular junction. Maximal twitches elicited every 10 seconds. A, acetylcholine; S, suxamethonium; C_{10}, decamethonium. Note increased block in B following acetylcholine injection.

alteration in this chain length reduces blocking activity, presumably because the drug molecule fits less well on to the receptor. Methonium compounds also block transmission across autonomic ganglia but, in this case, the optimum number of carbon atoms in the chain is five or six, a strong suggestion that the nicotinic receptors at this site and at the neuromuscular junction are not identical (see Fig. 7.7).

The depolarizing block and paralysis produced by the methonium compounds at the neuromuscular junction are the result of prolonged depolarization. This might be expected to produce a sustained tetanic spasm limited only by the refractory period of the membrane, but, in fact, this only occurs in slow-contracting multiply-innervated muscles.

The flaccid paralysis that occurs has been studied in the cat gracilis muscle and it is found that depolarization by decamethonium extends slightly beyond the region of muscle from which the end-plate potentials can be recorded. After applying decamethonium there is a brief increase in end-plate sensitivity but it then becomes less sensitive as does the region around the end-plate.

This loss of excitability may be due to inactivation of the sodium carrier in the membrane leading to the development of a 'zone of inexcitability' round the end-plate. A muscle action potential evoked at one end of the muscle fibre cannot then propagate across this zone. The block is very similar to that obtained with persistent cathodal stimulation.

A second important class of neuromuscular blocking drugs act in a very different way. They do not depolarize the postsynaptic membrane and they have no direct effect on the membrane potential, but they do prevent the action of depolarizing drugs.

Their blocking action may often be overcome by any procedure which increases the amount of transmitter in the vicinity of the end-plates. Tetanization of the motor nerve and the addition of an anticholinesterase will achieve this.

An example of this type of non-depolarizing blocking drug is **curare,** which is a South American arrow poison prepared from various species of plant. There are three varieties, known as pot-curare, tube-curare, and calabash-curare, named after the vessels in which they are kept. Tubocurarine is the

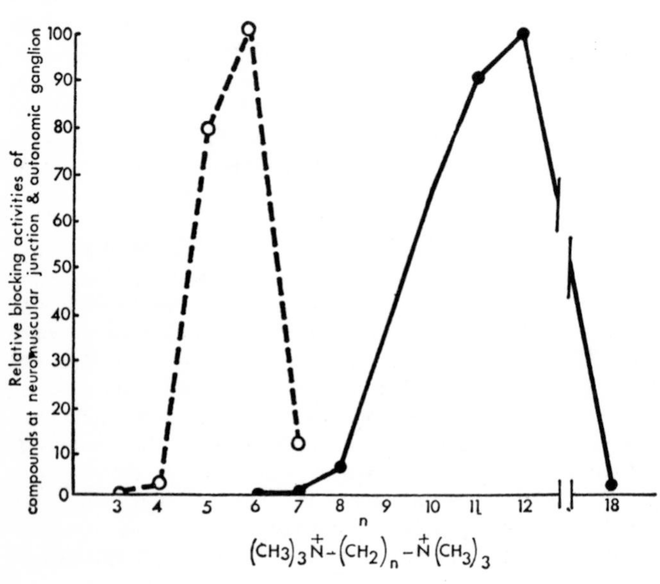

Fig. 7.7. The effect of altering the length of the methylene chain in methonium compounds on their ability to block transmission at the neuromuscular junction and at the autonomic ganglion. ●——●, neuromuscular junction (cat tibialis). ○– – –○, autonomic ganglion (cat superior cervical ganglion). (From data of Paton and Zaimis (1949 and 1951) *Brit. J. Pharmacol.* **4,** 381, and **6,** 155.)

dextroisomer of a pure alkaloid, obtained from tube-curare and from plant extracts.

Tubocurarine is not absorbed when taken orally and must be injected, but once in the plasma it disappears rapidly, so that the concentration is reduced by half every 13 minutes. About one-third of the dose is excreted in the urine, while the remainder is inactivated in the body in a few hours. The rapid rate at which the drug disappears ensures that its action lasts only a few minutes and that it is relatively ineffective when slowly absorbed.

The rat phrenic nerve–diaphragm preparation (p. 73) is a convenient method for the assay of tubocurarine.

The nerve is stimulated every 5–10 seconds and the resulting contractions remain constant for hours unless a drug is added to the bath.

The effect of curare is reversible; doses can be applied every 10 minutes, and standard and unknown solutions compared with one another.

Tubocurarine is still one of the most widely used neuromuscular blocking drugs and has played a part in balanced anaesthesia for many years. It is also used in the management of tetanus and has, in the past, been used in the diagnosis of myasthenia gravis.

Other neuromuscular blocking agents include **gallamine, dihydro-β-erythroidine,** and **benzoquinonium;** these are described on page 88.

DRUGS WHICH PRESERVE ACETYLCHOLINE

Drugs which inhibit or inactivate cholinesterase are called **anticholinesterases** and their action prevents the destruction of acetylcholine and so potentiates its effect. These drugs have a variety of uses as insecticides, as 'nerve gases', and as therapeutic agents.

They may be divided into two major groups, the reversible anticholinesterase drugs and the organophosphorus compounds which permanently inactivate cholinesterase. Both classes of drug react with cholinesterase in much the same way as does the natural substrate. If acetylcholine is the substrate then the molecule is bound to an active unit of the enzyme at an anionic and an esteratic site. From this choline is split off leaving an acyl group attached to the enzyme. The latter reacts with water to produce acetic acid and the regeneration of the enzyme.

This reaction is theoretically reversible but in practice moves rapidly to the state where acetylcholine is hydrolysed.

A weak anticholinesterase such as **edrophonium** produces a reversible inhibition of the enzyme by combining with it only at the anionic site thus blocking the attachment and subsequent destruction of acetylcholine.

More potent anticholinesterases like **physostigmine** and **neostigmine** form attachments at both sites and they are then hydrolysed in the same way as acetylcholine. The difference between this reaction and that with acetylcholine is that hydrolysis of the acyl enzyme is about a million times slower than the hydrolysis of the acetyl enzyme. These compounds therefore act as anticholinesterases because they form alternative substrates for the enzyme and are hydrolysed extremely slowly.

The organophosphorus anticholinesterases such as **diisopropylfluorophosphonate** (DFP) only bind with the enzyme at the esteratic site but the reaction then proceeds as it does with other anticholinesterases. In this case, however, the resultant phosphorylated enzyme is extremely stable and if isopropyl groups are involved virtually no hydrolysis or regeneration of the enzyme occurs. Cholinesterase activity will then only return as new enzyme is synthesized.

The negligible reactivation of phosphorylated forms of cholinesterase can be greatly speeded up if oximes are used to react with the enzyme instead of water. The best example of these compounds is **P–2–AM** (pralidoxime, PAM). The rate of combination of this type of compound is greatly helped by electrostatic forces between the quaternary nitrogen and the anionic site on the enzyme.

This type of enzyme reactivator will protect against otherwise lethal doses of anticholinesterases but phosphorylated cholinesterase 'ages' rapidly and, in a matter of minutes or hours, may become completely resistant to reactivators. The process of 'ageing' is likely to be due to the splitting off of an alkyl group leaving a more stable monoalkyl phosphorylated compound.

The pharmacological effects of the anticholinesterases are largely due to the accumulation of acetylcholine that they cause at all cholinergic synapses in the body.

Some of the anticholinesterase agents, particularly the quaternary ammonium compounds like neostigmine, have their own direct action on cholinoceptive sites. Neostigmine has a direct depolarizing action on the neuromuscular junction, an effect which is not surprising in view of the fact that it reacts efficiently with the same enzyme as acetylcholine.

The actions of anticholinesterases at autonomic effector cells, and to some extent in the CNS, are antagonized by atropine and at the neuromuscular junction and autonomic ganglia some antagonism may be effected by curare-like drugs and hexamethonium respectively.

The therapeutic uses of the anticholinesterases are limited to effects on the pupil and the intestine, and to the treatment of myasthenia gravis.

When applied locally to the eye the anticholinesterases cause pupil constriction and spasm of accommodation. Intraocular pressure falls because the miosis allows the reabsorption of aqueous humour.

Anticholinesterases, particularly neostigmine, increase motor activity in the small and large bowel and this action can be used to overcome atonic conditions.

THE AUTONOMIC GANGLION

Transmission at autonomic ganglia is not unlike that at the neuromuscular junction, acetylcholine is the transmitting chemical at both parasympathetic and sympathetic ganglia and the main receptors are nicotinic. There is some evidence to suggest that muscarinic-type receptors exist on the postganglionic membrane but their physiological function is not yet clear.

Small spontaneous potentials, similar to mepps at the neuromuscular junction, can be recorded from the postsynaptic ganglionic neurones and it is likely that when a large number of them occur simultaneously, a full ganglion spike potential will be generated.

The site which has been most fully studied is the cat superior cervical ganglion, because it can easily be perfused through its artery or studied *in vitro*. It contains no interneurones and transmission across the synapses can be measured by recording electrically from the postganglionic fibres or by measuring contractures of the nictitating membrane which it innervates. The stimulant and paralysing actions of nicotine on the ganglion and the effect on the nictitating membrane are illustrated in Fig. 7.8.

The evidence for cholinergic transmission at the ganglion is good. Choline acetyltransferase is present, cholinesterase is present, applied acetylcholine depolarizes the postsynaptic membrane, and acetylcholine is released from the stimulated preganglionic terminals.

The synthesis and turnover of acetylcholine in the preganglionic terminal have been studied in some detail and, as at the neuromuscular junction, choline and glucose are essential for synthesis. As might be expected, hemicholinium, triethylcholine, calcium and magnesium ions, and botulinum toxin all affect the synthesis and release of acetylcholine in apparently the same way as at the neuromuscular junction.

The effect of stimulating transmission through autonomic ganglia is best considered in relation to nicotine, acetylcholine, and TMA, which all work by depolarizing the postganglionic cell bodies.

Nicotine is readily absorbed from all mucous membranes, and more slowly on subcutaneous injection, or through intact skin. It causes excitation followed by inhibition at all sympathetic and parasympathetic ganglia. The first phase is the result of depolarization of the postganglionic membrane and the second phase results from the persistent de-

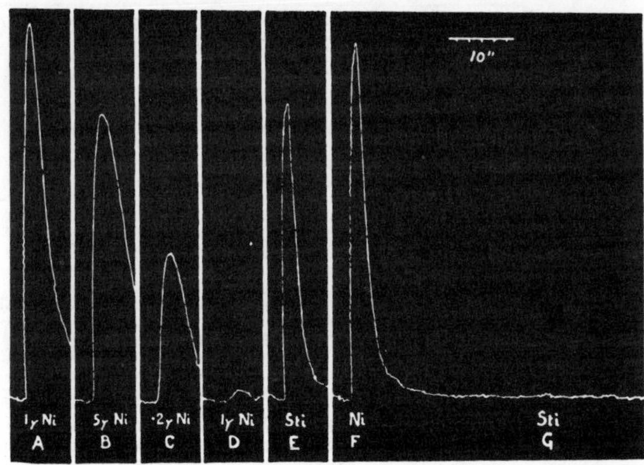

Fig. 7.8. The effects of nicotine on a sympathetic ganglion. The tracing shows contractions of the nictitating membrane of a cat. The superior cervical ganglion was perfused with Locke's solution. A–D show the stimulant action of small doses of nicotine injected in the perfusion fluid; E and G show the effect of stimulating the cervical sympathetic. The injection of a large dose of nicotine (0·05 mg) at F caused a contraction followed by paralysis of the ganglion. (From Feldberg and Vartiainen (1934) *J. Physiol.* (*Lond.*) **83,** 120.)

polarization of the membrane, probably by inactivation of the sodium carrier mechanism.

The peripheral responses to nicotine are complicated, because not only are there the excitatory and depressant effects, but also sympathetic and parasympathetic ganglia are equally affected. It imitates the effects of muscarine by stimulating the ganglia from which cholinergic nerves arise. It also imitates the actions of catecholamines by stimulating sympathetic ganglia and by causing a release of adrenaline from the adrenal medulla.

Nicotine is the most important pharmacological constituent of tobacco and the smoke from an average-sized cigarette may contain 6–8 mg of nicotine. Attention has been focused in recent years on the hazards of tobacco smoking and a strong association between the incidence of carcinoma of the lung and tobacco smoking has been established. This is not the only hazard, however, because there is evidence that the action of nicotine, particularly on the cardiovascular system, can be deleterious when taken over long periods. The effects of cigarette smoking may include peripheral vasoconstriction, a rise in systolic and diastolic blood pressures, the occasional initiation of premature systoles, and attacks of atrial tachycardia. Smoking also causes bronchial irritation and the long-term addict can usually be recognized by his wheezing and dyspnoea. He is often subject to upper respiratory infections and may suffer chest pains. Most of these symptoms disappear if smoking is discontinued.

Despite the unpleasant and sometimes fatal side-effects of smoking which are now recognized and publicized, the use of tobacco shows only slight signs of declining. This is likely to be partly due to the addictive nature of the whole smoking ritual and to the pleasant central effects that nicotine has for many individuals.

Other effects of nicotine include the stimulation of respiration, vomiting by an action on central and peripheral receptors, antidiuresis by stimulating the release of ADH, and an increase in tone and motor activity of the bowel due to parasympathetic stimulation.

The ganglion-stimulant action of nicotine, acetylcholine, and related compounds may be clearly illustrated in the whole animal by the effect of acetylcholine on the blood pressure of the cat (Fig. 7.9).

A small dose of acetylcholine produces a dramatic fall in the blood pressure because the muscarinic effects of acetylcholine (see p. 83) slow the heart and cause peripheral vasodilatation. If atropine is now given to block this action and a higher dose of acetylcholine

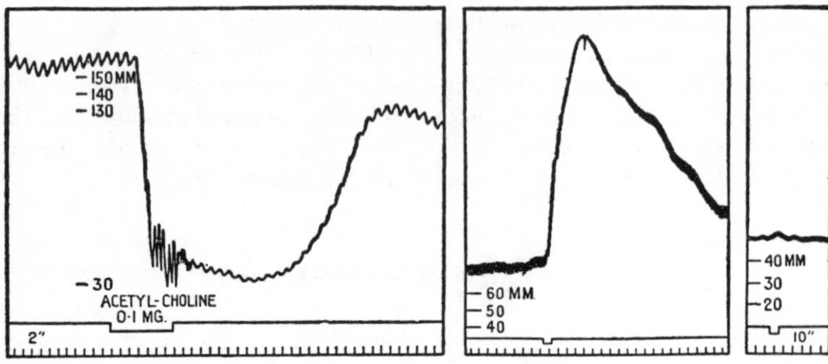

Fig. 7.9. Cat's blood pressure. Left—muscarine action of acetylcholine (0·1 mg). Vasodilatation and slowing of heart. Middle—nicotine action of acetylcholine (5 mg) after 1 mg of atropine, which antagonizes muscarine actions. The rise of blood pressure is partly due to the liberation of adrenaline and partly due to the stimulation of sympathetic ganglia. Right—after 30 mg of nicotine, the nicotine action of 5 mg of acetylcholine disappears. (From Dale (1914) *J. Pharmacol.* **6,** 152.)

is injected, the nicotinic actions are unmasked and revealed as a rise in blood pressure. This is the result of ganglion stimulation causing activity in postganglionic vasoconstrictor fibres and the release of adrenaline from the adrenal medulla. The former effect may be abolished by giving a ganglion blocking compound.

Tetramethylammonium (TMA), like acetylcholine and nicotine stimulates all autonomic ganglia and causes a rise in the cat blood pressure after atropine because the effect of stimulating the sympathetic ganglia then predominates. It has only very weak muscarinic activity and it excites the ganglia in much lower concentrations than it does the neuromuscular junction.

Other drugs with ganglion stimulating actions include **lobeline** (p. 64) and **dimethyl-4-phenylpiperazium** (DMPP).

The stimulant action of nicotine, choline esters, and related compounds is often followed by a block of transmission due to persistent depolarization but there are other drugs which block ganglionic transmission by a nondepolarizing antagonism. These drugs, like curare at the muscle end-plate, do not alter the ganglion cell potentials nor do they interfere with the release of acetylcholine. They paralyse all autonomic ganglia and so have a variety of effects in all parts of the body. The paralysis of sympathetic ganglia dilates blood vessels and so a general fall in blood pressure occurs. This effect has been made use of clinically in cases of hypertension but because all ganglia are affected, there are numerous side-effects associated with this treatment. In addition, cardiovascular reflexes will be abolished and this may result in postural hypotension.

Paralysis of parasympathetic ganglia reduces gastric secretion, causes a dry mouth, paralysis of the iris and ciliary muscles, paralytic ileus, retention of urine, etc. These side-effects limit the clinical usefulness of the compounds.

Tetraethylammonium (TEA) was the first drug to be used clinically to block ganglia but it is not very active or specific and has now been replaced by other compounds.

It is interesting that TMA stimulates the ganglion by depolarization but substitution of the methyl groups by ethyl groups produces a compound which blocks transmission by a non-depolarizing action.

Although the ammonium salt TEA has ganglion blocking activity, it was only with the development of the bisonium compounds that the sustained and specific action necessary for extensive clinical use could be obtained.

The bisonium compound **hexamethonium** has a highly specific action on ganglia, but, like most antagonists, in very large doses it will have other actions; these include atropine-like and curare-like effects.

It was employed in the treatment of hypertension but is now replaced by drugs with fewer side-effects that can be given orally. It is still used to produce hypotension during anaesthesia.

Other compounds which block transmission at autonomic ganglia include **pentolinium, pentamethonium,** and the orally active hypotensive agents, **pempidine** and **mecamylamine** (Fig. 7.16).

MUSCARINIC RESPONSES

The action of acetylcholine and acetylcholine-like drugs on 'muscarinic' receptors resembles the effect of stimulating the parasympathetic nervous system. These muscarinic actions are postganglionic and are exerted on the heart, the exocrine glands, and smooth muscle. They include:

1. Heart—slowing.
2. Eye—constriction of the pupil, contraction of the ciliary muscle (for near vision).
3. Blood vessels—most blood vessels have muscarinic receptors and acetylcholine will produce vasodilatation.
4. Exocrine glands—stimulation of secretion from sweat glands, salivary glands (watery secretion), mucous glands, lacrimal glands. Gastric, intestinal, and pancreatic secretions are also increased.
5. Stomach and intestine—increase in motility and tone, relaxation of sphincters.
6. Gall-bladder and ducts—contraction.
7. Bladder—contraction of detrusor and relaxation of sphincter.

Drugs which produce these effects include **acetylcholine, carbachol, pilocarpine, muscarine, arecoline, methacholine,** and the **anticholinesterases.**

All the muscarinic actions of these drugs are abolished or reduced by atropine and atropine-like compounds.

The postganglionic fibres of the parasympathetic nervous system innervate smooth muscle effector cells, and release acetylcholine on to muscarinic receptors. Very much less is known about these neuromuscular junctions than about skeletal muscle junctions because the nerve terminals are not so easy to define and the muscle cells are small and hard to pierce with electrodes. There is, however, good evidence to suggest that acetylcholine is the only excitatory transmitter released when these nerves are stimulated.

The arrangement of nerve and muscle fibres is quite different from that existing in skeletal muscle; there is no organized end-plate and the nerves ramify widely over the muscle fibres. The action of acetylcholine, whether produced by stimulation of the nerves or by local application, is slow, and the tension developed by the muscle is graded continuously up to a maximum.

The electrical events associated with smooth muscle cells have been investigated with intra- and extracellular electrodes and the resting potential, which is rather variable, has been found to be lower than in skeletal muscle, about -50 mV, and to be altered by changes in the tension applied to the muscle. The state of membrane polarization determines the rate of muscle action potential discharge and therefore the activity of the contractile mechanism. When acetylcholine and other drugs interact with the muscarinic membrane receptors a state of membrane depolarization is produced with a consequent increase in spike frequency and muscle tension.

As with the end-plate on skeletal muscle, the action of acetylcholine on the post-junctional membrane appears to be associated with changes in membrane permeability to sodium and potassium ions.

The muscarinic receptors on smooth muscle are specifically stimulated by muscarine and this action is antagonized by atropine and by atropine-like compounds which compete for the receptor sites.

A rather different situation exists at the junction between postganglionic vagal parasympathetic fibres and the heart. As at smooth muscle parasympathetic junctions the transmitter is acetylcholine but it acts as an inhibitory transmitter and the effect of its release is primarily to produce a slowing of the heart rate. The acetylcholine acts on muscarinic receptors and its action is abolished by atropine, but unlike all other peripheral cholinergic sites in the body, except those of the secretory glands, the response to acetylcholine is a hyperpolarization of the membrane with a consequent reduction in membrane excitability.

In 1953 it was shown that the resting potential of the cat auricle fibres was increased (hyperpolarization) in the presence of acetylcholine and parasympathetic drugs. This effect was greatest when the diastolic membrane potential was furthest from the equilibrium potential for potassium ions (−90 mV) and it was suggested that the effect was mediated by a large selective increase in membrane permeability to potassium, this ion passing out of the cell.

When the inhibitory action of acetylcholine on the heart is compared with its excitatory action at the neuromuscular junction it may be seen that both effects are essentially the same. They both involve a fall in membrane resistance, the difference being in the species of ions whose movement is facilitated. At the neuromuscular junction there is a non-selective increase in cation permeability while at cardiac muscle the increase is largely restricted to potassium ions (Fig. 7.10).

Drugs which act as agonists at muscarinic receptor sites have the actions described on p. 83. If the drug also has nicotinic activity then these effects will be superimposed on the muscarinic action. The individual compounds with muscarinic stimulating activity are described on pp. 91–2.

Drugs which antagonize the action of cholinergic drugs at muscarinic receptors are known as antimuscarinic or **atropine-like compounds.** Except in high doses, their action is specific and clinically their main use has been for premedication before operations in order to prevent excessive salivary and bronchial secretions.

The drugs in this group have many pharmacological properties in common and these

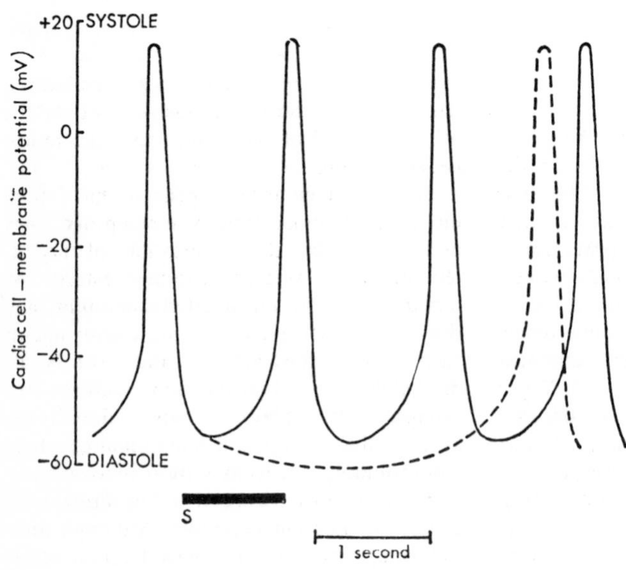

Fig. 7.10. Intracellular recording from a fibre of the sinus venosus of the frog heart. At S the vagus was stimulated at 20/s and the dotted line shows the effect of the liberated acetylcholine on the membrane potential. The continuous line shows the membrane potential in the unstimulated sinus venosus.

are well illustrated by considering the characteristics of atropine.

Various plants, including deadly nightshade (*Atropa belladonna*), contain the alkaloids **l-hyoscyamine** and **l-hyoscine.** Racemization occurs easily and the racemic *dl*-hyoscyamine is known as **atropine.** These compounds all have some actions on the CNS but their most important actions are concerned with their antagonism at peripheral muscarinic receptors.

Most of the actions of atropine can be deduced from a knowledge of the effect of muscarine-like drugs. It stops secretion, including tears, sweat, and saliva, and the secretions of the pancreas and mucous glands in the alimentary canal and respiratory passages but has no effect on the secretion of bile, milk, or urine. It abolishes vagal action, dilates the bronchi, and inhibits the emptying of the bladder. It dilates the pupil and paralyses accommodation so that the eye is focused for distant objects.

Atropine is a reversible antagonist of muscarine-like drugs and its effect can usually be overcome if the agonist concentration is made sufficiently high.

Atropine is used to reduce salivary and bronchial secretions during anaesthesia, to protect the heart from vagal inhibition, and to reduce the muscarinic actions of any anticholinesterases that may be given. It is sometimes given to reduce the pain of renal and intestinal colic. It is used locally in the eye when a prolonged mydriatic effect is required.

A person poisoned by atropine has a dry mouth and finds it difficult to swallow or speak; he has a dry skin, a rash like that of scarlet fever, and a high temperature; his pupils are dilated and owing to the action on the CNS he may be restless and even have convulsions followed by paralysis. The convulsions can be controlled by a general anaesthetic and the subsequent paralysis by central stimulants and warmth. The peripheral effects of atropine are comparatively harmless.

A large number of other atropine-like compounds have been discovered or synthesized. Some of these are described on pp. 92–4 and include **hyoscine, homatropine, dibutoline, methantheline, propantheline,** the longer-acting drug **lachesine,** and the irreversible antagonist **benzilylcholine mustard** (Fig. 7.17).

MIXED RECEPTOR SITES

THE SPINAL CORD

The synapses between collateral fibres from the motor axon and Renshaw cells in the spinal cord are of particular interest because it is at these sites in the CNS that evidence for the identity of the transmitting chemical is most complete. The transmitter is almost certainly acetylcholine and much of the evidence for this has been obtained by the microelectrophoretic application of cholinergic agonists and antagonists to the Renshaw cell. When the blood–brain barrier is circumvented, as it is with the electrophoretic technique, there are no anomalous features in the response of Renshaw cells to these compounds (Fig. 7.11).

In addition, acetylcholine has been shown to be released by the motor axon collaterals when they are stimulated just as it is from the other terminal of the same axon, the motor nerve terminal.

The Renshaw cells appear to have both nicotinic and muscarinic-type receptors. They are excited by the application of acetylcholine and related choline esters, by nicotine, and by tetramethylammonium and they are weakly excited by muscarinic agents such as muscarine and acetyl-β-methylcholine. Transmission across the synapse is blocked by dihydro-β-erythroidine, tetraethylammonium, hexamethonium, and weakly by d-tubocurarine, and the actions of acetylcholine are potentiated by anticholinesterases. Although muscarinic agents excite only weakly, their action

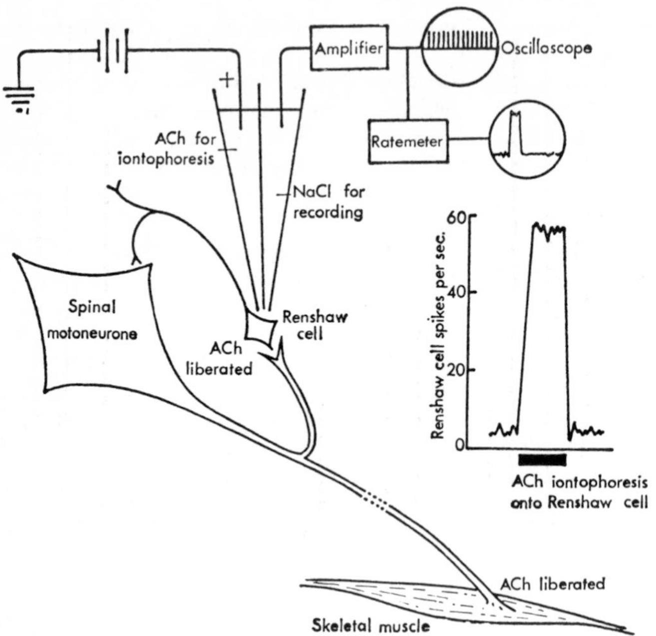

Fig. 7.11. Block diagram of the method used to investigate the action of iontophoretically applied drugs on Renshaw cells.

is resistant to block by nicotinic antagonists but is blocked by atropine, thus indicating the presence of muscarinic-type receptors.

Many attempts to find cholinergic synapses elsewhere in the spinal cord have failed.

THE BRAIN

When it was realized that acetylcholine was a transmitter at peripheral synapses Sir Henry Dale suggested it might also have this role in the CNS. Although there is still no direct evidence for cholinergic synapses in the brain there is abundant indirect evidence to suggest that, at a small proportion of synapses, it does have an important role as a transmitter.

Acetylcholine, choline acetyltransferase, and cholinesterase are all present in the brain and acetylcholine is released from the brain and the rate of this release and also the acetylcholine content are associated with nervous activity and the level of consciousness (Fig. 7.12). Microelectrophoretic techniques have located cholinoceptive neurones in many parts of the brain including the cerebral cortex, the cerebellum, thalamus, hippocampus, reticular formation, and medulla. In the cortex the receptors appear to be predominately of a muscarinic type although nicotinic agonists and antagonists sometimes have weak actions. In the thalamus and lower parts of the brain the cholinoceptive cells appear to have a mixture of nicotinic and muscarinic properties, and in the brain stem, for instance, there is evidence that the 'muscarinic' neurones are inhibited by acetylcholine whereas the 'nicotinic' cells are excited.

It seems likely that some of the cholinergic synapses in the brain are associated with major specific and non-specific ascending pathways from the reticular formation and from specific thalamic nuclei and are concerned with the maintenance of consciousness and the level of arousal in the mammalian brain.

From a consideration of all the cholinergic mechanisms discussed it is evident that, at the periphery, the receptors are relatively simple and may be clearly divided into those with

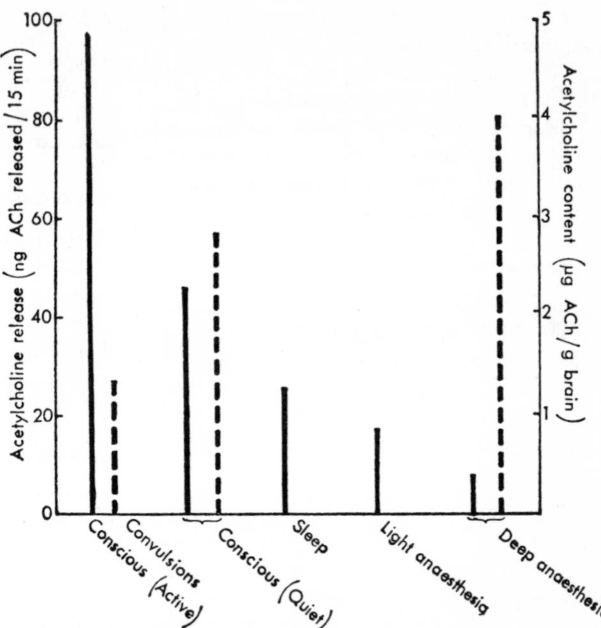

Fig. 7.12. The relationship between nervous activity and central acetylcholine content and release. Acetylcholine content measured in cerebral cortex of rats (dotted lines). Acetylcholine release measured from cerebral cortex of rabbits (full lines). As activity in the brain falls (deep anaesthesia) so the acetylcholine content rises and the release falls. This suggests that less is being liberated from cholinergic nerve terminals in the cortex.

nicotinic and those with muscarinic characteristics. As one proceeds centrally, so the characteristics of the postsynaptic membranes become more complicated with a variable ratio of muscarinic and nicotinic properties. There is certainly much still to be learnt about these receptor systems and the significance of their distribution and function in the nervous system.

INDIVIDUAL CHOLINERGIC DRUGS AND THEIR ANTAGONISTS

Drugs which block neuromuscular transmission by depolarization:

Nicotine

Like acetylcholine, nicotine depolarizes the neuromuscular junction end-plate but it is not destroyed by cholinesterases, so even in small doses, after an initial twitch, a depolarizing block will appear.

Suxamethonium (succinylcholine)

Suxamethonium depolarizes the end-plate and is hydrolysed by pseudocholinesterase, but its action is sufficiently prolonged to make it clinically useful as a neuromuscular blocking drug. It is used in short operations where profound muscle relaxation is required for a few minutes. It can be used for longer operations by repeating the dose or by giving infusions.

A few patients suffer prolonged apnoea after the injection of suxamethonium and many of these people have been found to have a reduced level of plasma cholinesterase, usually due to a genetic factor or, more rarely, to hepatic disease or a nutritional deficiency.

Suxamethonium blocks by depolarization but, like acetylcholine, its first effect may be to produce fasciculations which can result in post-operative muscle pains. It has no action on the CNS and unlike acetylcholine it has no muscarinic activity and so does not affect the autonomic nervous system.

When large doses are given, the initial block by depolarization gives way to a non-depolarizing curare-like block, which is relieved by anticholinesterase. This phenomenon is known as 'dual block' and may lead to prolonged muscle paralysis.

Decamethonium (C10)

Decamethonium is not destroyed by cholinesterase so its paralysing action is more prolonged than that of suxamethonium. There is no antidote which may be used safely. The mechanism of its blocking action is similar to that of suxamethonium (above).

Carbachol

Carbachol is an ester of choline with an action like acetylcholine except that its effect is more prolonged because it is not hydrolysed by cholinesterases. It has both muscarinic and nicotinic actions.

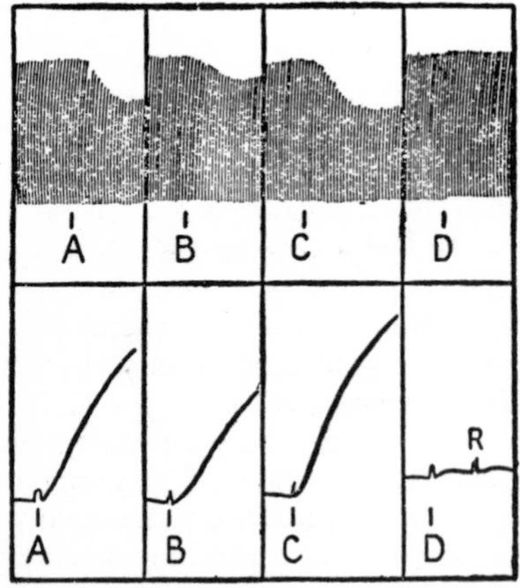

Fig. 7.13. Above—isolated frog's heart (Straub's method). Below—leech muscle sensitized with eserine. A—fluid from perfused sympathetic ganglion collected during stimulation. D—control fluid (no stimulation). B and C—acetylcholine (15 and 30 ng per ml.). A caused effects between those due to B and C on both preparations. This quantitative agreement between two tests suggests the identification of the active substance in A as acetylcholine. (From Feldberg and Gaddum (1934) *J. Physiol.* (*Lond.*) **81,** 314.)

Dihydro-β-erythroidine (DHE)

This compound contains only one atom of nitrogen in its molecule and is active orally.

It is an effective and highly specific antagonist at nicotinic receptors.

Benzoquinonium (*Mytolon*)

Benzoquinonium is a non-depolarizing blocker but has rather pronounced anticholinesterase properties in mammals, about one-tenth the activity of neostigmine. This may result in bradycardia and increased bronchial and salivary secretions. These are the result of the enhanced action of acetylcholine at muscarinic receptor sites and may all be abolished by atropine.

Because of its anticholinesterase activity it is only weakly antagonized by neostigmine and so it is not considered safe to be used clinically.

Gallamine

Gallamine is a synthetic compound which acts like tubocurarine but is about five times less active. It is widely used clinically to produce muscle relaxation during surgery. It may also be used in small doses to augment the effects of light anaesthesia in minor operations.

ANTICHOLINESTERASES

Edrophonium (*Tensilon*)

Edrophonium has a direct cholinergic action on nicotinic receptors and is a weak cholinesterase inhibitor.

It has a short duration of action and is used to antagonize curare-like drugs, and for the diagnosis of myasthenia gravis. Unlike neostigmine, a large dose of edrophonium produces nicotinic effects with muscle fasciculations leading to paralysis.

Neostigmine (*Prostigmin*)

Neostigmine has similar anticholinesterase properties to physostigmine but like edrophonium it also has a direct action on

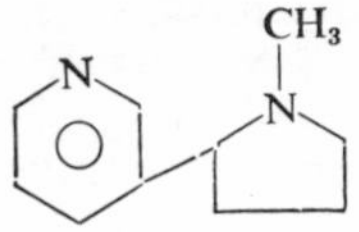

Nicotine

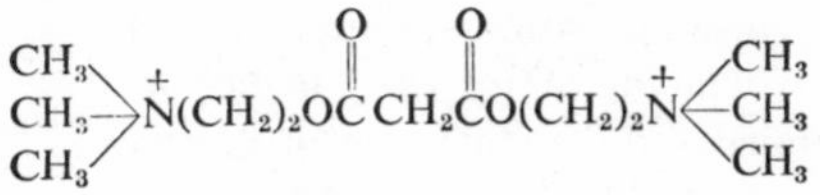

Suxamethonium

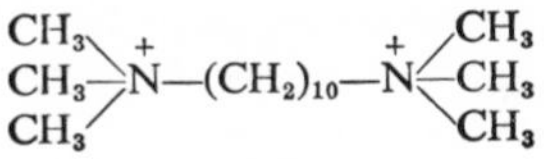

Decamethonium

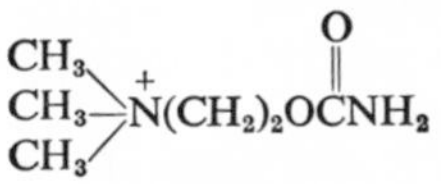

Carbachol

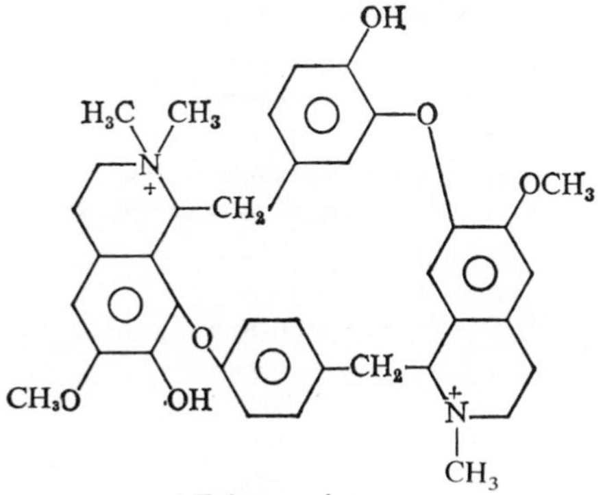

d-Tubocurarine

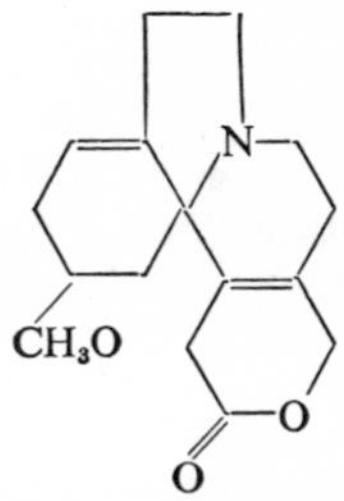

Dihydro-β-erythroidine

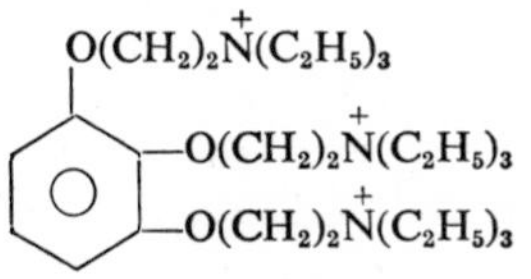

Gallamine

Fig. 7.14. Agonists and antagonists at the neuromuscular junction.

cholinergic receptors. It is used to antagonize the actions of curare-like drugs and in the treatment of atony of the bladder, myasthenia gravis, glaucoma, and sinus tachycardia. It is usually administered with atropine so that its muscarinic actions are reduced.

Physostigmine (eserine)

This was the first anticholinesterase to be used clinically. It is absorbed well whether injected or swallowed. Most, if not all, of the actions of eserine are due to the inhibition of cholinesterase. Physostigmine potentiates all the nicotinic and muscarinic actions of acetylcholine and it is a useful drug for increasing the sensitivity of biological assay preparations to acetylcholine and is widely used for this purpose.

Dyflos (diisopropylfluorophosphonate, DFP)

Dyflos reacts with cholinesterase and loses fluorine. A phosphorylated enzyme is formed which is stable for a week or more. If a choline ester, or a reversible inhibitor such as eserine, is present the active site on the enzyme is occupied and the enzyme is protected from inactivation by organic phosphorus compounds. Dyflos causes a prolonged and powerful constriction of the pupil and is used in glaucoma to reduce intraocular pressure. This last effect is due to contraction of the pupil allowing reopening of the canal of Schlemm in the filtration angle of the eye.

Organo-phosphorus compounds with similar actions to dyflos include the following compounds:

Phospholine	Used to treat glaucoma.
Mipafox	Insecticide and selective inhibitor of pseudocholinesterase.
Sarin	Toxic nerve gas.
Tetraethylpyrophosphate TEPP)	Early insecticide. Occasionally used in glaucoma and myasthenia gravis.

DRUGS WHICH BLOCK TRANSMISSION AT AUTONOMIC GANGLIA

Pentamethonium

The actions of pentamethonium are identical to, but slightly less potent than, those of hexamethonium (p. 82). Pentamethonium is not now used clinically.

Pentolinium

Pentolinium has similar properties to those of hexamethonium but it is more potent.

Mecamylamine

Mecamylamine is a secondary amine and was developed as an orally active hypotensive agent. It has a prolonged action of 8–12 hours and is at least as active as hexamethonium. It suffers from the disadvantage that, unlike quaternary methonium compounds, it enters the CNS with comparative ease and may cause tremor and/or psychoses.

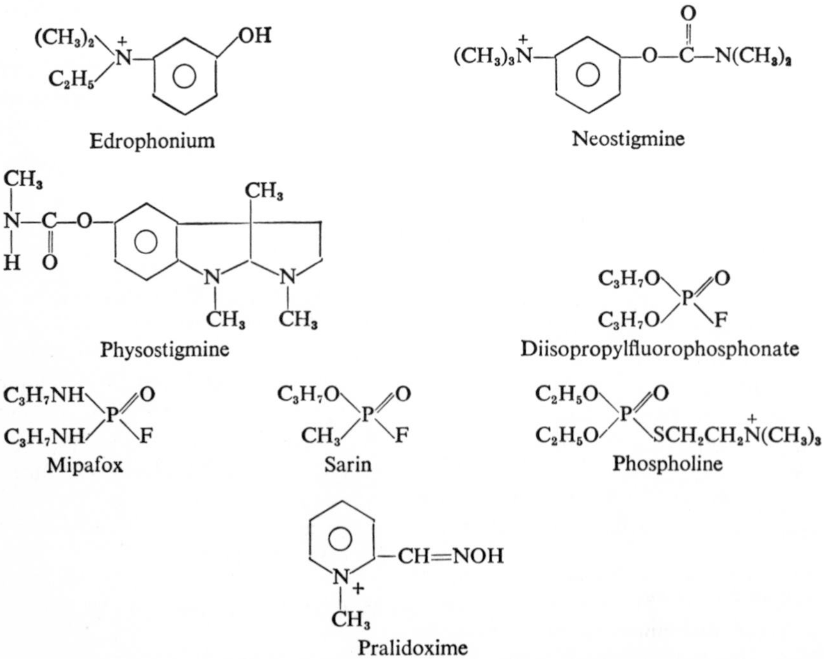

Edrophonium

Neostigmine

Physostigmine

Diisopropylfluorophosphonate

Mipafox

Sarin

Phospholine

Pralidoxime

Fig. 7.15. The structures of some anticholinesterases and a cholinesterase reactivator.

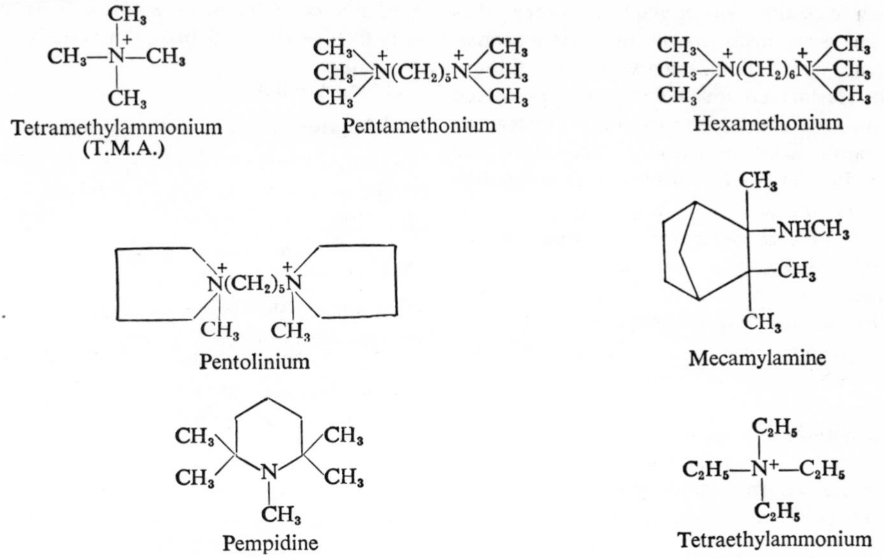

Tetramethylammonium (T.M.A.)

Pentamethonium

Hexamethonium

Pentolinium

Mecamylamine

Pempidine

Tetraethylammonium

Fig. 7.16. The structures of drugs which act on the autonomic ganglion.

It has side-effects similar to those exhibited by other ganglion blocking drugs.

Pempidine

Pempidine resembles mecamylamine in being absorbed when given orally but has a shorter duration of action. Pempidine is used in the treatment of all types of hypertension but is unsuitable for producing controlled hypotension during anaesthesia because of its prolonged action.

The ganglion blocking activity of mecamylamine and pempidine depends on the presence of a methyl group adjacent to the nitrogen; loss of this methyl group reduces activity.

AGONISTS AT MUSCARINIC RECEPTORS

Muscarine

Muscarine was taken as the substance typical of a class of drugs because it was thought to have an action exclusively on pure muscarinic receptors. This is now known not to be entirely true. It is a very stable and active substance and is excreted unchanged in the urine.

Muscarine stimulates the postganglionic parasympathetic receptor and so reproduces the effects of stimulating parasympathetic nerves (see p. 83). All its actions are antagonized by atropine. It is not used clinically.

Acetylcholine

Acetylcholine produces all the effects which are obtained by stimulation of the parasympathetic nervous system and, in addition, it stimulates nicotinic receptors at the skeletal neuromuscular junction, autonomic ganglion, and the adrenal medulla. Because it is quickly hydrolysed by cholinesterases its action is transient unless anticholinesterases are present.

Small alterations in the acetylcholine molecule produce profound changes in muscarinic activity. The size of the charged cationic head is important for activity, methyl groups being necessary for activity and substitution with more than one ethyl group considerably reduces muscarinic activity.

Replacing the acetyl group by others in the series always leads to a fall in muscarinic activity and homologues higher than butyrylcholine are even found to be acetylcholine antagonists. The changes in nicotinic activity of these substituted compounds do not follow the changes in muscarinic potency (Chapter 1).

If the choline part of the molecule is altered in length, again the muscarinic activity is reduced as in acetylnorcholine which has only weak muscarinic activity.

The introduction of asymmetry into the molecule by the addition of a branched methyl group to the chain also affects activity. Methacholine, in which the β carbon in acetylcholine has been methylated, has only half the muscarinic activity of acetylcholine and no nicotinic actions.

Methacholine

Methacholine has actions similar to the muscarinic actions of acetylcholine and it is more stable, being hydrolysed by acetylcholinesterase at only one-third the rate of acetylcholine. It is not hydrolysed by pseudocholinesterase. It is a safer drug than carbachol because of its lack of nicotinic effects. Its main actions are to slow the heart and dilate peripheral blood vessels while intestinal tone is raised and salivation and sweating are increased.

Choline

Choline has both nicotinic and muscarinic actions but these are about 1000 times weaker than those of acetylcholine.

Pilocarpine

Pilocarpine has muscarinic actions but no significant nicotinic activity. It produces marked sweating and the secretion of gastric juices. It is only used clinically to reduce intraocular pressure in the treatment of glaucoma.

Arecoline

The pharmacological actions of arecoline resemble those of pilocarpine. Arecoline is the chief alkaloid in betel nuts and has been used by natives of the East Indies from early times to produce euphoria.

Anticholinesterases

These compounds have actions resembling those which result from parasympathetic stimulation because they prevent the destruction of liberated acetylcholine.

The administration of physostigmine produces constriction of the pupil, stimulation of the intestine, and inhibition of the heart. If it is placed in the eye there is constriction of the pupil, spasm of accommodation, and a reduction of intra-ocular pressure (see p. 79).

ANTAGONISTS AT MUSCARINIC RECEPTORS

Hyoscine (scopolamine)

The peripheral actions of hyoscine resemble those of atropine but it is more effective in stopping secretions.

The central actions of hyoscine differ from those of atropine. They do not produce excitement at any stage but only depression, especially of the motor areas. It is an effective drug against motion-sickness and it is used for this purpose and as a sedative and to prevent secretions during operations.

Homatropine

This is a synthetic derivative closely allied to atropine in chemical structure. It has weaker antimuscarinic actions than atropine and its effect on the eye lasts for only hours instead of for days as with atropine.

Dibutoline

Dibutoline has some structural similarity to carbachol but has antimuscarinic properties. It is less potent than atropine and has ganglion blocking activity in high doses. It has a brief and rapid action and is therefore used for ophthalmic purposes.

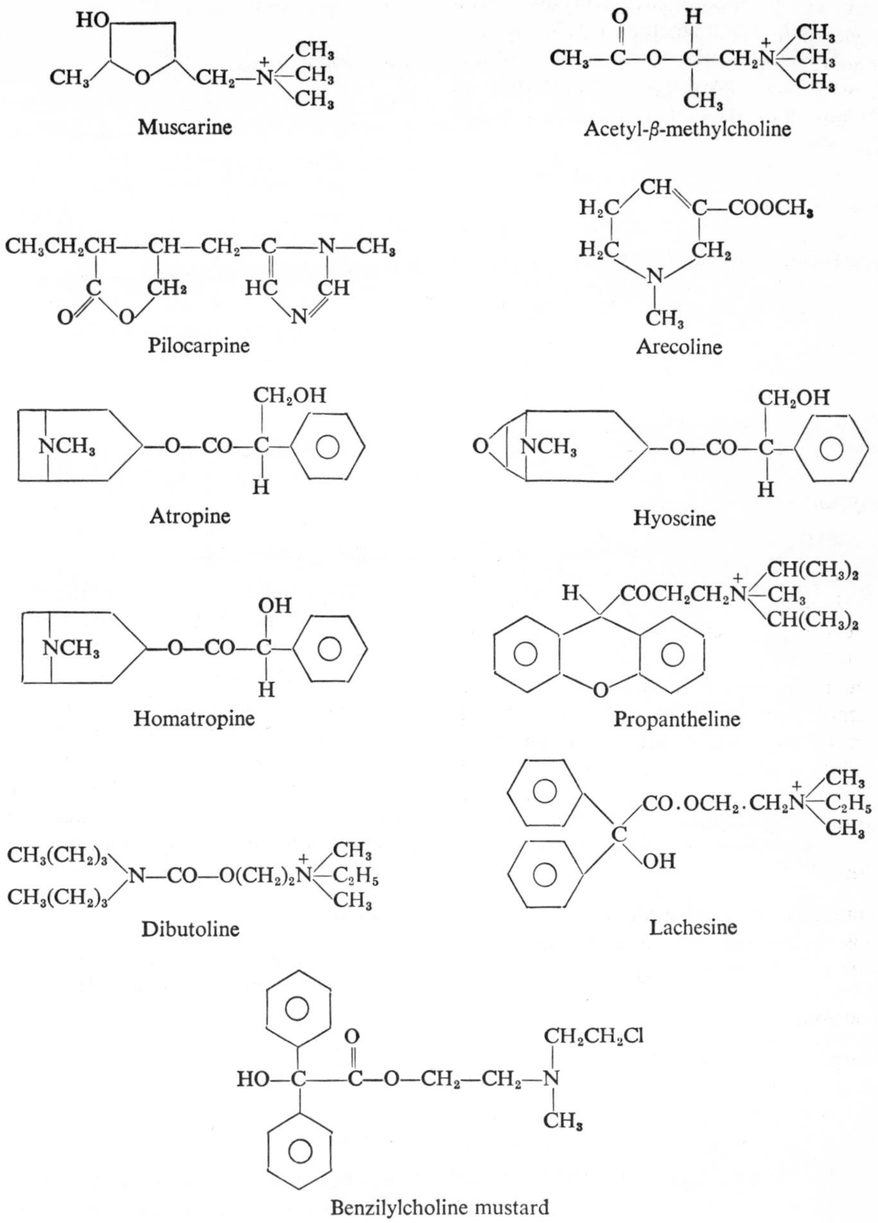

Muscarine

Acetyl-β-methylcholine

Pilocarpine

Arecoline

Atropine

Hyoscine

Homatropine

Propantheline

Dibutoline

Lachesine

Benzilylcholine mustard

Fig. 7.17. The structures of agonists and antagonists at muscarinic sites.

Lachesine

Lachesine has obvious structural similarities to acetylcholine but blocking activity is conferred by the presence of the bulky terminal ring structures. The drug is a mydriatic and antispasmodic. Its other pharmacological properties are similar to those of atropine except that, unlike atropine, it produces sedation.

Benzilylcholine mustard

In 1966 Gill and Rang, in Oxford, discovered an irreversible blocker of muscarinic receptors. It is a β-haloalkylamine which cyclizes in solution to give an ethyleneiminium derivative. It is a very specific and potent antagonist of muscarinic activity and has no blocking action at the neuromuscular junction or autonomic ganglion.

It produces an irreversible block in a similar way to dibenamine (p. 106) by alkylation of a receptor group with the formation of a very stable, covalent bond. It is found that the degree of irreversible muscarinic block is proportional to the concentration of ethyleneiminium ions present in solution.

Methantheline (*Banthine*)

This is a synthetic quaternary ammonium compound which has a wide clinical use. It differs from atropine in having relatively strong ganglion blocking activity compared to its antimuscarinic activity. The ganglion blocking activity may be apparent even in therapeutic doses.

Propantheline (*Pro-Banthine*)

This is a synthetic compound closely related to methantheline. It is about three times as active as methantheline as an antimuscarinic agent and its ganglion blocking activity is also greater. It was developed in an effort to produce a drug which would inhibit gastric motility and secretion without the undesired side-effects of atropine. Propantheline is used for this purpose either alone or with barbiturates in the treatment of peptic ulcers.

FURTHER READING

Birks, R. I. and Macintosh, F. C. (1961). Acetylcholine metabolism of a sympathetic ganglion, *Can. J. Biochem.* **39,** 787.

Bowman, W. (1962). Mechanisms of neuromuscular blockade, *Progr. Med. Chem.* **3,** 88.

Brown, G. L., Dale, H. H., and Feldberg, W. (1936). Reactions of the normal mammalian muscle to acetylcholine and eserine, *J. Physiol.* (*Lond.*) **87,** 394.

Burnstock, G. and Holman, M. (1966). Effect of drugs on smooth muscle, *Ann. Rev. Pharmacol.* **6,** 129.

Castillo, J. del and Katz, B. (1957). A study of curare action with an electrical micro-method, *Proc. R. Soc. B* **146,** 339.

Chang, H. C. and Gaddum, J. H. (1933). Choline esters in tissue extracts, *J. Physiol.* (*Lond.*) **79,** 255.

Collier, B. and Mitchell, J. F. (1967). The central release of acetylcholine during consciousness, and after brain lesions, *J. Physiol.* (*Lond.*) **188,** 83.

Curtis, D. R. (1966). Synaptic transmission in the central nervous system and its pharmacology, in *Nerve as a tissue*, ed. Rodahl, K., and Issakutz, B., New York.

DeFeudis, F. V. (1974). *Central cholinergic systems and behaviour.* Academic Press, London.

Dixon, W. E. (1907). On the mode of action of drugs, *Med. Mag.* (*Lond.*) **16,** 454.

Katz, B. (1967). *Nerve, muscle and synapse*, London.

Koelle, G. B. (ed.) (1963). Cholinesterase and anticholinesterase agents, *Handb. exp. Pharmak.* Suppl. 15, Berlin.

Krnjević, K. and Phillis, J. W. (1963). Pharmacological properties of acetylcholine-sensitive cells in the cerebral cortex, *J. Physiol.* (*Lond.*) **166,** 328.

McLennan, H. (1970). *Synaptic Transmission*, 2nd ed., Philadelphia.

Mitchell, J. F. (1963). The spontaneous evoked release of acetylcholine from the cerebral cortex, *J. Physiol.* (*Lond.*) **165,** 98.

Mitchell, J. F. (1966). Acetylcholine release from the brain, *Wenner-Gren International Symposium*, Stockholm.

Paton, W. D. M. (1959). The pharmacology of ganglion blocking agents, in *Hypertension*, ed. Moyer, J. H., Philadelphia.

Phillis, J. W. (1970). *The Pharmacology of Synapses*, Oxford.

8

ADRENERGIC SYSTEM

The peripheral sympathetic nervous system is derived from neurones arising in the lateral horns of the grey matter of the spinal cord. These neurones synapse mainly on ganglion cells located in the sympathetic chains which run on either side of the vertebrae, although some ganglion cells are also found in the autonomic nerves going to the peripheral structures innervated, and in some cases also in these tissues. The presynaptic nerves to the adrenal medulla synapse directly upon the medulla cells which are thus homologous to the postsynaptic neurone. The transmitter at these synapses is acetylcholine as it is in the entire cholinergic system. The postsynaptic neurone, on the other hand, contains catecholamines, which can be demonstrated by a brown colour produced by treatment with dichromate, and these cells are therefore called chromaffin cells. The presence of catecholamines can be more selectively demonstrated by a fluorescence technique in which the tissue is treated with formaldehyde vapour and the catecholamines converted to dihydroxydihydroisoquinolines which give a strong green fluorescence (Fig. 8.1). In the sympathetic neurones this is concentrated in granules collected in little varicosities along the length of the nerve, and it is particularly in these regions that the transmitter, which is noradrenaline (arterenol), is liberated when the nerve is stimulated.

Similar granules are present in very large numbers in the adrenal medulla cells and in this case the transmitter is mainly the *N*-methyl catecholamine adrenaline (epinephrine). These granules can be isolated by homogenizing the tissue and then separating the granule fraction by centrifuging in a sucrose gradient. The particles contain as much as 7 per cent catecholamine together with adenine nucleotides, proteins, and lipids. Present evidence suggests that the major part of the catecholamine in the nerve is present in these storage particles and that when catecholamines are liberated in response to nerve stimulation, the nucleotides and protein contained in the granule are liberated too. This suggests that liberation occurs as a result of fusion of the granule membrane with the cytomembrane, and discharge of the contents without their coming into contact with the cell cytoplasm. It is known that, as with acetylcholine transmitter release in response to nerve stimulation, release is dependent on the presence of calcium in the external medium, and it is believed that calcium entry into the nerve is responsible for the granule fusion and discharge.

The reserpine group of alkaloids have a selective action on storage of catecholamines in the granules, probably by increasing the permeability of the lipoprotein envelope of the granule. This causes release of the catecholamine into the neuronal cytoplasm where it is largely metabolized so that pharmacologically inactive degradation products are released into the extraneuronal space. The nerve may become almost wholly depleted of noradrenaline and hence unable to release transmitter on stimulation.

Noradrenaline is synthesized in the neurones from tyrosine which is first hydroxylated in the 3 position by tyrosine hydroxylase to give DOPA (dihydroxyphenylalanine; 3-hydroxytyrosine), which is then decarboxylated by DOPA decarboxylase to give dopamine (3-hydroxytyramine) and finally a β-hydroxyl group is introduced by dopamine β-oxidase to give noradrenaline (Fig. 8.2). The rate-limiting step in this biosynthetic sequence is the formation of DOPA. In the adrenal medulla a further step, *N*-methylation of noradrenaline to give adrenaline, occurs, catalysed by phenylethanolamine-*N*-methyl transferase. By injecting tyrosine or DOPA labelled with ^{14}C or tritium into an animal, the biosynthe-

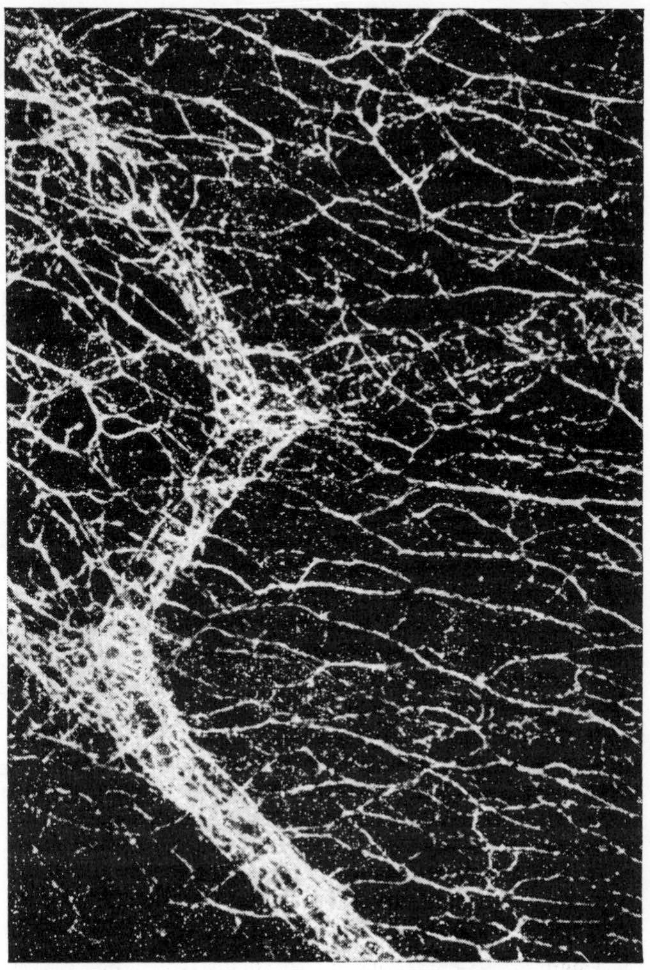

Fig. 8.1. Fluorescence micrograph of rat iris after treatment with formaldehyde. The sympathetic neurones appear as beaded structures with a green fluorescence. The dense mat of sympathetic neurones on the left of the picture surround an arteriole. (Malmfors, T. (1965) *Acta physiol. scand.* **64,** Suppl. 248.)

tic pathway can be studied *in vivo.* Because the conversion of tyrosine to DOPA is rate limiting, higher rates of biosynthesis can be achieved if DOPA is supplied, than with tyrosine.

There is some evidence that the level of free noradrenaline in the system is controlled by noradrenaline acting as a feedback controller of tyrosine hydroxylase. Inhibitors for several of these biosynthetic enzymes are known, for instance **α-methyltyrosine** and **3-iodotyrosine** are potent inhibitors of tyrosine hydroxylase and lead to a reduction of the noradrenaline content of the nerves. Inhibitors of DOPA decarboxylase such as **methyldopa** do not appear to reduce noradrenaline synthesis appreciably because the availability of DOPA dominates the rate of over-all biosynthesis. Dopamine-β-hydroxylase is inhibited by the copper chelater **disulfiram** leading to a relative accumulation of dopamine in the nerves. The enzymes in the biosynthetic pathway are not wholly specific and thus methyldopa is a substrate for dopadecarboxylase and leads to the formation of α-methyldopamine which is β-hydroxylated to α-methylnoradrenaline. This is stored in granules in the same way as

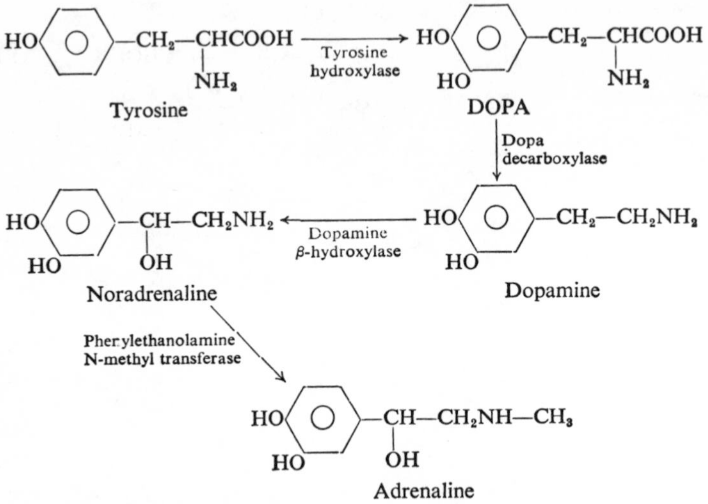

HO–C₆H₄–CH_2—CHCOOH(—NH_2) —Tyrosine hydroxylase→ HO(HO)–C₆H₃–CH_2—CHCOOH(—NH_2)

Tyrosine → DOPA

DOPA —Dopa decarboxylase→ Dopamine

HO(HO)–C₆H₃–CH_2—CH_2NH_2 (Dopamine) —Dopamine β-hydroxylase→ HO(HO)–C₆H₃–CH(OH)—CH_2NH_2 (Noradrenaline)

Noradrenaline —Phenylethanolamine N-methyl transferase→ HO(HO)–C₆H₃–CH(OH)—CH_2NH—CH_3

Adrenaline

Fig. 8.2. The biosynthesis of noradrenaline and adrenaline.

noradrenaline and replaces part of the noradrenaline, thus decreasing the content of the latter in the tissue. Similarly tyramine can be β-hydroxylated to **synephrine** (octopamine) which is also stored and replaces noradrenaline (Fig. 8.4).

Two major metabolic pathways exist for the degradation of catecholamines. These are the 3-*O*-methylation by the enzyme catechol-*O*-methyl transferase (COMT) which leads to the formation of **normetanephrine** and **metanephrine**. This enzyme appears to be localized exclusively outside the neurone but in close proximity, and is

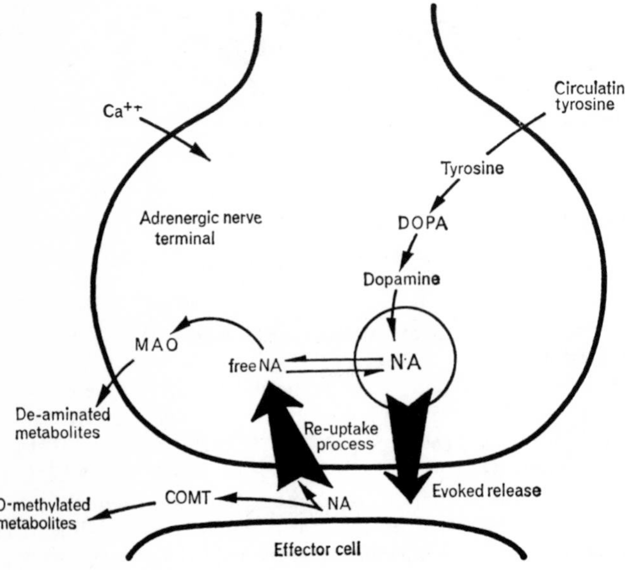

Fig. 8.3. Processes concerned in the synthesis, storage, release, and metabolism of noradrenaline (NA) in sympathetic nerves. MAO, mono-amine oxidase; COMT, catechol-*O*-methyl transferase.

Fig. 8.4. Formation of modified transmitters that can be stored in sympathetic nerves.

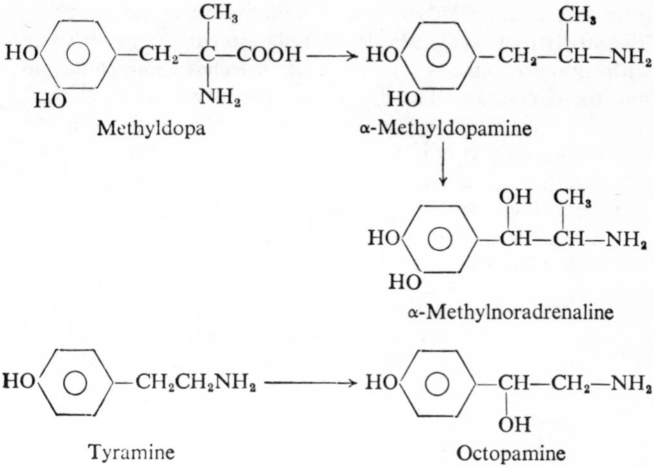

also found in large amounts in the liver and kidneys. The enzyme may be inhibited by the competitive substrates pyrogallol, tropolone, and dopacetamide, none of which is very potent. The second pathway for metabolism is by oxidative deamination by the enzyme monoamine oxidase (MAO) which is found in large amounts in the mitochondria of the sympathetic neurones as well as in the liver, intestine, and elsewhere (Fig. 8.3). Inside the cell noradrenaline is protected from MAO by segregation in the granules and probably also by other intracytoplasmic membranes. A large number of powerful inhibitors of MAO are known, the most important of which are the hydrazines (e.g. phenelzine). Because of the operation of these two enzymes the main metabolites of catecholamines excreted in the urine are 3-methoxy-4-hydroxy mandelic acid and 3,4-dihydroxymandelic acid (Fig. 8.5).

The metabolic pathways are *not* the major

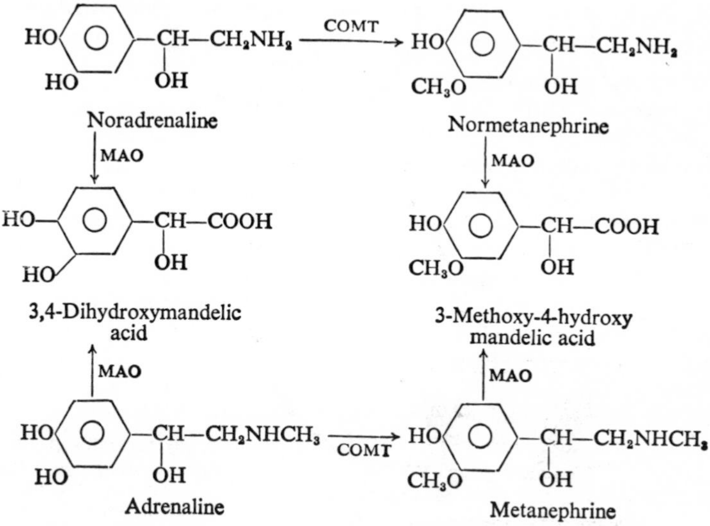

Fig. 8.5. The metabolic fate of noradrenaline and adrenaline.

processes dealing either with noradrenaline liberated from sympathetic stimulation or with noradrenaline or adrenaline injected into the circulation. The dominant process is uptake of catecholamine into the sympathetic endings which occurs in two stages: (1) active transfer through the cytomembrane; and (2) storage in the catecholamine granules.

This conclusion has been reached from the following observations:

1. If tritium-labelled noradrenaline is injected intravenously the major portion can be recovered from the tissues as unchanged noradrenaline and a minor part as metabolites.
2. Inhibitors of MAO and COMT *do not* significantly potentiate the actions of injected noradrenaline or of sympathetic stimulation.
3. The uptake process may be inhibited by **cocaine, desipramine,** and **phenoxybenzamine,** and the use of these drugs increases and prolongs the response to sympathetic nerve stimulation and to injected noradrenaline, and also increases the amount of noradrenaline that can be collected in perfused preparations. Present evidence suggests that 80–90 per cent of the noradrenaline released by nerve stimulation is reaccumulated in the nerve terminals.

This behaviour of the sympathetic transmitter contrasts with the parasympathetic transmitter acetylcholine which is wholly destroyed by hydrolysis by cholinesterase.

The re-uptake mechanism is not very specific and can take up related amines; one of the most interesting of these is 6-hydroxydopamine (3,4,6-trihydroxyphenylethylamine) which is highly toxic to the neurone and causes degeneration. Within a few days the sympathetic nerve endings disappear and with them the tissue noradrenaline. After intraventricular injection 6-hydroxydopamine causes degeneration of most of the noradrenergic nerves in the brain.

Noradrenaline may be released from sympathetic nerves in yet another way. This is by the action of certain sympathomimetic amines such as **tyramine.** When tyramine is injected into an animal it produces effects very much like noradrenaline except that the effects are slightly delayed and more long-lasting and also much larger doses are required.

Certain differences are found on more detailed examination:

1. The effects of repeated does gradually become less (tachyphylaxis); this does not happen with noradrenaline.
2. The effects are greatly diminished by section of the sympathetic nerves and subsequent degeneration. The effects of noradrenaline, on the other hand, are increased due to denervation hypersensitivity.
3. The effects are also diminished by pretreatment with doses of reserpine sufficient to deplete the nerves of noradrenaline.
4. The effects of tyramine are also diminished by uptake inhibitors (e.g. cocaine) which, at the same time, potentiate noradrenaline.
5. Successive doses of tyramine cause a progressive depletion of the noradrenaline content of the nerves.
6. In perfused organs noradrenaline can be detected in the perfusate following injection of tyramine.

This evidence is conclusive in showing that the major action of tyramine is to cause release of noradrenaline from the nerves as noradrenaline and not as metabolites (cf. reserpine) and that it is the released noradrenaline that produces the pharmacological effects. It is not certain how the release occurs. There is evidence favouring a displacement of noradrenaline from storage granules with protection from the action of MAO by substrate competition, but also some evidence suggestive of activation of the nerve membrane in a manner comparable to that produced by physiological nerve stimulation. This action is important and sympathomimetic drugs may be divided into *direct acting*, i.e. having actions like noradrenaline, *indirect acting* i.e. acting through release of noradrenaline, and *mixed acting*, i.e. in which both direct and indirect actions are playing a part.

Finally there is a group of drugs that interferes with the release of noradrenaline from sympathetic nerve terminals (Fig. 8.6). This action was originally found quite unexpectedly in **xylocholine** which produced a selective blockade of the effects of stimulating postganglionic sympathetic nerves without affecting the response to noradrenaline or adrenaline. Xylocholine has some nicotinic actions as might be expected from its structure, but these are absent from β-methylxylocholine. Subsequently high activity was found in other quaternary ammonium compounds of which **bretylium** is the most active. Bretylium does not deplete the sympathetic neurones of noradrenaline but is itself highly concentrated in these neurones. Since bretylium and related substances are local anaesthetics it has been suggested that they block conduction in the sympathetic nerve filaments, and are selective owing to the specially high concentration in these nerves. Direct evidence that they block conduction is absent. **Guanethidine** also blocks release of noradrenaline in a similar way to bretylium, but in addition causes depletion of the noradrenaline content. Bethanidine and debrisoquine are related guanidine derivatives.

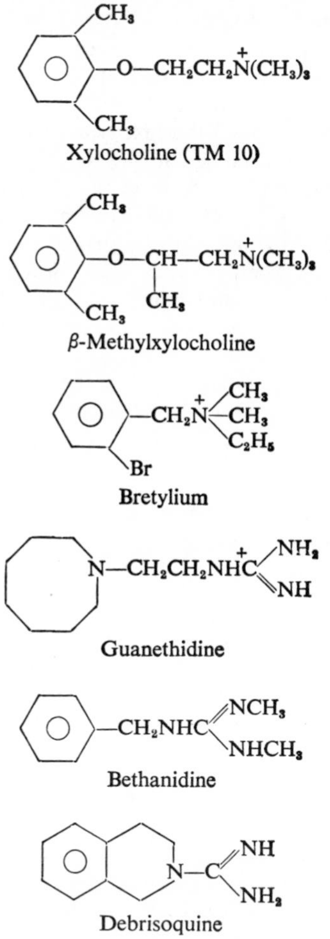

Xylocholine (TM 10)

β-Methylxylocholine

Bretylium

Guanethidine

Bethanidine

Debrisoquine

Fig. 8.6. The structures of drugs which interfere with the release of noradrenaline.

The adrenergic neurone blocking drugs do not enter or affect the central nervous system but the compound 6-hydroxydopamine is taken up by adrenergic nerve terminals where it will produce permanent degeneration and loss of catecholamines. It acts on both noradrenergic and dopaminergic structures in the central nervous system providing it is introduced directly into the brain or cerebrospinal fluid. This compound therefore produces complete and permanent chemical denervation and is proving a useful tool in the study of catecholamine pathways.

Burn and Rand have produced a large amount of evidence suggesting that noradrenaline is not directly released by the nerve impulse but that acetylcholine release is the primary event and that this leads secondarily to noradrenaline release. This is referred to as a 'cholinergic link'. Most pharmacologists are unwilling to accept this thesis while admitting that most sympathetic nerves are mixed (i.e. contain cholinergic as well as the predominant adrenergic fibres) and that release of acetylcholine may alter the amount of noradrenaline released.

A substance stimulating the growth of sympathetic neurones has been found in tumours, snake venom, and mouse salivary glands by Levi-Montalcini and her collaborators. It is a protein which, if given to young animals, leads to overgrowth of certain parts of the sympathetic nervous system specifically. It has little or no effect on the adrenal medulla. Antisera against the nerve growth factor can be prepared and, when injected into young animals, cause a selective loss of sympathetic neurones, for instance, in the rat the heart can lose up to 95 per cent of its noradrenaline content.

THE EFFECTS OF SYMPATHETIC NERVE STIMULATION AND OF NORADRENALINE AND ADRENALINE

When sympathetic nerves are stimulated they cause increase of tone in some varieties of smooth muscle and relaxation in others, as well as increasing the rate and force of the heart and stimulation of the secretion of some glands (Table 8.1) and also effects on carbohydrate and lipid metabolism.

Qualitatively similar effects are produced by noradrenaline and adrenaline. However, the intensity of the effects produced by these two drugs is not similar, the inhibitory cardiac, and metabolic effects being greater with adrenaline. Since the chemical difference between adrenaline and noradrenaline is the presence of the *N*-methyl group in adrenaline, it is interesting that if this group is made larger as in *N*-ethyl noradrenaline or isoprenaline (*N*-isopropyl noradrenaline, isoproterenol) these latter effects are further intensified and the excitor effects on smooth muscle become very weak. The different order of potency, i.e. **noradrenaline** $<$ **adrenaline** $\gg$ **isoprenaline** for the excitor actions, and **noradrenaline** $<$ **adrenaline** $\ll$ **isoprenaline** for the inhibitory, cardiac, and metabolic actions is most easily explained if these are mediated by two distinct receptors—this was first pointed out by Ahlquist who named the first type of receptor α and the second β. Strong support for this hypothesis has come from the discovery that antagonists of the catecholamines have a selective action on these two classes of response. The older established antagonists ergotamine, phentolamine, and phenoxybenzamine are selective α-blockers totally without effects on the β-responses. On the other hand, propranolol, iproveratrine, and dichloroisoprenaline block β-responses and have no effect on α-action. It is interesting to note

Table 8.1. Distribution of adrenergic receptors

Organ	Effects	Receptor type
Heart	Increased heart rate, contractibility, and excitability	β
Coronary arteries	Decreased blood flow	α
	Increased blood flow	β (predominant)
Skeletal muscle arterioles	Increased blood flow	β
Skin arterioles	Decreased blood flow	mainly β
Spleen	Contraction	α
Iris (radial muscle)	Pupil dilated	α
Smooth muscle of gut	Relaxed rhythmic activity inhibited	β
Bladder	Sphincter contracted	α
	Detrusor relaxed	β
Salivary glands	Secretion	α
Metabolism (liver, fat, heart)	Increased	β

that whereas all the β-blockers so far described are closely related in structure to isoprenaline, the α-blockers bear a less obvious chemical resemblance to the catecholamines. Although the β-actions of noradrenaline are weaker than those of adrenaline it appears that the effects of sympathetic neurones terminating on β-receptor areas are due to the liberation of **noradrenaline;** this is the case for the heart, liver, and intestine to mention just a few areas.

BIOPHYSICAL AND BIOCHEMICAL ACTIONS OF CATECHOLAMINES

On smooth muscle where α-excitation occurs, sympathetic stimulation causes depolarizing junction potentials which, if they are suprathreshold, lead to propagating action potentials. Applied catecholamines similarly lead to depolarization. This is probably produced by an increase in sodium permeability. In the heart, on the other hand, there is little change in either resting or action potential to account for the large positive inotropic action. Under rather abnormal conditions (i.e. raised Mg concentration) catecholamines will increase the magnitude and duration of the action potential probably by increasing entry of both sodium and calcium. In nodal tissues the action of the sympathetic is clearer, depolarizing junctional potentials are produced together with a greater rate of diastolic drift in the resting potential and these are responsible for increasing the rate of impulse discharge. Again the effects are probably mediated by an increase in sodium permeability. Undoubtedly the main part of the positive inotropic effect in the ventricles is unaccounted for by obvious ionic changes and much interest has recently been centred on biochemical changes.

The starting-point of this new approach was the discovery that the amount of the cyclic nucleotide, 3′,5′-adenosine monophosphate (cyclic AMP) in the heart was markedly increased when the heart was stimulated by catecholamines. Further study has shown that this is due to an activation of the enzyme adenylcyclase that forms cyclic AMP from ATP. It was also found that cyclic AMP is destroyed by an intracellular phosphodiesterase which can be inhibited by theophylline; this can also raise the level of cyclic AMP. Since theophylline produces inotropic effects in the heart very similar to those of catecholamines it is interesting that both effects are mediated by a rise in cyclic

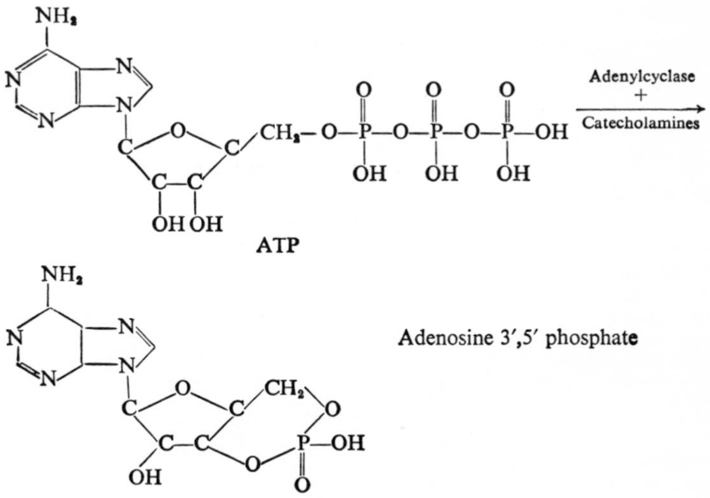

ATP

Adenylcyclase + Catecholamines

Adenosine 3′,5′ phosphate

Fig. 8.7. Cyclic AMP.

AMP. Subsequently it was found that adenylcyclase and cyclic AMP are involved in a very wide range of hormone actions, including the lipolytic effects of adrenaline and insulin on fat cells, the action of corticotrophin on the adrenal cortex, the action of catecholamines on cerebellar neurones, the action of parathormone on the kidney, and most interesting, on gene expression in bacteria. It is also the hormone causing colony formation in the free swimming forms of the cellular slime moulds. In nearly every case the action of the initiating hormone can be mimicked in whole or in part by addition of cyclic AMP itself or its more stable, lipid-soluble derivative, dibutyryl cyclic AMP.

The actions of cyclic AMP appear to be due to a general action in which proteins are phosphorylated by the cyclic AMP and thereby change their activity. This class of enzyme is generally referred to as a protein kinase and is responsible for various reactions involving phosphorylation. A well-known example is phosphorylase which catalyses the equilibrium between glycogen and phosphate on the one hand and glucose 1-phosphate on the other. As mentioned earlier theophylline, by inhibiting phosphodiesterase, potentiates actions involving cyclic AMP; other xanthines such as caffeine and 8-chlorotheophylline are also active.

THE ACTION OF SYMPATHOMIMETIC SUBSTANCES

The action of sympathomimetic substances (Fig. 8.8) depends on their relative activity on α- and β-receptors, the proportion of direct and indirect action, as well as on their metabolic handling.

Noradrenaline

Noradrenaline is more active on α-receptors than on β-receptors, but is by no means devoid of β-action. It is rapidly taken up by sympathetic neurones, is a good substrate for COMT but not a particularly good substrate for MAO. Noradrenaline is practically inert when given by mouth because of extensive metabolism in the gut wall and liver.

Adrenaline

Adrenaline is more active on β-receptors than on α-receptors, is less well taken up by neurones and in consequence a higher proportion is metabolized. As with noradrenaline, absorption from the gut is slight.

Isoprenaline

Isoprenaline has a very powerful β-action but is almost devoid of α-actions. Its duration of action is greater than either of the preceding due to its failure to be taken up by

(Ring positions 2–6)—CH—CH—NH

	2	3	4	5	β	α	N
Phenylethylamine	H	H	H	H	H	H	H
Noradrenaline	H	OH	OH	H	OH	H	H
Adrenaline	H	OH	OH	H	OH	H	CH_3
Isoprenaline	H	OH	OH	H	OH	H	$CH(CH_3)_2$
Methoxamine	OCH_3	H	H	OCH_3	OH	CH_3	H
Methoxyphenamine	OCH_3	H	H	H	H	CH_3	CH_3
Isoxsuprine	H	H	OH	H	OH	CH_3	$CH(CH_3)CH_2O\langle\bigcirc\rangle$
Tyramine	H	H	OH	H	H	H	H
Octopamine	H	H	OH	H	OH	H	H
Metaraminol	H	OH	H	H	OH	CH_3	H
Ephedrine	H	H	H	H	OH	CH_3	CH_3
Amphetamine	H	H	H	H	H	CH_3	H
Methamphetamine	H	H	H	H	H	CH_3	CH_3
Salbutamol	H	CH_2OH	OH	H	H	H	$C(CH_3)$

Fig. 8.8. Sympathomimetic amines.

neurones and its resistance to MAO. It is active by mouth when given in large doses as is sometimes done in treating Stokes–Adams attacks (intermittent heart block), although it is more usually given by the sublingual route by which absorption is more rapid and complete.

Salbutamol

Sulbutamol differs from isoprenaline mainly in having a hydroxymethyl group in the 3-position in place of a hydroxy group; this weakens the action on the heart without affecting the bronchodilator action. Salbutamol may thus be used in asthma with a lower risk of cardiac side-effects. The selective effects of salbutamol and of some β-blockers have led to a subdivision of β-receptors into β_1 receptors on the heart and β_2 receptors on smooth muscle. The hydroxymethyl group also renders salbutamol insensitive to COMT and this gives it a longer duration of action than isoprenaline. Soterenol has a similar pharmacology.

Methoxamine

Methoxamine has nearly pure α-actions, though it has some weak β-blocking action. Being already *O*-methylated it cannot be inactivated by COMT and like other substances derived from isopropylamine and other secondary amines is not attacked by MAO. For these reasons it has a long duration of action. The chemically related **methoxyphenamine** and **isoxsuprine** are selective β-stimulators.

Tyramine

Tyramine is the archetypic indirectly acting amine. It is low in activity in part because tyramine is an excellent substrate for MAO. Tyramine is found in many foods (notably in mature cheese, broad beans, yeast extract, yoghurt, and wine) but is destroyed by MAO in the gut and liver. However, when MAO inhibitors are administered the tyramine reaches the systemic circulation and causes noradrenaline release which may result in dangerous hypertension and cerebral oedema or haemorrhage. In the presence of MAO inhibitors tyramine is also protected from the intracellular attack of MAO in sympathetic neurones and the preserved tyramine is partially converted to octopamine by dopamine β-oxidase and this leads to partial replacement of noradrenaline by octopamine in the granules.

Metaraminol

Metaraminol is a highly active mixed sympathomimetic agent—it has a strong direct action and is also a noradrenaline releaser. It is taken up and stored in the granules. It is not a substrate for either COMT or MAO and has a long duration of action.

Ephedrine

Ephedrine acts almost wholly indirectly and, as expected from such an action, shows rather a rapid development of tolerance. Because of its resistance to MAO it is active by mouth and is still much used as an orally acting bronchodilator in asthma. Its main disadvantage is a pronounced central action leading to jitteriness and wakefulness.

Amphetamine and methamphetamine

Amphetamine and methamphetamine have mainly central actions which have a complicated basis. They are directly sympathomimetic, are releasers of noradrenaline and inhibitors of uptake, and are also inhibitors of MAO. Their central actions are discussed in Chapter 5.

These drugs are also used to reduce appetite and hence food intake in the treatment of obesity.

α-BLOCKERS
(Fig. 8.9)

Ergot alkaloids

These compounds are dealt with in detail in Chapter 10. They are rarely used as pharmacological tools because the strong direct stimulation of smooth muscle complicates their actions. These actions are reduced in the dihydrogenated alkaloids.

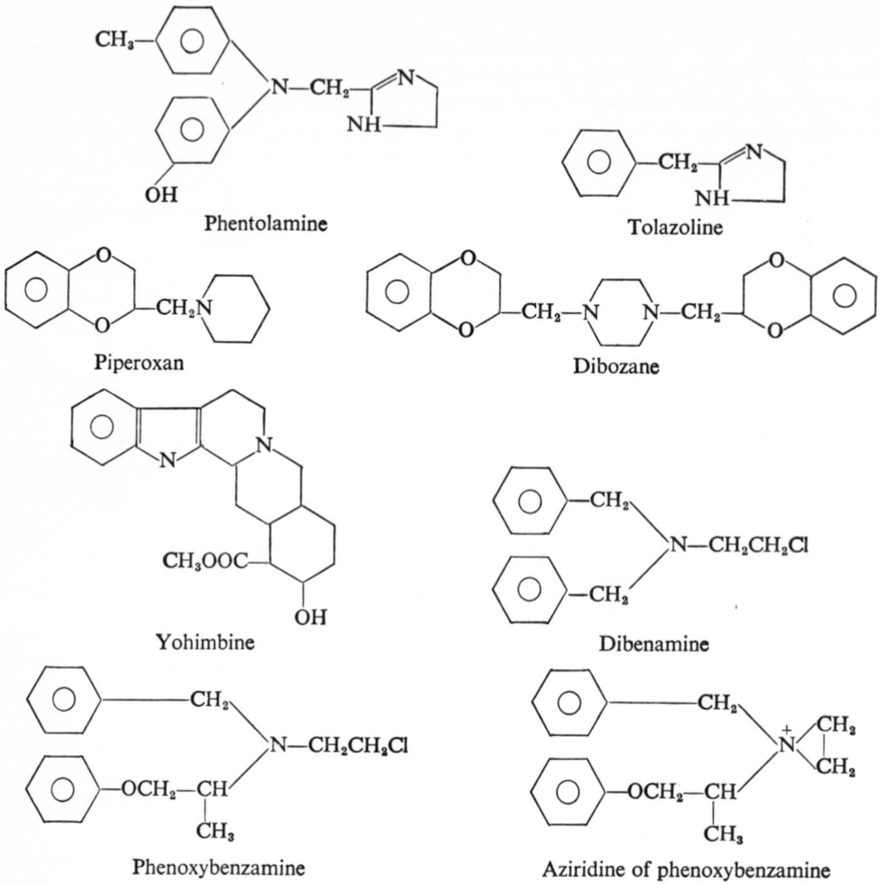

Phentolamine

Tolazoline

Piperoxan

Dibozane

Yohimbine

Dibenamine

Phenoxybenzamine

Aziridine of phenoxybenzamine

Fig. 8.9. α-blocking drugs.

Phentolamine and tolazoline

Phentolamine and tolazoline are substituted imidazolines which are highly selective α-blockers but which also are directly depressant on smooth muscle. They also have some direct sympathomimetic action on the heart Their action is transient and they are used in the diagnosis and treatment of phaeochromocytoma, a tumour of adrenal medullary cells which secretes noradrenaline and adrenaline often in a paroxysmal fashion.

Piperoxan and dibozane

These are α-blockers in addition to having direct actions on smooth and cardiac muscle. Toxic effects have made them unsatisfactory for therapeutic use. **Azapetine** is a dibenzazepine with actions rather similar to tolazoline.

Yohimbine

Yohimbine is related to both ergot and reserpine and is another α-blocker with relatively pure action.

Haloalkylamines

The first of these compounds to be studied was **dibenamine.** This produces a very prolonged block of α-receptors which takes days to recover. The effects develop slowly due to the necessity of forming the intermediate aziridine (ethyleneiminium) which occurs as in the nitrogen mustards (p. 225) by elimination of halogen. The three-membered ring is strained (i.e. bond angles are abnormal so that orbital overlap is imperfect and hence the bonds are weakened) and acts as an alkylator which reacts covalently with some group in the α-receptor. Selectivity is presumably achieved by preliminary non-covalent complex formation determined by the fit of the molecule for the receptor. Recovery from block is dependent on the rate of hydrolysis of the ester bond formed with the group in the receptor.

Phenoxybenzamine

Phenoxybenzamine is both more potent than dibenamine and more selective and has supplanted it in use. Both agents are able to block histamine receptors and muscarinic receptors in higher doses as well as probably having direct actions on cell membranes. Phenoxybenzamine is a very potent irreversible blocker of noradrenaline uptake into neurones and therefore has the property of potentiating β-actions of noradrenaline and of sympathetic stimulation.

The main clinical use of phenoxybenzamine is in controlling hypertensive episodes due to phaeochromocytoma as a preliminary to operation. It has a limited use in traumatic shock as it reduces visceral vasoconstriction provided that perfusion rates are maintained by adequate plasma expansion.

β-BLOCKERS

A study of the order of potency of a series of sympathomimetic amines on different test objects revealed marked differences between adrenaline, noradrenaline, and isoprenaline. This suggested the existence of more than one type of adrenoceptor and initially two types were distinguished known as α and β. It was then discovered that dichloroisoprenaline (DCI) selectively blocked the types of responses classified as β but this compound was a partial agonist, first stimulating and then blocking the receptors. Pronethalol, on the other hand, is free of stimulant action and is more potent as a β-receptor blocker.

Using the relative potencies of agonists on different test systems and and the effects of antagonists it became clear that, while the α-receptor formed a relatively homogeneous population, the β-receptors did not. A subclassification for β-receptors has now been developed based on the effectiveness of agonist compounds in eliciting various types of β responses. Two main types of β-responses can be elicited; one includes cardiac stimulation and lipolysis and receptors mediating these effects are known as β_1. Relaxation of the smooth muscle of blood vessels and bronchi and glycogenolysis are mediated via β_2-receptors. Selective blockers have been developed for β_1- and β_2-receptors and they can be regarded as derivatives of isoprenaline in which modifications have been made to the aromatic part of the molecule.

The β-blockers have found important roles in medicine and these are described for the particular drugs.

Propranolol (inderal)

Propranolol replaced pronethalol as a β blocker since the latter, although a pure antagonist, had pronounced central nervous side-effects and produced thymic tumours in mice. Propranolol has a prolonged competitive blocking action and has been widely used to treat angina pectoris by blocking the effects of the increased sympathic drive in exercise, so minimizing the increase in cardiac work and hence allowing greater exercise before pain develops. However, if the heart is in occult failure and the cardiac output is being maintained by sympathetic drive β-blockers may precipitate overt failure and, in a corresponding way, they may exacerbate bronchoconstriction in asthmatic patients. β-blockers are potent antiarrhythmics; this is partially due to blocking the excitatory

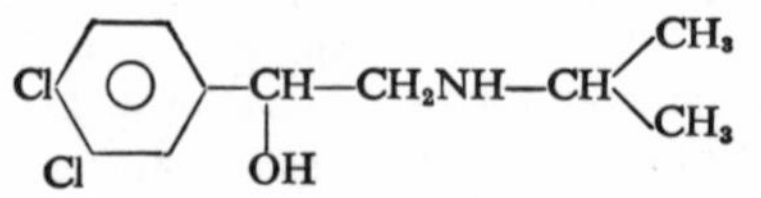

Dichloroisoprenaline (DCI)

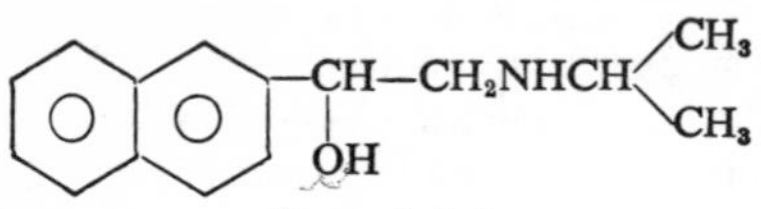

Pronethalol

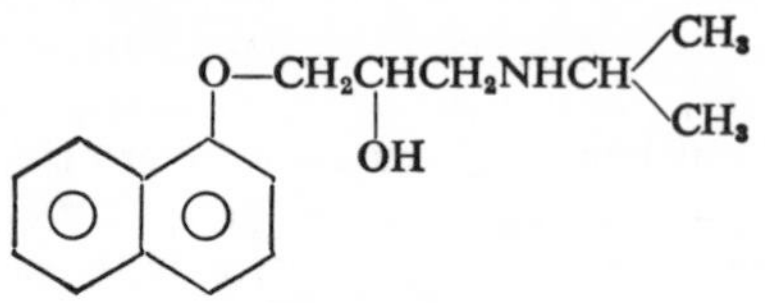

Propranolol

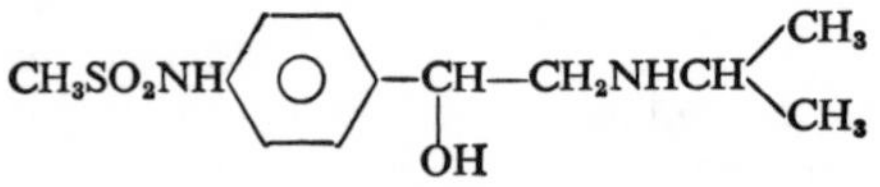

Sotalol

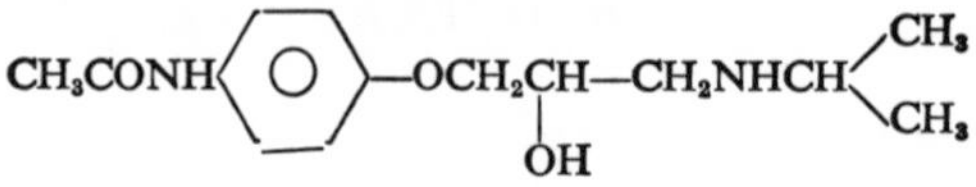

Practolol

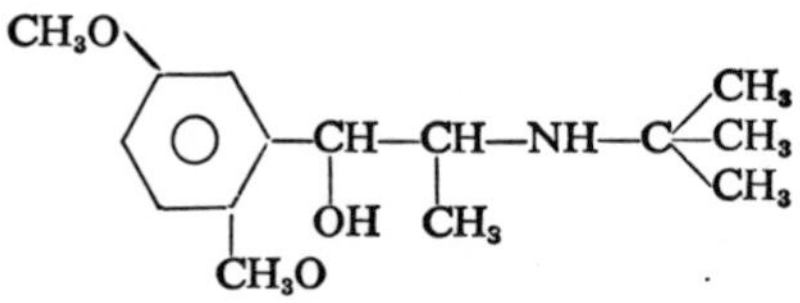

Butoxamine

Fig. 8.10. β-blocking drugs.

effects of catecholamines, but also to an anti-arrythmic activity which is analogous to that of quinidine and lignocaine.

One of the most unexpected actions of β-blockers is that they suppress the symptoms of hyperthyroidism in a considerable proportion of patients and are especially useful in thyrotoxic crises. This is interesting because so many of these symptoms are mimicked by administration of adrenaline. β-Blockers are also of considerable value in combating the effects of excessive catecholamine release from adrenal medullary tumours (phaeochromocytoma).

Oxprenolol, alprenolol, sotalol, and pindolol are other β-receptor blockers which affect both β_1- and β_2-receptors.

Practolol (eraldin)

Practolol, unlike propranolol, has some degree of specificity for β_1-receptors on the heart and has a reduced action at β_2-receptors in smooth muscle, and is therefore less likely to cause bronchoconstriction. It binds strongly to plasma proteins and has a prolonged action, but adverse responses including skin and ocular reactions have limited its use. Tolamolol and acebutalol are also drugs with a cardioselective action.

Butoxamine

Butoxamine has little blocking action on the classical β-response to adrenaline but is effective in preventing increases in blood glucose and free fatty acids following the administration of adrenaline.

DRUGS AFFECTING NORADRENALINE RELEASE

Guanethidine

Guanethidine blocks sympathetic transmission both by depleting the noradrenaline content and by interfering with neurally evoked release. This process does not discriminate between nerve endings in α and β receptive sites. With the usual doses administered therapeutically block develops slowly over several days and also passes off slowly when administration is stopped. Hypersensitivity to noradrenaline develops as it does after surgical denervation. Guanethidine is used almost exclusively as a hypotensive. The major side-effects are diarrhoea, tremors, weakness, mental depression, parotid pain, nasal stuffiness, and failure of ejaculation. **Bethanidine** acts more rapidly and has a shorter duration so that adjustment of dosage is simpler; diarrhoea is also less common. **Guanoxan** and **guanochlor** are related compounds.

Reserpine

Reserpine is a central sedative, acting probably by depleting serotonin and noradrenaline from central neurones; it also depletes peripheral neurones. Effects develop slowly unless very large doses are given. Effects wear off over several days. It has been used both in hypertension and in treating psychoses, but is liable to produce severe depression which may lead to suicide.

Methyldopa

Methyldopa also blocks sympathetic neurones as referred to above, but the mechanism of action is still uncertain. It is likely that its major action is to replace noradrenaline by **α-methylnoradrenaline** (nordefrin) which is less active on the receptors. It has a number of important, unwanted actions, of which weakness and headache are common, as is the development of hypersensitivity.

The action of MAO inhibitors is considered in Chapter 5.

INHIBITORS OF NORADRENALINE UPTAKE

Noradrenaline uptake is inhibited by **cocaine** but not other local anaesthetics, by **phenoxybenzamine,** and by the antidepressants of the tricyclic group (p. 58) including **imipramine, desipramine amitriptyline,** and **nortriptyline.**

FURTHER READING

Acheson, G. H. (1965). Second catecholamine symposium, *Pharmacol. Rev.* **18,** 1.

Anden, N. E., Carlsson, A., and Häggendal, J. (1969). Adrenergic mechanisms, *Ann. Rev. Pharmacol.* **9,** 119.

Boura, A. L. A. and Green, A. F. (1965). Adrenergic neurone blocking agents, *Ann. Rev. Pharmacol.* **5,** 183.

Iversen, L. L. (1967). *The uptake and storage of noradrenaline in sympathetic nerves,* Cambridge.

Iversen, L. L. (ed.) (1973). Catecholamines. *Br. Med. Bull.* **29,** 130.

Moran, N. C. (1967). New adrenergic blocking drugs: their pharmacological, biochemical and clinical actions, *Ann. N. Y. Acad. Sci.* **139,** 541.

Vane, J. R. (1960). *Adrenergic mechanisms,* London.

9

PEPTIDES, HISTAMINE, AND PROSTAGLANDINS

PHARMACOLOGICALLY ACTIVE PEPTIDES

Drug receptors are mostly proteins and the great variety of drug receptor sites is due to the enormous potential of proteins for generating topologically distinct sites—this is due both to the size of the structures so that the groups comprising the site can be arranged in three dimensions, and also to the diverse nature of the amino acids which enable them to contribute basic groups (histidine, lysine, arginine, terminal amino), acidic groups (glutamate, aspartate, terminal carboxyl), hydrophilic groups (serine, threonine, glutamine, asparagine), hydrophobic groups (leucine, valine, phenylalanine, tryptophane, etc.), and sulphydryls into the site. Very similar merits of diversity of action and potential specificity apply to proteins and peptides as drugs, and indeed just as the native folded state of a protein is due to interaction of parts of the peptide sequence, we would expect that exogenous peptides might well interact with a suitable protein in a similar manner. Furthermore, just as the folding of the peptide chain in a protein is determined solely by the sequence of amino acids, so the interaction of a pharmacologically active peptide would be expected to follow the same rule. Indeed, the 'shape' of a peptide drug is not fixed since peptides are very flexible molecules. Presumably, when the peptide is fixed to its receptor it will have a well-defined shape, but we do not know what this shape is for any active peptide at the present time. Because the length and sequence of a peptide is the only way of characterizing peptide drugs, this has not yet attained the familiarity with which, after a little experience in chemistry, one can pick out the salient features of, say, a steroid or a penicillin.

Knowledge about peptides as drugs has developed rather slowly since the first peptide hormone, secretin, was discovered in 1902 and insulin extracted in 1923. Indeed it was not until 1953 that the structure and synthesis of a peptide hormone, oxytocin, was reported by du Vigneaud. The reasons for the delay were that the chemistry of peptides and proteins was not sufficiently advanced, nor were methods for extraction, purification, and characterization. As the technology has advanced so an increasing number of biologically active peptides have been characterized and synthesized until at least one major new type of compound is being discovered each year. Although synthesis remains a rather difficult and costly business for any except rather short peptides, this has now developed sufficiently that the beginning of structure–activity relationships are appearing for a few peptides so that genuine drugs as opposed to hormones are appearing.

Oxytocin and vasopressin

These are two closely related nonapeptides isolated from the pituitary and hypothalamus. They both have actions on smooth muscle and an antidiuretic action of different intensity. Vasopressin contracts vascular smooth muscle and raises the blood pressure, but in excessive dose the pressure falls because constriction of the coronary vessels is produced which leads to anoxic hypodynamism of the myocardium. Vasopressin produces a marked antidiuresis in doses much less than those needed to produce a pressor effect. The mechanism of action on the kidney is still a matter of debate; it appears most likely that it is due to a control of water permeability, possibly involving an intermediate cyclic nucleotide.

When the secretion of vasopressin (ADH) fails because of lesions in the hypothalmus or pituitary, the urine flow becomes very large, the condition being called diabetes insipidus. This condition can be controlled by administration of ADH. It has recently been found that a synthetic analogue, DDAVP (1-desamino-8-D-arginine vasopressin) is much more effective, lasts longer, and has few side-effects, so that a single dose per day administered by intranasal aerosol will control the disease.

Both vasopressin and oxytocin will contract the non-pregnant uterus. Sensitivity of the immature uterus is low and can be markedly increased by prior treatment with oestrogen. During pregnancy the sensitivity of the uterus to oxytocin increases very much, especially as parturition approaches. Small doses of oxytocin will initiate contraction or increase the force and frequency of a pre-existing rhythm. In larger doses it causes a sustained increase in tone.

Oxytocin may be used to initiate labour, to stimulate a flagging uterus in the second stage when the cervix is well dilated, and also in the third stage to cause expulsion of the placenta and contraction down of the uterus to control post-partum bleeding.

For these purposes, oxytocin is frequently administered by a continuous intravenous infusion. It also contracts the smooth muscle in the trabeculae of the mammary gland and can cause milk expulsion; this is important in many domestic animals and is known as milk let down.

The structure of oxytocin and arginine vasopressin are shown in Table 9.1 and Fig. 9.1. They are both cyclic nonapeptides and differ only in the amino acids in position 2 and position 8. In oxytocin these are Ile and Leu respectively, whereas in arginine vasopressin these are the Phe and Arg. The selectivity of action on the uterus and in blood vessels (and kidney) can be seen. The vasopressin from the pig has lysine at position 8 (LVP) and it is not very different in its pattern of activity from AVP. In birds and amphibia a single peptide called vasotocin which combines oxytocic and pressor activity is found in the hypothalmus—it has Ile^2 and Arg^8 and so is structurally a compromise between oxytocin and AVP. The difference in the structural requirements for these two actions thus seems to be that if the hydrophobic group at 2 is large and there is a hydrophilic group at 8 pressor activity is favoured.

Both oxytocin and AVP have only a brief half-life in the plasma due to the action of peptidases which remove the terminal glycinamide residue, producing a virtually inactive material. This peptidase activity is greatly increased in the latter part of pregnancy. They are also destroyed by the proteolytic enzymes in the gut and are thus not active when given by mouth. Because of the short biological half-life oxytocin and LVP have a very short duration of action when given intravenously. The duration is greater when they are given subcutaneously, and can

Table 9.1. Oxytocin and Vasopressin

	1	2	3	4	5	6	7	8	9		*Uterus*	*Pressor*
Oxytocin	Cys	Tyr	*Ile*	Glu	Asn	Cys	Pro	*Leu*	Gly	NH_2	100	1·5
AVP	Cys	Tyr	*Phe*	Glu	Asn	Cys	Pro	*Arg*	Cly	NH_2	4	100
LVP	Cys	Tyr	*Phe*	Glu	Asn	Cys	Pro	*Lys*	Gly	NH_2	1	70
Vasotocin	Cys	Tyr	*Ile*	Glu	Asn	Cys	Pro	*Arg*	Gly	NH_2	27	60
Orn^8Oxy	Cys	Tyr	*Ile*	Glu	Asn	Cys	Pro	*Orn*	Gly	NH_2	40	70
DesAmino-Oxy	*TP**	Tyr	*Ile*	Glu	Asn	Cys	Pro	*Leu*	Gly	NH_2	180	0·4
2-PheOxy	Cys	*Phe*	*Ile*	Glu	Asn	Cys	Pro	*Leu*	Gly	NH_2	7	0·1
3-TyrOxy	Cys	Tyr	*Tyr*	Glu	Asn	Cys	Pro	*Leu*	Gly	NH_2	0·02	0·003

* TP = 2-mercaptopropionic acid.

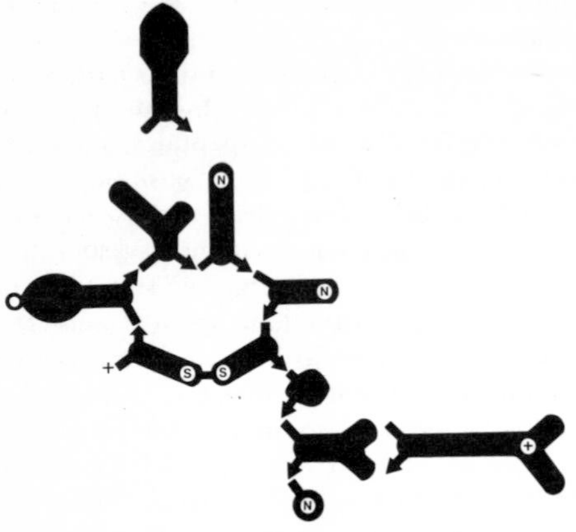

Fig. 9.1. Structure of oxytocin and lysine vasopressin. The main structure shows a representation of the peptide structure of oxytocin. The side chains are shown approximately to scale. The symbol N indicates an amide group, S a sulphur and + a positive charge. The two extra outlines indicate the changes at positions 3 and 8 to produce lysine vasopressin. The substitution of *Phe* at position 3 increases the bulk, the substitution of *lys* at position 8 increases bulk and makes the molecule more hydrophilic.

be prolonged still further when given in the form of a salt such as pitressin tannate suspended in oil.

Angiotensin

Saline extracts of kidney when injected intravenously cause a rise of blood pressure that develops rather slowly and is sustained. The activity of the kidney extract is destroyed by boiling. On the other hand, if the kidney extract is mixed with plasma and allowed to stand at room temperature for a few minutes and then injected, the pressor effect is immediate and furthermore this activity is not destroyed by boiling.

The mechanism of this action is as follows, in the extract of kidney there is a proteolytic enzyme *renin* that splits a decapeptide angiotensin-I off a precursor plasma protein belonging to the α_2 globulin class which is called angiotensinogen (or angiotensin precursor). Angiotensin I is itself quite inactive but the terminal two amino acids are split off by another peptidase called the 'converting enzyme' to give the highly active octapeptide, angiotensin II. The converting enzyme is widely distributed, but the lungs are particularly rich in it. Angiotensin is readily attacked further by peptidases yielding less active products; this occurs most readily through the action of carboxypeptidases which remove the terminal Phe.

Angiotensin II is a powerful smooth muscle stimulant acting especially on the arterioles but also on the gut and uterus. It can be used by intravenous injection to restore blood pressure in traumatic shock. Angiotension II also has a powerful action on the adrenal cortex causing the release of the mineralocorticoid, aldosterone, and its physiological function is believed to reside in its ability to control the release of aldosterone.

Evidence exists that the renin mechanism is involved in some cases of hypertension and for this reason its structure–activity relationships have been much studied. Asp^1 is not essential and if replaced by sarcosine leads to a more stable peptide, but Phe^8 cannot be replaced without great loss of activity—indeed replacement by Ala or Ile leads to powerful antagonists, and if this is combined with the replacement of Asp^1 by Sar^1 gives even more potent and long-lasting antagonists of angiotensin II. These substances have negligible effect on normal blood pressure, but will reduce the blood pressure in experimental acute renal hypertension and also in some cases of human hypertension. An alternative approach to this problem is to attempt to inhibit the converting enzyme, thus preventing the conversion of angiotensin I to angiotensin II. A nonapeptide first found in viper venom (pyr-Trp-Pro-Arg-Pro-Gln-Ile-Pro-Pro) is a powerful inhibitor and lowers blood pressure in acute renal hypertension. It is also useful in experimental haemorhagic shock where the endogenous release of angiotensin is excessive and deleterious.

A simple inhibitor of the converting enzyme has recently been reported (SQ1422S; D-2-methyl-3-mercapto propionyl-L-pioline) which is highly active by month.

Kinins

In a manner analogous to that for angiotensin, the extracts of various tissues, such as the pancreas and salivary glands, as well as saliva and urine when injected intravenously cause a *fall* of blood pressure. This is due to the release of a nonapeptide bradykinin due to the action of proteases in these tissue extracts on plasma α_2 globulins which are referred to as kininogens. The enzymes which are poorly characterized are referred to as kallikreins (=pancreas). In this case also there is a precursor peptide kallidin which has an extra amino acid (Lys) at the NH_2-terminal end. This amino acid is very readily split off by plasma aminopeptidase activity.

Bradykinin is a very potent vasodilator, having an especially strong effect on the skin vessels, but it will dilate all small blood vessels. On local injection increased permeability of the small vessels occurs with plasma protein extravasaton and whealing; a strong local flush is produced but usually no flare. The injection is painful and bradykinin will produce intense pain elsewhere, for instance when injected into joints. Bradykinin will also produce bronchoconstriction.

The pain produced by kinins is relieved by aspirin and other members of the antipyretic class. Recent evidence suggests that bradykinin activates the prostaglandin system and it is these agents that are directly algesic. Aspirin is then seen to act by inhibiting prostaglandin synthesis.

It seems likely that kinins play an important role in generating the local phenomena of inflammation particularly the vasodilatation, oedema, and pain. It has also been suggested that they are responsible for most of the 'work' vasodilatation in secreting tissues. When plasma is placed in glass containers, bradykinin is released due to the surface activation of one of the clotting factors (Hagemann factor) and is also activated on dilution of plasma. In carcinoid tumours which are tumours of argentaffin cells, one of the prominent features is intense flushing of the skin; this is due to the release of kinins as well as serotonin. No effective antagonists of bradykinin are known but the formation of kinins can be suppressed by a large peptide extracted from bovine parotid glands, called trasylol.

Other kinins with homologous structures have been isolated from the venoms of bees and hornets, and from the skin of amphibia. The venom of some snakes contains powerful kallikreins.

Substance P

Substance P is an undecapeptide that has been extracted from brain and which was originally found to contract the smooth muscle of the intestine and the uterus. The peptide is present in a variable distribution in the central nervous system, the maximum concentration being about micromolar. Its distribution has recently been studied in detail by immunohistology and can be seen to be in neurone cell bodies and axons. It has a powerful depolarizing action on motor neurones and has generally established a good case to be regarded as a primary neurotransmitter. The peripheral actions are mainly on smooth muscle which it relaxes although there is also a stimulant action on some glands. Substance P is also found in smaller amounts in the gut. Peptides with sequence homology are *eledoisin* isolated from octopus salivary gland and *physalaemin* from toad skin; these peptides are about ten times as active as substance P on motor neurones. Note that these peptides share the same terminal tripeptide. Shorter peptides retain some activity. No specific antagonists are known.

Table 9.2. Activity of Substance P and related substances on spinal neurones

Substance P	Arg	Pro	Lys	Pro	Gln	Gln	Phe	Phe	Gly	Leu	Met	NH_2	100
Physalaemin	Pyr	Ala	Asn	Pro	Asn	Lys	Phe	Try	Gly	Leu	Met	NH_2	750
Eledoisin	Pyr	Pro	Ser	Lys	Asp	Ala	Phe	Ile	Gly	Leu	Met	NH_2	1000
						Lys	Phe	Ile	Gly	Leu	Met	NH_2	400

Ergot (Fig. 9.2)

Ergot is a fungus (*Claviceps purpurea*) which grows on rye so that the infected ears turn dark. Ergot contains many interesting substances but we are concerned here only with the characteristic alkaloids which are all amides of lysergic acid. We have previously referred to methysergide, the *N*-methyl lysergic butanolamide. Ergometrine (ergonovine) is the closely related lysergic propanolamide. Ergometrine stimulates smooth muscle in blood vessels and hence causes a rise of blood pressure with reflex bradycardia, contracts smooth muscle of the gut, ureter, biliary tract, and the uterus. It is the action on the latter that provides the main use for ergot.

Ergometrine will contract the uterus even when not oestrogen-primed, but the sensitivity of the uterus is greatly increased in the latter stages of pregnancy. Ergot produces a great increase in the rhythmic activity rather than of tone. It is given routinely by most obstetricians at the beginning of the third stage of labour to aid the expulsion of the placenta and blood clots. It has a long duration of action.

Ergot alkaloids are also used in the treatment of migraine which is a paroxysmal dilatation of vessels related to the internal and external carotid arteries leading to severe throbbing headache, and often visual disturbances. Ergot alkaloids are effective by virtue of their vasoconstrictor actions. Ergometrine and methysergide are most frequently used.

The main toxic effect of the alkaloids is due to their powerful and prolonged effect on arteries, which may lead to peripheral gangrene, particularly of fingers or toes. It was this action which was recognized in the Middle Ages as St. Anthony's Fire after the shrine where people sought a cure. Other toxic effects include nausea, vomiting, diarrhoea, dizziness, and confusion. The side-effects unfortunately frequently make it impossible to give adequate doses to migraine sufferers.

Histamine

Histamine was first isolated from ergot (in which it is a contaminant) due to the action of bacteria on histidine. Later it was found in a variety of fresh animal tissues. Its concentration in the tissues is related to the concentration of mast cells (basophils) in these tissues, the mast cells having an extremely high concentration of histamine of the order of several mg/g. In mast cell tumours and in the collections of mast cells in the skin in the disease urticaria pigmentosa similar high concentrations are found.

Histamine is synthesized in the tissues by decarboxylation of histidine by the pyridoxal-requiring enzyme histidine decarboxylase. This enzyme may be inhibited in isolated preparations by semicarbazide.

Histamine is readily released from mast cells by mechanical trauma, such as a firm stroke of the skin, by heat, cold, and ultraviolet radiation. Release is also produced

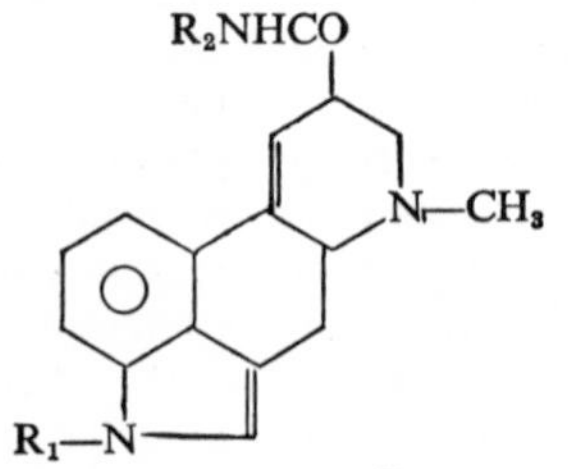

R_2NHCO

$N—CH_3$

$R_1—N$

	R_1	R_2
Ergometrine (ergonovine)	H	$—CH(CH_3)CH_2OH$
Methysergide	CH_3	$—CH(C_2H_5)CH_2OH$
Lysergic diethylamide (LSD)	H	$(C_2H_5)_2$

Fig. 9.2. Ergot alkaloids.

by many common chemicals and drugs (notably bases) including morphine, atropine, tubocurarine, and stilbamidine. Especially effective is a substance known as 40/80 which is an oligomeric condensation product of 4-methoxyphenylethylmethylamine with formaldehyde. Some polymers also cause release of histamine, for instance dextran and ovomucoid in the rat and polyvinylpyrrolidone in the dog. Small doses of histamine liberators cause the discharge of granules from the mast cells, larger doses cause disintegration of the cells. Other substances are also released including serotonin, heparin, and slow-reacting substances. It has been known for a long time that the action of releasers was dependent on calcium and it has recently been shown that calcium ionophores (such as A23187) , which permit net calcium entry into the mast cells, also cause histamine release.

Mast cell destruction and histamine liberation also result from the immediate type of hypersensitivity reaction. This is seen if an animal is sensitized by giving it an injection of a foreign protein such as ovalbumin and then 10 days later challenged with a second injection of the same protein. Histamine is released and the complex pharmacological effects of histamine are observed. The mechanism of this reaction is that the foreign protein induces the development of antibodies, one class of which (IgE) become attached to the mast cell surface, and when the antigen is provided on the second occasion it combines with the IgE and sets in train a complex series of reactions involving plasma factors (complement). This activates a phospholipase in the cell membrane and hence leads to an increase in permeability and, if intense enough, to lysis. These reactions can be demonstrated on isolated tissues such as bronchi, uterus, and intestine, as well as in the whole animal. The allergic reaction in the respiratory tract caused by allergens in pollen acts through the same mechanism. Considerable amounts of histamine are also found in the stinging hairs of nettles and are responsible for the whealing and itching they cause.

Histamine is rapidly metabolized in the body by two routes. First it is ring methylated to give 1-methylhistamine which has very low pharmacological activity and secondly the aliphatic amino group is oxidatively removed by diaminooxydase (which can be inhibited by aminoguanidine or by isoniazid) to give imidazole acetic acid. There are considerable amounts of these enzymes present in the gut wall and in the liver, these metabolize histamine so effectively that it is quite inactive when given by mouth. This is important because many bacteria produce histidine decarboxylases so that free histidine in the gut is rapidly decarboxylated to histamine. A further safeguard is that the bacteria can also metabolize histamine further, mainly by acetylation to give *N*-acetylhistamine which is inactive.

Pharmacological actions

Histamine causes contraction of the smooth muscle of the intestine and bronchi. Its action on the smooth muscle of the blood vessels depends on the species studied. In man, histamine relaxes the arterioles and small venules but constricts the larger veins. The net effect on the circulation is a fall in arterial blood pressure with reflex tachycardia. Histamine has a positive inotropic effect on the isolated heart but it is doubtful if any direct effect on the heart contributes to the circulatory changes. In man the effects on the cutaneous circulation are a reddening and increase in temperature of the skin, especially in the blush area of the head and neck. With large doses of histamine the profound fall of blood pressure is due in part to a decrease in plasma volume arising from an increase in permeability of the small venules. The impermeability of the normal venule to plasma protein depends on the continuity of the endothelial cell layer. Histamine causes the endothelial cells to separate from each other so that plasma protein can escape and extravasate into the extracellular space and so cause oedema.

When histamine is injected intradermally the triple response of Lewis results. This consists of (1) a localized bluish-red area around the site of injection in the centre of which (2) an area of oedema develops, and (3) an irregular area of reddening called the flare. The site of injection is itchy. The first two responses correspond to the action on vessels already described, but the third is due to stimulation of sensory nerve fibres (the same fibres causing the sensation of itch) whose branches liberate an unknown vasodilator substance which dilates the arterioles some distance from the site of injection. The flare is abolished by chronic sensory denervation. As mentioned earlier the circulatory effects of histamine in other animals are not the same as in man. In the rabbit the arterioles are constricted and, because of the resulting rise in peripheral resistance, the blood pressure rises and the heart rate is reflexly slowed. In the cat systemic blood pressure falls, but the pulmonary blood pressure rises, both changes being due to a selective constriction of the pulmonary arterioles. In the dog there is also a fall of blood pressure, but in this instance due to constriction of the hepatic vein causing pooling of blood in the portal circulation.

One of the symptoms of histamine administration in man is a throbbing headache due to a combination of dilatation of cerebral vessels and a rise in intracranial pressure.

Histamine is a very powerful gastric secretagogue and leads to the secretion of juice of high hydrochloric acid content. The effects on the uterus are rather variable; it contracts the uterus in most species (the guinea pig is typical) but relaxes the rat uterus and has little effect on the human uterus. Histamine also has little or no effect on the smooth muscle of the bladder or the iris.

Antihistamines

A large number of antihistamines are known which are based on a diarylalkylamine structure (Fig. 9.3). They are effective in antagonizing the effects of histamine on vascular smooth muscle and on capillary permeability, but are totally without effect on gastric secretion, or on the relaxing effect of histamine on the rat uterus. This was a puzzle for many years. The beginning of a solution came from the study of the activity of methyl derivatives of histamine. It was noted that 4-methyl histamine was almost without activity on blood vessels but had an action on gastric secretion nearly as great as that of histamine itself, whereas 2-methyl histamine was much less active on gastric secretion than on vascular smooth muscle. This differential agonist activity suggested that there were distinct receptor types responsible for the action of histamine on these two groups of tissues and that the aralkylamine antagonists were able to block only one group. These receptors were called H_1. Black and his colleagues used the clue given by the methylhistamines to develop antagonists for the second histamine (H_2) receptor. **Metiamide** and **cimetidine** are such H_2 antagonists and their derivation from histamine itself is obvious.

The H_1 antagonists find their major uses as antihistamines in combating allergic rhinitis and urticaria. Their major disadvantages are that they tend to cause drowsiness and incoordination—an especial problem for car drivers. Their central actions are put to use in the control of motion sickness and some antihistamines are of value in treating paralysis agitans (Parkinsonism). A large number of H_1 antagonists are in use, far more than are justified by their usefulness. **Promethazine, phenindamine, chlorcyclizine, diphenhydramine,** and **mepyramine** (Fig. 9.3) are amongst those most commonly used.

The actions of the H_2 antagonists are still being explored but it is already evident that they are very effective in blocking the effect of histamine on gastric secretion as well as blocking the effect of pentagastrin. The latter is of considerable interest because it had been postulated many years ago that gastrin acted by causing local liberation of histamine in the gastric mucosa—these results support this theory. They are also important in that gastrin plays an important role in controlling gastric acid secretion and H_2 antagonists have been found to be very effective in reducing resting and postprandial secretion, in consequence they are useful both in symptomatic treatment of peptic ulcer and in accelerating

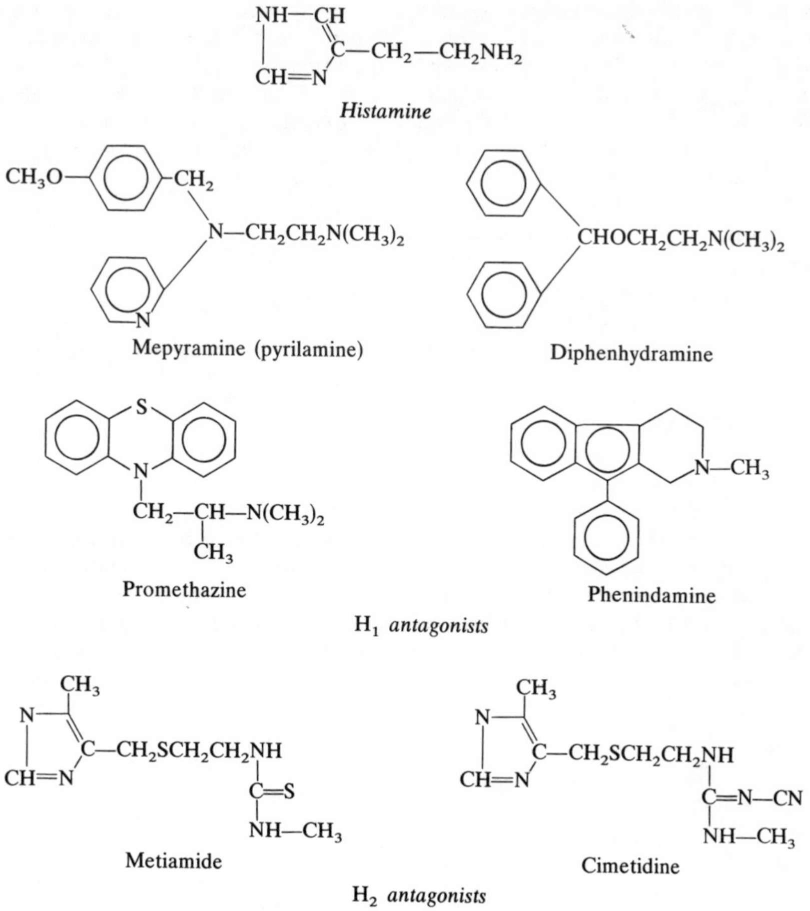

NH—CH
C—CH_2—CH_2NH_2
CH=N

Histamine

CH_3O— —CH_2
N—$CH_2CH_2N(CH_3)_2$
N

Mepyramine (pyrilamine)

$CHOCH_2CH_2N(CH_3)_2$

Diphenhydramine

S
N
CH_2—CH—$N(CH_3)_2$
CH_3

Promethazine

N—CH_3

Phenindamine

H_1 *antagonists*

CH_3
N
C—$CH_2SCH_2CH_2NH$
CH=N
C=S
NH—CH_3

Metiamide

CH_3
N
C—$CH_2SCH_2CH_2NH$
CH=N
C=N—CN
NH—CH_3

Cimetidine

H_2 *antagonists*

Fig. 9.3. Histamine and antihistamine.

the healing of ulcers. The Zollinger–Ellison syndrome is a condition in which a tumour develops that secretes very large amounts of gastrin, with resulting gross overstimulation of the gastric mucosa—H_2 antagonists have a dramatic effect in improving this condition. The availability of H_2 antagonists has demonstrated that rather few effects of histamine are pure H_1 and that, for instance, the vascular effects and focal oedema are more effectively antagonized by a combination of H_1 and H_2 antagonists than by H_1 alone. It is likely that H_2 antagonists will find other uses than just the control of gastric acid secretion.

Cromoglycate (cromolyn, intal)

The allergic response with the release of histamine and other mediators can be suppressed by cromoglycate. This substance prevents the combination of reagin (monovalent antigens such as are present in pollen) with the specific IgE on the cell surface, leading to mediator release; it has been suggested that activation of calcium entry no longer occurs. Cromoglycate does not suppress the effects of chemical or physical histamine releasers.

Cromoglycate is a very effective drug in hay fever and asthma, and in milk allergies in

Fig. 9.4.

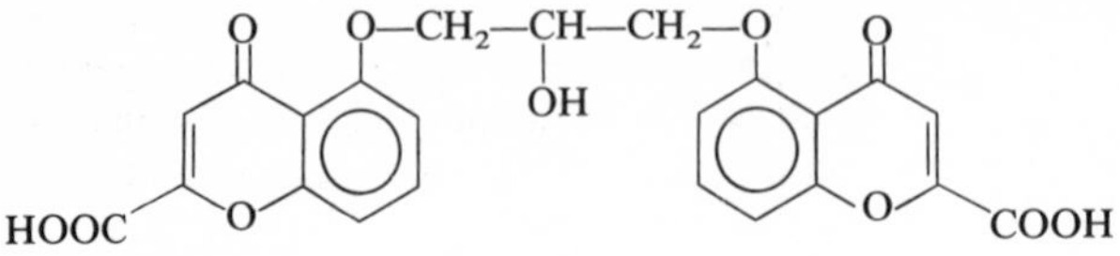

Cromoglycate

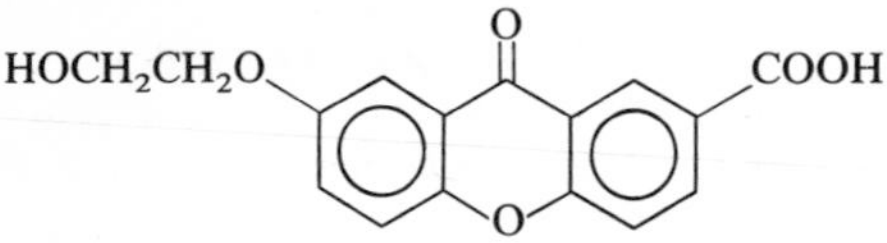

AH 7725

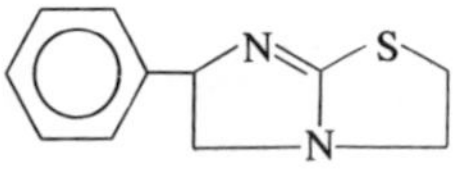

Levamisole

babies. It is not absorbed from the gut and is administered by inhalation as an aerosol in the nose and respiratory tract, or applied locally (e.g. to the conjunctiva). A related compound AH 7725 (see Fig. 9.4) is active by mouth and is undergoing clinical trials.

Levamisole

Levamisole was introduced into medicine as an anthelminthic especially useful for nematodes. Recently it has been found to have remarkable effects in enhancing immune responses. It will rapidly restore immune responses in patients with immunodeficiency or senile anergy. In experimental tumours it has increased the immune suppression of a sarcoma. It has also produced encouraging early effects in improving rheumatoid arthritis. The mechanism is still not clear, but while no definite effects have been shown or peripheral lymphocytes, it does enhance phagocytosis by macrophages.

Prostaglandins

Extracts of seminal fluid and of the vesicular gland may contract or relax smooth muscle or cause a fall of blood pressure when injected intravenously. The active substances were named prostaglandins by von Euler, who showed that they were lipid acids that could be divided into two classes according to whether they were extractable by ether (the E series) or not (the F series). Further work on these compounds did not proceed until the chemical structures of prostaglandin E_1 and prostaglandin $F_{2\alpha}$ were elucidated in 1962. They were shown to be fatty acids with a peculiar cyclopentane ring part way down the chain and with hydroxyl or keto functions; the basic skeleton is called prostenoic acid. It was also shown that prostaglandins were readily synthesized by incubating a homogenate of sheep vesicular glands with polyunsaturated fatty acids such as arachidonic and dihomo-γ-linolenic acid. The study of prostaglandins has become an extremely active and exciting field of research. Much is now known about the stages in synthesis of these substances, and a bewildering number of variants of the original substances have been identified.

The basic synthetic route from arachidonic acid is indicated in Fig. 9.5 and by the action of fatty acid cyclo-oxygenase (loosely referred to as prostaglandin synthetase) ring closure occurs between carbons 8 and 12 while two oxygens are introduced between carbons 9 and 11 as an endoperoxide, and a peroxide group is introduced at position 15—this molecule is now referred to as prostaglandin G_2 (PGG_2). By the successive action of

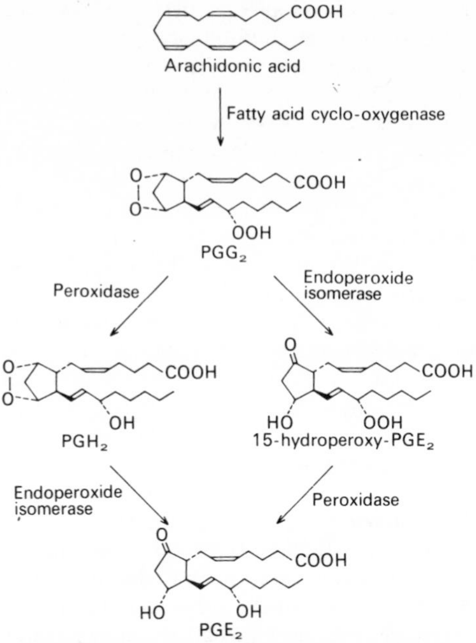

Arachidonic acid

Fatty acid cyclo-oxygenase

PGG_2

Peroxidase

Endoperoxide isomerase

PGH_2

15-hydroperoxy-PGE_2

Endoperoxide isomerase

Peroxidase

PGE_2

Fig. 9.5. Pathways in the biosynthesis of PGE_2 from arachidonic acid.

peroxidase and endoperoxide isomerase, the peroxide is reduced and the endoperoxide opened to give PGE_2. Prostaglandins generally have short *in vivo* half-lives due mainly to a further metabolic change in which the double bond at 13,14 is reduced and the hydroxyl group at 15 oxidized to the ketone by the enzyme prostaglandin 15-dehydrogenase. The terminology of prostaglandins is rather complicated—the letter after the initial PG designates the state of the cyclopentane ring and is shown in Fig. 9.6, and the subscript refers to the number of double bonds in the side chains.

An action on smooth muscle is a very general property of prostaglandins, and in general they contract intestine longitudinal muscle, and may produce cramps or diarrhoea. Variable effects are produced on the non-pregnant uterus, but PGE_1 and $PGF_{2\alpha}$ systemically contract both the pregnant and non-pregnant uterus, and may be used to produce abortion or to help evacuate products of conception. They relax small blood vessels and hence increase the blood flow to the kidney and other organs. On intradermal injection PGE_1 and $PGF_{2\alpha}$ cause a wheal and a flare and local pain. They also irritate the conjunctiva. PGE_1 relaxes bronchial tone but its potential use as a bronchodilator in asthma is limited by its tendency to irritate the bronchal mucosa. A variety of effects have been reported after the injection of PGE_1 into the cerebral ventricles, the most striking of which is fever, and evidence has been advanced that release of PGE_1 and PGE_2 is a necessary intermediary in fever produced by bacterial pyrogens. Stupor, catatonia, and other behavioural effects may also result.

Numerous effects on endocrine systems have been reported, including increased release of insulin and adrenal steroids, but the

Fig. 9.6.

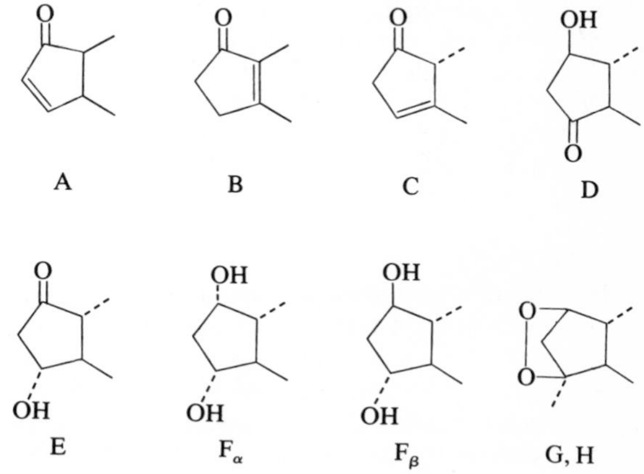

A B C D

E F_α F_β G, H

most dramatic is the effect possessed in highest degree by $PGF_{2\alpha}$ of causing regression of the corpus luteum with depression of progesterone release. Comparatively high affinity receptors for prostaglandins of type A, E, and F have so far been detected and it appears that in most, if not all, tissues the activation of these receptors is somehow involved in the activation of adenyl cyclase, so that cyclic AMP has a role in the mediation of prostaglandin effects.

The synthesis of prostaglandins by the tissues can be depressed by drugs of the aspirin group, of which **indomethacin** and **naproxen** are especially effective. A non-metabolizable analogue of arachidonic acid, **5,8,11,14-eicosatetraynoic acid** in which all four double bonds are replaced by triple bonds is also an active inhibitor of the fatty acid cyclo-oxygenase. It is also curious that some amineoxydase inhibitors such as tranylcypromine and phenelzine are also inhibitors. Antagonism to some prostaglandins at the receptor level is produced by the analogue **7-oxa-13,14-prostynoic acid.**

Prostaglandins are so widely distributed in tissues and have such a variety of actions that it is very likely that they have important physiological functions. However, since their synthesis can be reduced to very low levels by clinical doses of indomethacin and related drugs it is clear that they are not essential to survival. The most clear-cut functions are in connection with painful responses—the effects are peripheral and seem to be due to sensitizing pain endings to the action of bradykinin and possibly other locally released agents. There is also very well-documented evidence in relation to organ blood flow, where it appears that prostaglandins have a place in autoregulatory processes. The role in reproductive functions is still not clear but it has been suggested that they may be responsible for the initiation of parturition.

The estimation of prostaglandins in body tissues and fluids is a matter of considerable difficulty both because of the small amounts present and their multiplicity. More or less selective bioassays are available, as an immunoassays and gas-chromatographic and mass spectrometric methods.

PGE_2 and $PGF_{2\alpha}$ are released by blood platelets during aggregation and this has encouraged the investigation of their biosynthesis in these structures. PGE_2 itself aggregates platelets, whereas PGE_1 is a powerful inhibitor of aggregation. Arachidonic acid also causes aggregation, and it was found that the two intermediate endoperoxides PGG_2 and PGH_2 were also active. A further group of compounds have recently been isolated which do not have the prostanoic skeleton but are clearly derived from the prostaglandin endoperoxides; these have been called **thromboxanes** (Fig. 9.7) and are very active in causing aggregation. Most recently an enzyme has been found in the endothelium of blood vessels which converts PGG_2 and PGH_2 into a very powerful antiaggregator PGX (prostacyclin).

It is clear that the prostaglandins represent an extremely important development in pharmacology that is at present in a state of flux and ferment. It will be surprising if important new therapeutic agents are not discovered in relation to this group.

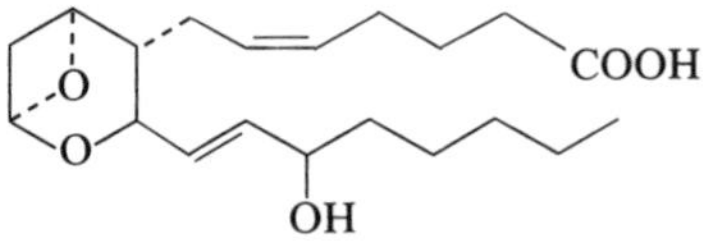

COOH
O
O
OH

Thiomboxane A_2

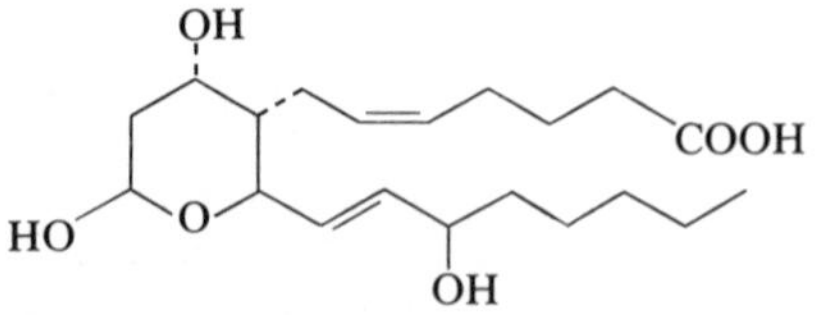

OH
COOH
HO
O
OH

Thiomboxane B_2

Fig. 9.7.

FURTHER READING

Black, J. W. *et al.* (1972). Definition and antagonism of histamine H_2 receptor. *Nature, Lond.* **236,** 385.

Cuthbert, M. F. (ed.) (1973). *The prostaglandins,* Philadelphia.

Hamberg, M., Svensson, J., and Samuelson, B.

(1975). Thromboxanes, *Proc. Nat. Acad. Sci. U.S.A.* **72,** 2994.

Heffter, A. (1966). Histamine and Antihistamines, *Handbook exp. Pharmacol.* Vol. XVIII/1.

Heffter, A. (1968). Neurohypophysial hormones, *Handbook exp. Pharmacol.* Vol. XXIII.

Heffter, A. (1970). Bradkinin, kallidin and kallikrein. *Handbook exp. Pharmacol.* Vol. XXV.

Heffter, A. (1974). Angiotensin. *Handbook exp. Pharmacol.* Vol. XXXVII.

Horton, E. W. (1972). Prostaglandins, *Proc. R. Soc. B.* **182,** 411.

Kadowitz, P. J. Joiner, P. D., and Hyman, A. L. (1975). Physiological and pharmacological role of prostaglandins *Ann. Rev. Pharmacol.* **15,** 285.

Lewis, T. and Grant, R. T. (1924). Vascular reactions of the skin to injury. *Heart,* **11,** 209.

Paton, W. D. M. (1957). Histamine release by compounds of simple chemical structure. *Pharmacol. Rev.* **9,** 269.

Ramwell, P. and Shaw, J. E. (1971). Prostaglandins. *Ann. N.Y. Acad. Sci.* **180,** 1.

Rudinger, J. (1971). *The design of peptide hormone analogs* In: Arients, E. J. (ed.) *Drug design,* Vol. II, New York.

Samuelson, B. *et al.* (1975). Prostaglandins. *Ann. Rev. Biochem.* **44,** 669.

Walker, J. M. (ed.) (1971). *Pharmacology of naturally occurring polypeptides and lipid soluble acids.* Oxford.

10

CIRCULATION

DRUGS acting on the circulation may produce their primary effects on the heart or the vessels or more frequently on both but, because of the complex integration of the circulation, the final effects of drugs may be greatly modified by the homeostatic processes involved. For this reason, before we attempt to analyse drug actions, we will briefly describe the main circulatory control mechanisms.

The stroke output of the ventricles is primarily dependent on the filling pressure at the end of diastole, in that the more the ventricular muscle is stretched the greater is the stroke ejection. However, if the pressure is increased far enough the stroke output reaches a maximum and no longer responds to changes in filling pressure. The range over which there is a proportionality between filling pressure and stroke output is often referred to as the operating range. This is a very important regulator that has the effect of increasing the stroke output in response to the venous return and is the means by which the output from the two sides of the heart is balanced. The output curve is not invariant and can be modified, for instance, if the ventricular muscle is damaged or is anoxic the curve will be depressed and displaced so that to achieve the same stroke output the filling pressure must be increased or alternatively if the filling pressure remains unchanged the output is reduced and the emptying of the ventricles in systole is reduced.

The characteristic curve can be elevated by sympathetic stimulation or by catecholamines and certain other drugs and in these circumstances for any specified filling pressure the stroke output is increased and the ventricle more completely emptied in systole, or alternatively to maintain a specified stroke output a reduced filling pressure is needed. The effect of the sympathetic in speeding up the heart results in an even greater increase in minute output with respect to any reference filling pressure. This action of the sympathetic is of great importance in the regulation of heart action and its influence is seen in emotional excitement, in exercise, after blood loss, and, as a compensatory effect, in hypodynamism of the ventricular muscle in disease.

It has been emphasized that stroke output depends most directly on the diastolic filling pressure and this in turn depends on certain characteristics of the venous system. A part of the arterial blood pressure is transmitted through the capillaries to the small venules and it is the pressure difference between these vessels and that in the right atrium that drives blood back to the heart. However, the mean pressure within the venous system depends also upon the volume of blood contained in the venules and veins and the tone of the walls of these vessels; the veins are not merely passive vessels but are under tonic control of sympathetic nerves and are also susceptible to the effects of drugs. Thus if the venous tone is decreased the blood becomes pooled in the venous system, the pressure in the right atrium decreases and the stroke output diminishes, and on the contrary, if the venous tone increases the pressure gradient diminishes and the pressure in the right atrium will increase provided that venous tone does not increase so much that the resistance to flow in the veins, which is usually slight, becomes a limiting factor. It is clear that the venular pressure will also depend on the state of tone of the arterioles—if these dilate the venular pressure will rise and the venous return will increase. Finally the arterial blood pressure will depend both on the output of the left ventricle and the ease with which blood can leave the great arteries and pass through the capillary bed. This peripheral resistance is mainly controlled by the calibre of the arterioles which are affected both by

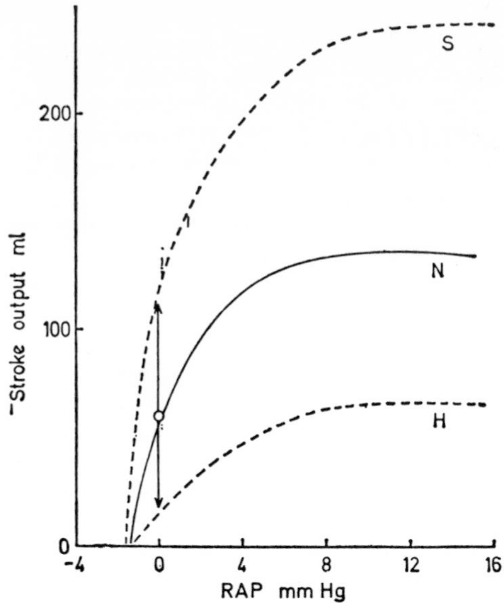

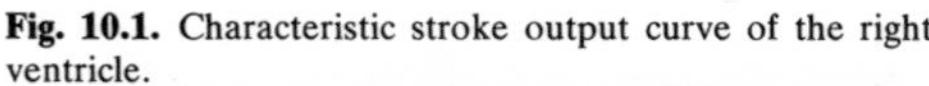

Fig. 10.1. Characteristic stroke output curve of the right ventricle.

N shows the relationship of stroke output of the normal ventricle at different values of right atrial pressure.
H those of the hypodynamic (i.e. depressed ventricle).
S those of the ventricle stimulated by sympathetic stimulation.

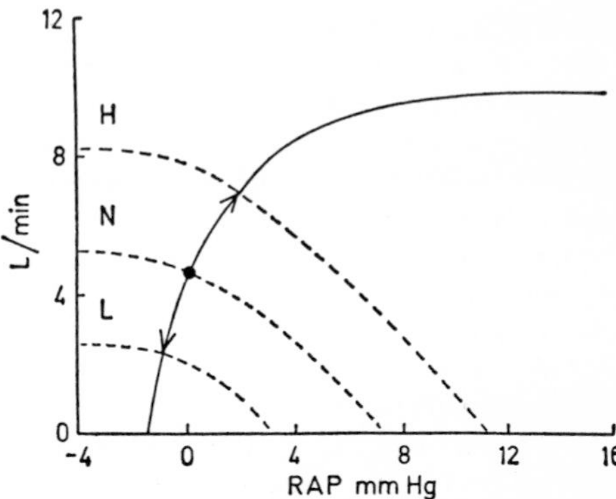

Fig. 10.2. The effect of venous return on minute output of the right ventricle.

N is the normal venous return curve—the operating point of the ventricle is at the intersection of this curve with output curve.
H high venous return (e.g. in exercise).
L low venous return (e.g. peripheral venous pooling).

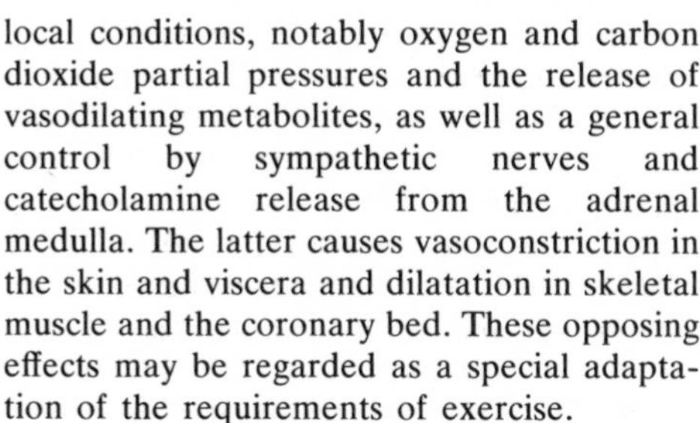

local conditions, notably oxygen and carbon dioxide partial pressures and the release of vasodilating metabolites, as well as a general control by sympathetic nerves and catecholamine release from the adrenal medulla. The latter causes vasoconstriction in the skin and viscera and dilatation in skeletal muscle and the coronary bed. These opposing effects may be regarded as a special adaptation of the requirements of exercise.

Set over the haemodynamic mechanisms we have described are various regulating systems of which the dominant is normally that exerted through the carotid-aortic pressor receptors. These structures are in the aortic arch and carotid artery and are sensitive both to the mean pressure within them and also to the dynamic pressure variation during the course of a cardiac cycle. A rise in pressure or an increase in pressure swing causes an increased rate of firing in the sino-aortic sensory nerves and this alters the state of activity of cells in the CNS, notably in the medulla, and leads to a decreased sympathetic discharge to the heart and peripheral vessels as well as an increase in the vagal discharge to the heart. The over-all effect is to reduce both the stroke output of the heart and the peripheral resistance and hence to lower the blood pressure, this minimizing the alteration in blood pressure which would have occurred if this compensation were inoperative. Other modifications of cardiovascular tone are produced through peripheral chemoreceptors and by alterations in central nervous activity.

Much has been learned of the way drugs act on the cardiovascular system by using simplified preparations, such as the heart perfused through the coronary vessels, perfused peripheral beds, isolated artery and vein strips, and heart–lung preparations and these remain invaluable objects for the study of drugs, but major advances in the understanding of how cardiovascular drugs act has come in recent years from new methods, particularly those that can be used in unanaesthetized animals and man, and include cardiac catheterization for measurement of pressures, Fick and dye methods for measurement of cardiac output, and the attachment of radiopaque markers to the ventricles for the measurement of ventricular contration.

We will now consider the action of some major groups of drugs on the cardiovascular system.

NORADRENALINE AND RELATED COMPOUNDS

Noradrenaline (Chapter 8) is a catecholamine acting predominantly on the sympathetic α-receptors and has in most species a relatively weak β-action. It produces a considerable increase in blood pressure and slowing of the heart with cutaneous vasoconstriction. The primary effects are to increase the stroke output (the positive inotropic action) and to increase the heart rate, and also to constrict arterioles in the skin and viscera while having little effect on the vessels in skeletal muscle. It is also venoconstrictor and hence raises left atrial pressure further augmenting the increase in stroke output. These effects are modified by the baroreceptors which in compensation increase vagal tone and so slow the heart but the vagus has little inotropic effect (there are few vagal fibres ending on the ventricular myocardium). There will also be a reduction in sympathetic tone to the vessels. The slowing of the heart tends to counteract the direct effects of noradrenaline tending to increase the minute output, so that over all the cardiac output may not be much changed.

Mexthoxamine which seems to be completely devoid of β-actions is without any direct effect on the heart but increases the blood pressure purely by its effect on peripheral resistance. A secondary bradycardia is produced through the baroreceptors.

The actions of **isoprenaline (isoproterenol)** are exerted almost entirely on the β-receptors. There will, therefore, be strong positive inotropic and chronotropic actions on the heart, but there will be no vasoconstriction in the skin and viscera, and marked vasodilatation in muscle, and some venodilatation too. The effects on the mean arterial blood pressure will therefore depend on the balance between the direct effects on the heart increasing stroke and minute output, and hence tending to raise the pressure, and the decrease in peripheral resistance and increase in venous capacity tending to reduce pressure. The balance of effects differs in different animals. In man the mean pressure is not much changed. In other animals there may be a precipitous fall in pressure or a modest rise. In all cases there is a tachycardia and an increase in pulse pressure. The chronotropic action of isoprenaline is made use of in intermittent heart block (Stokes–Adams syndrome) where the increase in excitability of the conducting tissue restarts impulse production.

The action of **adrenaline (epinephrine)** is intermediate between those of noradrenaline and isoprenaline. It acts effectively on both α- and β-receptors. This means that it has a strong cardiac inotropic and chronotropic action, but it has a mixed peripheral action. It constricts skin and visceral vessels, dilates muscle vessels, and constricts most veins. The over-all effect on the peripheral resistance is a modest reduction. The net effect on the blood pressure is a small rise and since the direct cardiac effects are strong and the stimulus to the baroreceptors rather slight, the direct positive chronotropic effect is not annulled by increased vagal tone.

The contrast between noradrenaline and adrenaline is an interesting one and has some relevance to the use of these agents in raising blood pressure in hypotension. Noradrenaline is the more reliable drug for this purpose and also causes a smaller increase in cardiac work for a given rise in blood pressure, because the cardiac output is lower. Both agents have the serious disadvantage of raising blood pressure at the cost of vasoconstriction in the viscera which may cause dangerous ischaemia. **Metaraminol** is sometimes used for the same purpose and has the advantage of a more prolonged action.

HYPOTENSIVE DRUGS

A wide variety of drugs can lower the blood pressure and we will deal here only with some of the more interesting ones.

Ganglion blockers

Ganglion blockers such as **hexamethonium, pempidine,** or **mecamylamine** (Chapter 7) cause a rapid and marked fall in arterial pressure with a moderate increase in heart rate. The fall in arterial pressure is mainly due to block of ganglia in the sympathetic vasoconstrictor path, with reduction in vasomotor tone and hence a fall in peripheral resistance.

This would increase the pressure in the small venules, but because of the simultaneous block of sympathetic tone in the veins, the venous capacity is also increased and the right atrial pressure falls, hence the cardiac output falls. This occurs despite the tachycardia due to block of vagal ganglia, which would otherwise tend to increase the minute output. The ganglion blocking drugs were the first drugs to be used in the treatment of hypertension but they are now little used owing to certain undesirable complications. One of these is the large fall in blood pressure that usually occurs in changing position from recumbency to standing. This is due mainly to pooling in the veins and the absence of any baroreceptor reflex consequent on the blocking of all the efferent paths of the autonomic system. The drugs retain a limited usefulness in treating acute hypertensive attacks and sometimes in malignant hypertension. The other unpleasant side-effects are due to the fact that these drugs block all autonomic ganglia including those in the gut causing constipation, in the eye affecting accommodation, and in the bladder causing difficulty with micturition, and in the salivary and lacrimal glands causing dryness of the mouth and eyes.

Sympathetic block

A more selective effect can be produced by blocking the sympathetic system alone. Direct α-blockade has proved rather ineffective in hypertension largely because although the peripheral resistance is decreased the cardiac sympathetic effects are not blocked so that an increase in heart rate and cardiac output occur. Curiously β-blockers, such as propranolol, do lower the blood pressure by reducing cardiac output and have a place in the treatment of mild hypertension. The details of this action will be described later.

Selective block of sympathetic action is, however, best produced by the agents interfering with noradrenaline biosynthesis and release, namely **guanethidine** and **bethanidine** and **methyldopa.** Because these drugs interfere with the sympathetic neurone rather than with the sympathetic receptor they are effective in blocking both α and β types of effect. They therefore reduce blood pressure by effects both on peripheral vessels and on the heart. Because they leave the vagal effects intact orthostatic hypotension is less marked due to this route of compensation being still available, and indeed there remains available a reduced but significant tachycardia in exercise. These three drugs are the most satisfactory ones available for the treatment of hypertension and are relatively free of side actions, except for rather frequent development of hypersensitivity to methyldopa.

Reserpine produces hypotension in part by its action on peripheral sympathetic neurones, interfering with the storage of noradrenaline, but since the drug is also a sedative it is quite likely that part of the hypotensive effect is due to a depression of the vasomotor centre.

Clonidine

Clonidine (dichlorophenylaminoimidazoline) is a very potent hypotensive substance. There is clear evidence from injection into the vertebral arteries and the cerebral ventricles that most of the hypotensive effect is central in origin and is due to a reduced sympathetic tone which acts through reduced tone in both resistance and capacitance vessels as well as reduced sympathetic drive to the heart. The drug is so powerful that less than a milligram in man or ten micrograms in a cat will produce substantial effects. In addition there are weak α-adrenergic effects peripherally and for this reason the blood pressure rises briefly after intravenous injection before the central effects have developed. Clonidine finds some use in the treatment of hypertension but has side effects in sedation and dryness of the mouth. It is also useful in some cases of migraine.

Veratrin alkaloids

The ester alkaloids from Veratrum species, of which **veratridine** may be taken as typical, have a complicated pharmacology. Their major action is to affect excitable structures, decreasing the threshold for discharge and often causing single impulses to be converted into bursts. Repetitive firing is associated with a large increase in the negative after-potential of the the spike which acts as a source of depolarization for excitation. The ionic mechanism of this change is apparently by an interference with the mechanism which shuts off sodium permeability after an action potential. The effects of veratrin can be reversed by lowering the external sodium concentration.

When veratridine is injected intravenously there is pronounced bradycardia and a fall of blood pressure. The bradycardia is vagal in origin and is abolished by atropine, which, however, does not affect the hypotension. The cardiovascular response is totally abolished by bilateral vagal section. This suggested that veratridine caused stimulation of vagal afferents. These have been localized by the demonstration that very small doses of veratridine injected into the coronary arteries or applied to the visceral pericardium produce the same cardiovascular effects as much larger amounts injected intravenously. The afferent fibres concerned originate mainly in the left ventricle and its overlying pericardium and the effect of veratridine on such fibres may be demonstrated by isolating single fibres from the vagal fibres coming from the heart. Some fibres show phasic activity, firing in systole and being silent during the rest of the cardiac cycle; after administration of veratridine, firing is continuous and at a high rate. The cardiovascular response to veratrin was first described by Bezold in 1867 and the receptors in the heart are therefore usually called Bezold receptors. This type of action is not confined to veratrin but is also found with a variety of phenylguanides and amidines and with serotonin. Veratrin is not used much therapeutically because of the small margin between the therapeutic and the side-effects, the most consistent of which is nausea and vomiting.

Hydralazine

Hydralazine produces general vasodilatation accompanied by tachycardia. Its mode of action is far from settled but appears to be in large measure due to a direct reduction of tone in arterioles, with some depression of vasomotor centre activity. The drug has been extensively used in hypertension but has been dropped mainly because of a wide range of serious side actions including jaundice, pancytopenia, polyneuritis, and a syndrome resembling chronic lupus erythematosus.

Nitrites and nitrates

Inorganic nitrites have a general relaxant effect on smooth muscle, and this applies to all elements of the peripheral vascular system. However, the veins and venules are particularly affected. The effect on the circulation is to cause a marked fall of blood pressure with tachycardia, cutaneous vasodilatation especially noticeable in the blush area where the skin temperature rises, arterial pulsation becomes marked, and a throbbing headache develops. The blood pressure and heart rate changes are accentuated in the upright posture and fainting may ensue. These changes follow mainly from the decrease in tone in the venules and veins increasing the capacity of this system, and hence causing peripheral blood pooling. Thus despite the arteriolar dilatation and hence greater transmission of arterial pressure to the veins the venous return to the heart is not increased in the supine position and is reduced in the upright position. The change in cardiac output follows the change in venous return. Because the peripheral resistance is reduced the cardiac work is also reduced.

The mechanism of action of the nitrite ion is uncertain, thus in common with cyanide and azide it reacts with cytochrome oxidase and it is of interest that these agents are also powerful vasodilators, and it may be that the interference with oxygen transfer in the cell is responsible for the pharmacological action. However, other factors must be involved as nitrites have a much smaller effect on general oxygen utilization otherwise they would not have their relative freedom from toxicity. Indeed, the main toxic effect of nitrites is due to oxidation of haemoglobins to methaemoglobin.

Qualitatively identical actions to those of inorganic nitrites are produced by aliphatic nitrites such as **amyl nitrite.** This is a volatile substance (b.p. 130° C) which can be inhaled and is rapidly absorbed from the lungs thus producing effects in a very short time. Other aliphatic nitrates such as **glyceryl trinitrate, pentaerythritol tetranitrate,** and **triethanolamine nitrate** have similar actions and are much more potent than inorganic nitrite. It was formerly believed that these substances must first be reduced to nitrites (by the enzyme, polynitrate reductase) before acting. Doubt is thrown on this both by the high activity and rapid action of the ester nitrates and the lack of correlation between the amount of nitrite produced and the intensity of action. There remains the possibility that the ester nitrates owe their high activity to rapid penetration into the target cells with local reduction to nitrites.

The ester nitrates have a prolonged duration of action, whereas sodium nitrite produces effects for less than 1 hour, the effects of pentaerythritol tetranitrate and triethanolamine nitrate (trolnitrate) last for about 6 hours.

Nitrites are a group of drugs to which marked tolerance develops in a few days and becomes maximal after a few weeks, but sensitivity is restored on withdrawal.

ANGINA PECTORIS

Angina pectoris follows the structural narrowing of one or more coronary arteries. In its milder form it is an angina of effort in that the pain develops when an extra task is carried out and ceases rapidly if rest is taken. In severe cases the effort that can be undertaken is very restricted. The pain is due to anoxia in the ventricles affecting directly or indirectly pain afferents in the myocardium. During exercise cardiac work is increased and if the myocardial blood flow cannot be increased in proportion to the oxygen utilization the oxygen tension will fall. Vasodilator drugs like the nitrites enable a patient to undertake more severe exercise before pain develops. Since nitrites can readily be shown to increase coronary flow in isolated perfused hearts it was assumed for many years that nitrites must be increasing exercise tolerance in angina by coronary dilation. However, since it has been shown in intact animals and in man that it is more common to see a small fall in coronary flow rather than any sustained rise when nitrites are administered, it is very doubtful if this is true. Furthermore, the pathological changes in the coronary artery system affected by atheroma lead to rigidity of the larger vessels which will not be dilatable by any drugs. The remaining possibility is further dilation of very small vessels and of collaterals. It is possible that these vessels may be dilated more by nitrites than by direct effects of anoxia and myocardial metabolites but the changes are probably marginal. If nitrites do not increase exercise tolerance by dilating the coronary vessels what alternative have we? We noted above that by the combination of action on peripheral venules and arterioles nitrites reduced peripheral resistance without normally increasing cardiac output, resulting in a diminution in cardiac work and hence in cardiac oxygen requirements. It seems likely therefore that nitrites act more by reducing the demand for oxygen by the myocardium than by increasing the supply.

Because of the brief duration of angina of effort there is little value in treating an attack with nitrites which therefore have their main use in prophylaxis, i.e. in enabling individuals to do more than they could otherwise. For this purpose tablets of **glyceryl trinitrate** are chewed, allowing rapid and efficient absorption from the buccal mucosa. By contrast, if the tablets are swallowed absorption is slower and much more irregular. The longer-acting nitrates (pentaerythritol tetranitrate and triethanolamine nitrate) are swallowed rather than chewed.

Recently it has been found that the β-adrenergic blocking agent **propranolol** is effective in angina. The mode of action of this drug is interesting; it does not dilate the coronaries, indeed there are suggestions that it may even reduce coronary flow, nor does it reduce peripheral resistance, but the increase in cardiac work in exercise is in large part mediated by the cardiac sympathetic nerves which increase heart rate, and contractility. By enabling exercise to proceed with a reduced increase in cardiac work propranolol increases exercise tolerance. Since the effects of nitrites are different these drugs are complementary and may be used with profit in combination. A third drug with some value in angina is **dipyridamole**. The present evidence suggests that this drug acts by potentiating the effects of normal metabolic products such as purine nucleotides which are natural coronary dilators.

THE CARDIAC GLYCOSIDES

The rational use of digitalis (foxglove) leaf in cardiac conditions is due to William Withering. He was struck by cases of dropsy (oedema) that had been improved by herbal remedies and came to the conclusion that the active ingredient was foxglove. He then systematically explored the use of the drug, the preparation and standardization of extracts, described many of the toxic effects, and recognized that the improvement of the patient was associated with an improvement in the pulse. He published his results in 1785 in a book entitled *An Account of the Foxglove, and Some of its Medical Uses.* The main active principle of purple foxglove is digitoxin, a glycoside of a sterol lactone, digitoxigenin, which is known as the aglycone. Similar substances with actions on the heart are found not only in *Digitalis* species, but in a number of *Strophanthus* species, and most curious of all, secretions of the skin of toads. The latter is the basis of a traditional Chinese remedy Ch'an su.

A large number of active glycosides have been isolated which differ in the substituent groups and position of unsaturated groups in the sterol, in the structure of the lactone, and in the sugar residues. The sterol skeleton is a peculiar one differing from that in adrenal steroids. In adrenal steroids the A and C and B and D rings are coplanar whereas in the cardiac glycosides the A and D rings are coplanar giving an over-all structure that is much less planar.

The actions of digitalis on the heart may be divided into ones on contractility (inotropic) and on rate and rhythm (chronotropic). The inotropic effct is readily shown under conditions in which the ventricular muscle is hypodynamic, i.e. producing less tension than usual. This can be seen in the ordinary Langendorff preparation in which the coronary arteries are perfused with Krebs salt solution, or when isolated papillary muscles from man or other animals are stimulated *in vitro.* With relatively large does of ouabain the effects are well developed in a few minutes, but with smaller doses the effects take rather longer to appear. The counterpart of this effect is seen in the intact animal or man when the ventricular contractility is low because of anoxia or muscle damage. The cardiac glycosides shift the filling curve up in the same way that adrenaline does, so that the stroke output and work rise for a given diastolic filling pressure, and also the maximum stroke work is increased. The alternative way of looking at this is to say that to maintain the same stroke ouput, a lower filling pressure is needed, and hence the pressure in the venous system falls and if oedema is present it will be removed. A more subtle effect on contractility is a consistent increase in the rate of development of tension in the ventricle and this is seen in the normodynamic as well as the hypodynamic myocardium.

The heart rate is slowed in the isolated beating heart, but the slowing is greater *in vivo* and this additional slowing is attributable to an increased rate of discharge of the vagal efferents to the heart, due to a direct action of digitalis on the vagal nucleus; a bradycardia dvelops when cardiac glycosides are applied directly to the floor of the fourth ventricle in the neighbourhood of the vagal nuclei. In addition to these effects the glycosides potentiate the effects of peripheral vagus stimulation. The vagal slowing of the heart by the glycosides can be removed by atropine administration but the direct effect remains. When digitalis is given in heart failure in therapeutic doses these effects on cardiac rate are not of significance as factors leading to improvement of cardiac function. Indeed, the slowing of the heart that is usually seen as heart failure improves is secondary to the improved function, with a consequent reduction in the sympathetic drive to the heart. However, with increased dosage chronotropic effects become important and these may evolve into partial and finally complete atrioventricular dissocation due to depression of the excitability of the nodal tissue of the atrioventricular bundle, In addition extra systoles arising from the ventricular muscle may occur, a characteristic form being bigeminy or coupled beats in which a normally conducted beat is followed at a short interval by an extra systole. With lethal doses the ventricle may fibrillate or be arrested in systole.

It was noticed by Mackenzie that digitalis was particularly effective in heart failure in which the atria were fibrillating and the ventricle was beating excessively fast. A marked slowing of the ventricular rate is produced due to a direct effect on the excitability of the bundle tissue reducing the passage of impulses arising in the subnormal phase of excitability; the direct effect on the atrium is usually to increase the rate of fibrillation.

The cellular mechanism of action of the cardiac glycosides is complex and still incompletely known. However, it is likely that all the actions will eventually be found to stem from the highly specific action of the glycosides on membrane bound ATPase. Membrane bound ATPase is an enzyme found in cell membranes which is activated by sodium and potassium ions; in intact cells enzyme activity depends on the sodium concentration inside the cell and the potassium concentration outside the cell, the enzyme is able to split phosphate from adenosine triphosphate although it is likely that its function in the cell is to transfer a group from ATP to some membrane component. This enzyme is inhibited by cardiac glycosides in the same range of concentrations required to produce the inotropic effect. Furthermore, there is a striking parallelism between the potency of the drugs as inhibitors of the enzyme and as positive inotropic agents. The cardiac glycosides also inhibit the active transport of sodium by cell membranes and it is therefore likely that these two actions are related either because the operation of ATPase supplies the energy for the sodium pump or because it combines both functions. The most obvious consequence of inhibiting the sodium pump is that the intracellular concentration of sodium rises and that of potassium falls. This may explain the small decrease in resting potential and decreased velocity of contraction, but it is hard to see how it could cause an increase in contractile response directly. On the other hand, it has been established that cardiac glycosides increase the rate of calcium entry with each beat and since there is good evidence that contractile force is dependent on intracellular calcium release, a plausible theory is that the rise in intracellular sodium secondarily facilitates calcium entry which is responsible for the inotropic effect. In fact, cardiac glycosides are known to depress a number of membrane processes which transport substances into cells and these processes are all dependent on extracellular sodium for activity. It should be noted that the effects of digitalis on ionic movements are not restricted to the heart but are exerted on all tissues. However, their effects on the physiological state of the tissue will be related to the turnover of ions in the tissue.

The glycosides that are in common use are

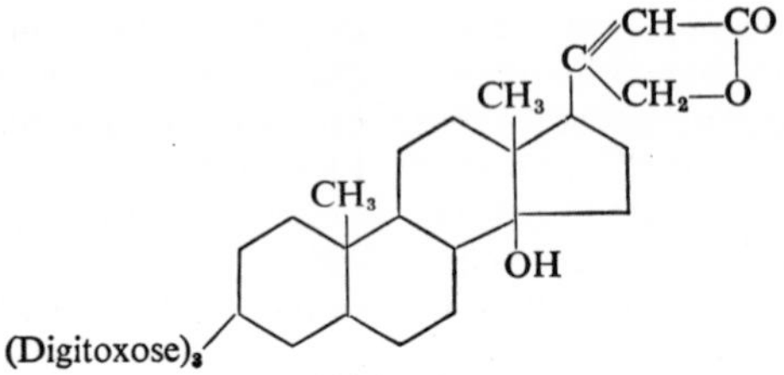

Digitoxin

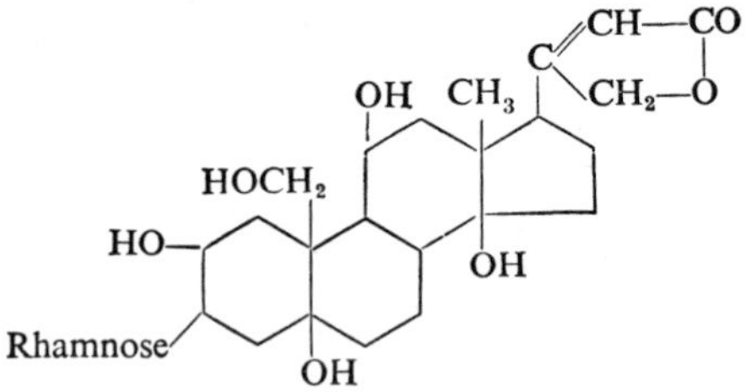

Ouabain (Strophanthin G)

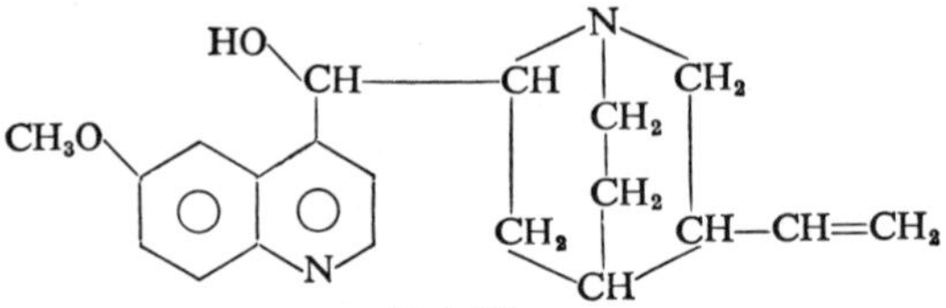

Quinidine

Fig. 10.3.

digoxin and **lanatoside C** from *Digitalis lanata*, **digitoxin** from *Digitalis purpurea*, and **ouabain** (strophanthin G) from *Strophanthus gratus*. They have very similar actions in very similar dosage and differ mainly in the rapidity with which effects come on and how long they last; in order of speed and shortness of action they range from ouabain, the fastest, through digoxin and lanatoside C to digitoxin which has effects lasting for about 2 weeks.

In therapeutic use the effects are produced by a loading dose given either by mouth or by injection followed by a daily maintenance dose which in the case of digoxin is about one-quarter of the loading dose.

It has been said that every patient who is on chronic administration of cardiac glycosides suffers from toxic effects at some time or another; this situation exists because the toxic effects of digitalis are those of overdose rather then hypersensitivity or cytotoxicity and in heart failure there is a natural tendency to obtain as much improvement in cardiac function as the drug is capable of giving. Nausea and vomiting are common and are mainly due to stimulation of the chemoreceptor trigger zone in the medulla; as mentioned above arrhythmias may occur and bigeminy is a sign of overdosage as is excessive slowing of the rate. Digitalis toxicity depends on the levels of potassium and calcium in the plasma, and thus toxic effects may be precipitated by a diuretic such as chlorothiazide which causes hypokalaemia; contrariwise the toxic effects may be antagonized by the cautious use of potassium salts. Propranolol has proved a useful agent in dealing with digitalis arrhythmias.

ANTIARRHYTHMIC DRUGS

Arrhythmias are due to the development of new pacemakers in the myocardium distinct from the normal pacemakers in the nodal tissue. In nodal tissue the membrane potential is not constant during diastole but gradully falls ('the diastolic drift') and at a critical potential level a regenerative response develops with the initiation of an action potential. In non-nodal tissue the diastolic drift is absent and no intrinsic rhythmicity is present. However, in injured myocardial tissue pacemaker activity may develop in non-nodal tissue and this may lead to a very high rate of discharge as in atrial or ventricular fibrillation, a lower rate as in flutter or paroxysmal tachycardia or isolated extrasystoles. These effects can be counteracted by agents which: (1) raise the threshold for excitation; and (2) prolong the refractory period.

The first effect means that a greater diastolic drift is needed for excitation, the second that the possibility of re-excitation from adjoining active areas of membrane is reduced. The agents that produce these effects are local anaesthetics and the effects are due mainly to a reduced sensitivity of the membrane sodium carrier to depolarization and a reduced ability to reload the sodium carrier. The effects of antiarrhythmic drugs are always accompained by a reduced contractility. The first agent to be used for this purpose was quinine but it was subsequently found that the stereoisomer **quinidine** was more effective and less toxic. **Procaine** was later found to be effective but suffered from the disadvantage of a very brief action and excessive central nervous actions. Replacement of the ester linkage in procaine by an amide grouping gave the stable substance **procainamide** with reduced central side-actions. **Lignocaine** administered by intravenous infusion is the most effective antiarrhythmic of all, and is particularly of use after cardiac surgery and myocardial infarction. More recently the β-blocking drug **propranolol** has been found to be a very effective antiarrhythmic agent. There does not appear to be any necessary connexion with β-blocking action as some β-blockers are devoid of antiarrhythmic action, and in the stereoisomers of propanolol while the (+) isomer is nearly devoid of β-blocking activity it is a potent antiarrhythmic. **Practolol** is also used. Recently it has been shown that **phenytoin** (*Dilantin*) is effective in ventricular ecotopic rhythms and in paroxysmal atrial tachycardia.

In summary, the desirable antiarrhythmics appear to be local anaesthetics with minimal central action.

Antiarrhythmics are used to control paroxysmal tachycardia, the showers of extrasystoles that may arise in cardiac infarction, and to convert atrial fibrillation and flutter to normal rhythm. In this case the heart rate is first controlled by doses of digitalis adequate to depress the bundle of His. Conversion is easiest in atrial arrhythmias of recent origin, but these also revert to the arrhythmia rather readily.

Quinidine is a rather dangerous drug due mainly to its marked tendency to cause hypersensitivity-type toxic reactions.

FURTHER READING

Dawes, G. S. (1952). Experimental cardiac arrhythmias and quinidine-like drugs, *Pharmacol. Rev.* **4,** 43.

Glynn, I. M. (1964). The action of cardiac glycosides on ion movements, *Pharmacol. Rev.* **16,** 381.

Pickering, G. W. (1961). *The Treatment of Hypertension*, Springfield, Ill.

Rowe, G. G. (1968). Pharmacology of the coronary circulation, *Ann. Rev. Pharmacol.* **8,** 95.

Sekeres, L. and Papp, J. G. (1968). Antiarrhythmic compounds, *Prog. drug Res.* **12,** 292.

Sonnenblick, E. H., Braunwald, E., and Morrow, A. G. (1965). The contractile properties of human heart muscle, *J. clin. Invest.* **44,** 966.

Stoll, A. (1949). The cardioactive glycosides, *J. Pharm. Pharmacol.* **1,** 849.

Trautwein, W. (1963). Generation and conduction of impulses in the heart, *Pharmacol. Rev.* **14,** 277.

Wilbrandt, W. (1963). *New Aspects of Cardiac Glycosides*, London.

11

BODY TEMPERATURE AND THE ANTIPYRETIC-ANALGESICS

ALTHOUGH it is generally recognized that body temperature is regulated it is less commonly recognized that the temperature of the body is not uniform; for instance, the skin temperature is variable over different parts of the body surfaces, being lowest at the extremities, and is in general much cooler than the core temperature measured in the interior of the thorax or abdomen. Furthermore, surface temperature will vary markedly with environmental conditions. It is difficult to know which should be adopted as the reference temperature of the body since, for example, liver temperature is influenced by the rate of metabolism in that organ and rectal temperature by bacterial metabolism in the rectal contents. There is a lot to be said in really accurate studies for measuring temperature at the ear drum by a thermocouple placed in the external auditory meatus. However, in experimental situations, rectal temperature is usually accepted as a reasonable measure of core temperature.

Heat is produced in the body as an inevitable by-product of metabolic processes and the mechanical work of muscular contraction. Heat is exchanged with the environment by the processes of radiation, convection and conduction, and by the evaporation of water from the skin and respiratory passages. In a resting individual whose temperature regulation mechanims are inactivated the body temperature remains constant if the environmental temperature is about 30° C, but at lower temperatures the body temperature cools at a rate proportional to the difference of temperatures from 30° C and conversely rises if the ambient temperature is above this level. In the normal individual, body temperature is conserved over a wide range of temperature by regulatory mechanisms affecting both heat production and heat loss. Heat production is increased in response to a fall in body temperature almost entirely by an increase in muscular activity in the form of involuntary shivering or by voluntary action such as swinging the arms, whereas heat loss is altered by change in surface temperature and blood flow and by sweating. In a cold environment the blood flow through the skin is reduced and blood is shunted into the deep vessels in the core of the limb; this reduced carriage of heat to the skin allows the skin temperature to fall while reducing heat loss from the body core—the converse occurs in hot environments where radiative and conductive losses are made more effective by a rise in skin temperature.

Temperatures are sensed both by central thermoreceptors in the hypothalamus and in the periphery where the sensitivity is mainly to the temperature gradient. Regulation is integrated by two interconnected centres in the hypothalamus, the more anterior of which brings in compensatory mechanisms for hot environments whereas the posterior region is concerned with heat conservation.

Little is understood of the mechanisms which determine that the core temperature is normally regulated at the level of 36–37·5° C. However, in fever the regulation is set to a higher level. At the onset of a fever shivering occurs, the skin is pale, and the individual feels cold, i.e. heat production has been increased and heat loss diminished and in consequence the temperature rises rapidly. As the temperature rises the usual heat loss mechanisms come into play, and the skin vessels dilate, but heat production remains high in part due to the increased rate of metabolism secondary to the rise in temperature. The subject feels hot at this stage. Fever is usually due to infection with microorganisms and can be reproduced by the injection of extracts of bacteria containing substances called pyrogens. These are of several kinds but the most active are lipopolysaccharides. They are of importance in pharmacology because solutions prepared for injections should be free of them. Pyrogen-free water is prepared by doubly distilling water and collecting under strictly aseptic conditions.

Body temperature is raised by drugs causing an increase in metabolism. Examples are **2,4-dinitrophenol** and **3,5-dinitro-orthocresol** (DNOC); the latter is a pesticide. These substances uncouple phosphorylation and stimulate tissue respiration. The result is an uneconomical process by which more oxygen and substrates are used and hence more heat produced with little return in the form of high energy phosphate compounds (ATP, ADP, phosphagen, etc). Many phenols have this property including salicylic acid which paradoxically increases body temperature in high doses. Thyroxine also raises temperature by increasing metabolism in part by an uncoupling action, but it has other actions on metabolism as yet ill defined.

Convulsants increase temperature secondary to the excessive muscular activity and hence increase in heat production; lesser rises in temperature result from drugs that cause restlessness, such as **adrenaline, amphetamine, cocaine,** and **β-tetrahydronaphthylamine.** In atropine poisoning hyperthermia may be present due to similar causes. Atropine in ordinary doses does not raise the body temperature except when the ambient temperature is high or during exercise when heat loss by sweating is dominant.

Body temperature is lowered by many drugs having central actions: for instance, in deep general anaesthesia temperature regulation is almost completely lost so that if the operating room temperature is low hypothermia can develop; equally the wraps covering the patient may interfere with heat loss. **Alcohol** also interferes with temperature regulation partly by its central action and also by causing vasodilatation of skin vessels. It is for this reason that alcohol gives the feeling of warmth while simultaneously lowering the temperature. This combination of properties can make it dangerous medication in severe cold weather. **Morphine** and other narcotic analgesics have a similar effect. More striking still is the fall of body temperature induced by **chlorpromazine** and some other phenothiazine drugs. This seems to be mainly due to vasodilatation in the skin but there is an undoubted central component. These actions have been of use in producing hypothermia for cardiac and intracranial surgery. If one attempts to cool an individual by surface cooling, the degree of cooling is restricted by the reactive vasoconstriction and increased metabolism; chlorpromazine largely eliminates these reactive effects and enables cooling to be smoother and more rapid. Naturally all these responses to hypothermic drugs are seen in heightened degree in pyrexial patients, and formerly opium and alcohol were both given to induce sweating and lower the body temperature.

A response of quite a different character is produced by the miscellaneous drugs of the antipyretic-analgesic group such as **acetylsalicylic acid (aspirin), acetanilide, paracetamol, phenacetin, phenazone,** and **phenylbutazone.** These substances do not lower the body temperature in normal individuals, indeed as pointed out earlier if the dose is large enough they may raise the temperature by increasing metabolism. However, in pyrexia, they produce peripheral dilatation, abundant perspiration, and a prompt fall of temperature. Identical effects are produced with fever due to injected pyrogens.

It is commonly said that these drugs can reset the thermostat when it is set too high by infection but this is merely conjuring with words and the mechanism of action is really not understood. Furthermore, while these drugs will make the fevered patient more comfortable it is still not clear whether they favour or retard recovery from the infection itself.

Salicylates

The salicylates are an example of a drug of very simple chemical structure but with complex and perplexing pharmacology.

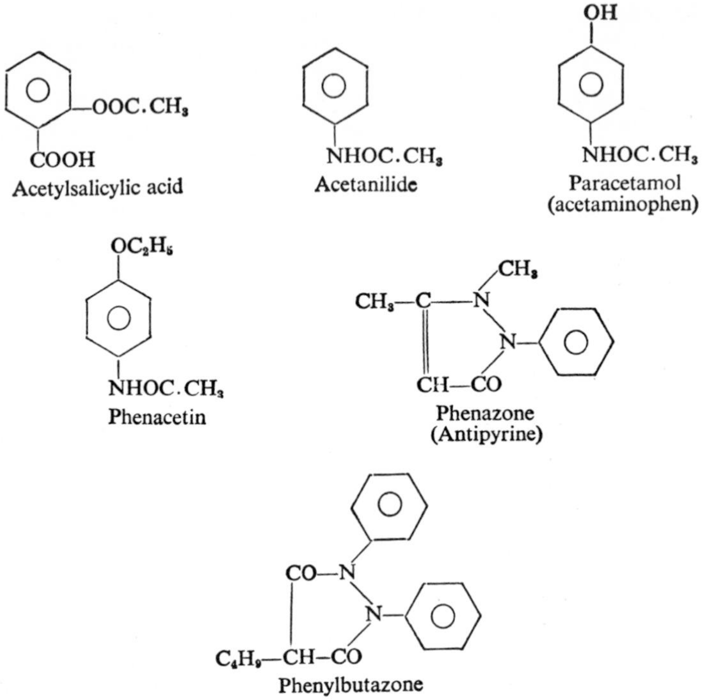

Acetylsalicylic acid

Acetanilide

Paracetamol (acetaminophen)

Phenacetin

Phenazone (Antipyrine)

Phenylbutazone

Fig. 11.1. Antipyreticanalgesics.

The antipyretic action of willow bark (*Salix alba*) was known to the ancients, and in the early nineteenth century a glucoside of salicylic acid, salicin, was isolated from it and this was followed shortly by the isolation of salicylic acid which was then shown to be antipyretic. Widespread use followed the recognition of its analgesic activity and the development of a cheap synthesis.

The analgesic action of salicylate is of a different character from that of the opiates, for whereas the latter do not truly eliminate the sensation of pain, but rather alter the psychological reaction to pain, so that the individual becomes indifferent to pain, the salicylates within their limitation cause a genuine analgesia. They are especially effective in aching low-grade pain, e.g. headache, toothache, joint pain and do not have much effect in visceral or wound pain.

There seems to be a ceiling to the intensity of pain that can be suppressed as there is also for opiates. As pointed out in Chapter 4, the experimental assessment of pain and analgesics is very unsatisfactory and this is especially the case with the salicylate type of analgesic. Almost the only test in which their analgesic action has been demonstrated unequivocally is tooth pain produced by electrical stimulation of the dental pulp. There is no question that salicylates are also effective in reducing the malaise accompanying infections and are widely believed to have a tranquillizing effect. However, analgesia by salicylates is not accompanied by any really striking changes of mood, especially not by euphoria, unlike that produced by the opiates. The paucity of overt central effects has led to the suspicion that at least part of the action is a peripheral one on sensory endings. In particular the anti-inflammatory action of salicylate and its effectiveness in countering some of the actions of bradykinin which is generally believed to have a significant role in the phenomena of inflammation have tended to support this proposition. However, it is rendered more dubious by comparison with paracetamol or acetanilide, on the one hand, which are good analgesics but practically devoid of anti-inflammatory action, and phenylbutazone, a poor analgesic, but a powerful anti-inflammatory agent, on the other hand. This does not suggest a close correlation between anti-inflammatory action and analgesia. The anti-inflammatory action is an important feature of salicylate action and leads to decrease in swelling and heat; in the inflamed joints of rheumatic fever, a similar and more powerful effect is produced by adrenal corticoids. It is interesting that although the action of salicylates in this disease has been a major part of therapy for more than 50 years it is still quite uncertain whether the evolution of rheumatic carditis is favourably influenced by it.

Salicylates have well-marked metabolic effects the most prominent of which is the uncoupling of oxidative phosphorylation, which raises the basal metabolic rate; it also has a hyperglycaemic action possibly mediated by adrenaline released through hypothalamic stimulation, and the formation of glycogen is reduced and the glycogen content of muscle and liver is depleted. This is not an unmixed effect and in some circumstances the blood sugar may be lowered; for this reason salicylates have been used in diabetes but are not very effective.

The commonly used preparations of salicylates are **aspirin** (acetylsalicylic acid) and **sodium salicylate,** although combinations with other drugs such as **phenacetin, paracetamol, codeine,** and **caffeine** are popular and it is now known that aspirin-like drugs probably owe their effect to an inhibitor of prostaglandin synthesis (see Chapter 9). There is little evidence of genuine potentiation in these mixtures, which can be replaced without loss by a larger dose of aspirin or paracetamol.

The pK of salicylic acid is 3·0 so that in the stomach much of the acid is in the non-ionized form. Since this is the form most readily absorbed, it would be expected that absorption from the stomach would be rapid. However, this is limited by the low solubility of the acid (0·3 per cent) so that absorption will be limited by the rate of dissolution; in the case of tableted preparations the rate of absorption is increased if the particles in the tablets are very small. A considerable part of the salicylate will be absorbed in the small gut despite the tiny proportion ($<$0·01 per cent) that is un-ionized. The major route of metabolism is by conjugation to give salicylglycine (salicyluric acid) and glycuronides. Conversion to gentisic acid (2.5-dihydroxybenzoic acid) is minimal. Of the total excreted in the urine more than half is in the form of unchanged salicylic acid.

Aspirin is absorbed in the same way as salicylic acid but it is rapidly deacetylated in the blood stream, so that after absorption it is equivalent to free salicylate.

The excretion of salicylates is such as to give a half-time of about 4–8 hours for the plasma concentration.

Toxic effects. Considering the enormous scale on which they are used (in the United States the average annual consumption is about 200 tablets per head) major toxic effects are uncommon, but minor toxic effects largely of gastro-intestinal type are very common.

Epigastric discomfort is common as is minor bleeding due to gastric erosion. If gastroscopy is undertaken after a dose of aspirin, injection and small haemorrhages may be seen in the neighbourhood of the undissolved aspirin particles deposited on the gastric mucosa. Occasionally major gastric bleeding occurs. With large doses there may be ringing in the ears, dizziness, deafness, drowsiness, and confusion. This syndrome is called salicylism and is similar to the pattern of toxicity produced by quinine. Salicylates may also produce allergic disorders and, for instance, may precipitate asthma in susceptible individuals. They may also produce renal damage as evidenced by increased urinary excretion of epithelial cells and leucocytes.

The major toxic effects of large doses of salicylates are due to disturbances of respiration and acid–base balance. Respiration is stimulated and air hunger may occur which is difficult to distinguish from that in diabetic ketosis, the overbreathing leads to a fall in the arterial p_{CO_2} and a respiratory alkalosis. Compensation occurs by bicarbonate loss in the urine so that the plasma bicarbonate falls. In addition lactic acid and keto acids accumulate in the blood due to interference with normal carbohydrate and fat metabolism. The patient will also be hyperthermic. The blood concentration of salicylate will usually be greater than 50 mg per cent (~4 mEq/l). The removal of the excessive body burden of salicylate is favoured by administration of sodium bicarbonate which increases the urinary excretion. Salicylates are not uncommonly taken in large amounts in suicidal attempts.

Phenacetin and paracetamol

These two drugs have the same application as salicylates to the relief of minor pain and malaise, are as effective and are less likely to cause gastric upsets, but they have their own toxic effects. In particular phenacetin is under a cloud at present owing to reports from Sweden, where the drug is very popular, of the development of interstitial nephritis with papillary necrosis. Paracetamol appears to be free from this toxic effect. Both of these drugs may cause cyanosis due to methaemoglobin formation and may shorten red cell life and hence lead to anaemia.

Mefenamic acid and **flufenamic acid** are recent drugs with aspirin-like activity whose usefulness is still to be determined. **Phenazone** (antipyrine) is little used because of its great liability to produce hypersensitivity reactions.

Phenylbutazone

The anti-inflammatory actions of phenylbutazone were discovered by accident when the drug was used to increase the solubility of amidopyrine. It is much more effective in rheumatoid arthritis and gout than salicylates but it is a poorly tolerated drug with a wide range of toxic effects, notably gastro-intestinal disturbances, including peptic ulceration, hypersensitivity reactions, and bone marrow disorders including fatal aplastic anaemia. It is reserved for cases that are unresponsive to other drugs and then used in short courses to reduce the risks.

Indomethacin has similar effects to phenylbutazone and similar indications. It also produces severe gastro-intestinal side-effects and vertigo but does not produce bone marrow depression.

FURTHER READING

Euler, C. von (1961). Physiology and pharmacology of temperature regulation, *Pharmacol. Rev.* **13,** 361.

Gross, M. and Greenberg, L. A. (1948). *The salicylates,* New Haven.

Hardy, J. D. (1955). Control of heat loss and heat production in physiologic temperature regulation, *Harvey Lect.* **49,** 242.

Newburgh, L. H. (ed.) (1949). *Physiology of heat regulation and the science of clothing,* Philadelphia.

Smith, M. J. H. (1959). Salicylates and metabolism, *J. Pharm. Pharmacol.* **11,** 705.

Smith, M. J. H. (1963). In *Salicylates,* ed. Dixon, A. St. J. *et al.,* London.

12

ALIMENTARY CANAL

GASTRIC SECRETION

GASTRIC juice has a high concentration of hydrogen and chloride ions. Hydrions are highly concentrated in the parietal cells of the stomach, the basic reaction being:

$$H_2O + CO_2 \rightarrow HCO_3^- + H^+$$

Because hydrions are being removed from the extracellular fluid, a surfeit of HCO_3^- is left behind and if gastric fluid is lost by vomiting, then a metabolic alkalosis will result.

The digestive properties of gastric juice are due mainly to the presence of pepsin and the secretion of gastric acid provides an environment of pH 1·5–4 which is optimal for pepsin activity.

The secretion of gastric acid and of pepsin is controlled by both humoral and nervous factors. Stimulation of the vagus nerve, or the action of muscarinic drugs, increases gastric secretion and, through this nerve, secretion is affected by various reflexes initiated by gustatory, olfactory, and other stimuli. The vagus is also important in controlling and potentiating the action of the hormone **gastrin** on the oxyntic acid-secreting cells and the pepsin secreting cells of the stomach.

Gastrin is secreted from the antral region of the stomach in response to the stimulus of food in the stomach and it has a powerful stimulating effect on gastric secretion.

Gastrin has been purified and found to consist of two polypeptides, known as gastrin I and gastrin II, both of which are potent stimulants of gastric secretion. The composition of gastrin I is Glu–Gly–Pro–Tyr–Met–Glu–Glu–Glu–Glu–Glu–Ala–Tyr–Gly–Tyr–Met–Asp–Phe(NH_2). Gastrin II is identical except for the addition of an —SO_3H group on the 12th amino acid (tyrosine).

Although these peptides are normally both stimulants of gastric acid secretion, they may, under some conditions, actually inhibit acid secretion but at the same time increase pepsin secretion, pancreatic secretions, and gastric tone. Whether these effects of gastrin are of physiological importance is not yet known.

Injected histamine is also a powerful stimulant of gastric acid secretion but it is not known whether endogenously released histamine plays a role in the excitation of oxyntic cells or whether gastrin stimulates histamine release near or within oxyntic cells to cause their secretion. The possibility of histamine being the final link in the excitation of oxyntic cells cannot be decided with our present meagre knowledge of the mechanism of action of, and interaction between, gastrin, histamine, and acetylcholine released from the vagus.

Peptic ulcers

Gastric juice, with its high acidity and high pepsin content, is highly corrosive, but normally the stomach and upper intestinal walls are protected from its action by a mucosal layer. The development of an ulcer does not appear to depend on any one clear factor but seems frequently to be precipitated by stress conditions occurring over long periods. The patient with a duodenal ulcer has a resting secretion of hydrochloric acid at least twice that of the normal person and the gastrin content of the antrum is also raised. In patients with gastric ulcers, however, the resting acid release is often below normal levels.

Despite much discussion, the usual primary treatment of peptic ulcers is with antacids. Undoubtedly antacids relieve the pain of the ulcer but this does not necessarily mean that the drug allows the ulcer to heal unless the gastric pH is constantly monitored and not allowed to fall lower than 4. The most effective antacids are the nonsystemic inorganic ones, particularly calcium carbonate and magnesium carbonate.

Since pepsin is probably involved in producing ulcers considerable work has been done to find specific anti-pepsin compounds. Some success has been obtained with a sulphated amylopectin and carbenoxolone, an extract of liquorice, appears to aid the healing of ulcers.

In more serious cases of ulceration other types of treatment are usually considered. A low protein content in the diet reduces secretogogue effects, and large meals, which would mechanically distend the stomach, should be avoided.

The use of anticholinergic compounds is controversial because of the side-effects accompanying any reduction in acid secretion, the most important of these is a reduction in gastric motility and emptying time and, while this may be an advantage in the case of a gastric ulcer, it does not speed the healing of a duodenal ulcer.

Drugs which antagonize H_2 receptors (Chapter 9) inhibit the gastric response to histamine and other secretory stimulants. Compounds such as burinamide, metiamide, and particularly cimetidine have been used to treat peptic ulcers and the results so far look most promising.

Surgical intervention in the form of vagotomy to reduce gastric secretion or antrectomy and gastric resection are only used in the most difficult cases.

Probably the most important advances in the treatment of peptic ulcers will result from our knowledge of the structure of gastrin and the synthesis of gastrin antagonists. Already a promising compound, thioacetamide, has been developed.

ANTACIDS

The normal concentration of hydrochloric acid in the gastric secretion is about 0·5 per cent. The volume secreted in 24 hours is about 1·5 litres and so there is no way to replace a deficiency in the acid of gastric juices by mouth. On the other hand, it is comparatively easy to neutralize the gastric acid, and pain which is due to hyperchlorhydria can be relieved in this way. Antacids are used for this purpose when the acid secretion is producing an irritant action or in order to allow the healing of damaged or ulcerated parts of the stomach, oesophagus, or duodenum. A good antacid should sufficiently neutralize free acidity but at the same time it should not cause systemic alkalosis or unpleasant side-effects such as the generation of very large quantities of gas. Food and milk are both useful non-systemic antacids.

Sodium bicarbonate is a systemic antacid used to secure quick relief from the discomfort of heartburn and dyspepsia. The reaction which occurs in the stomach is as follows:

$$NaHCO_3 + HCl \rightarrow NaCl + H_2O + CO_2$$

The neutralizing action does not last long and sodium bicarbonate is not usually the antacid of choice, especially if an antacid is to be administered for long periods. The evolved carbon dioxide distends the stomach and causes belching and protein digestion is impaired because pepsin is inactivated in alkaline and neutral solution. A more serious feature of prolonged sodium bicarbonate treatment is the possibility that large numbers of hydrions may be removed, causing systemic alkalosis.

Magnesium trisilicate acts as a non-systemic antacid and an adsorbent. As an adsorbent it is able to reduce the effects of acidity by forming a colloidal adsorbent gel in the stomach.

The hydrated silicic acid, formed in the stomach, passes into the intestine and its gelatinous nature may protect ulcerated tissue from attack by gastric acid. The antacid action of magnesium trisilicate is slow in onset but is prolonged and the stomach contents are usually stabilized at pH 4–6.

This compound is widely used in the treatment of peptic ulcers and it is non-toxic but may, in large doses, produce diarrhoea due to the action of soluble magnesium salts in the intestinal tract.

Other magnesium compounds used as antacids include **magnesium oxide** and **magnesium hydroxide.**

Aluminium hydroxide is widely used as an antacid or adsorbent in the form of a suspension, powder, or tablets.

After administration of this compound the pH of the stomach contents lies between pH 3·5 and 4·0. This is sufficient to inactivate pepsin. It is not absorbed through the intestine and so there is no risk of systemic alkalosis.

Aluminium hydroxide may cause constipation and is therefore often used in combination with magnesium hydroxide.

VOMITING

The act of vomiting is primarily protective and is designed to remove unwelcome substances from the stomach. Some animals, such as rodents, are not endowed with this faculty but in many animals, such as dogs and pigeons, it is well developed. Vomiting involves many parts of the body but is controlled by the vomiting centre in the medulla. The premonitory sensation, which is felt when this centre is being stimulated, but has not yet acted, is known as nausea. It is generally accompanied by salivation, bronchial secretion, sweating, and inhibition of gastric secretion, and many drugs have these effects in small doses and cause vomiting in large doses. In other words they act as sialagogues, expectorants, diaphoretics, and inhibitors of secretion in small doses and as emetics in large doses.

If the medullary vomiting centre is destroyed, vomiting cannot occur whatever stimulus is used. A second centre, known as the chemosensitive trigger zone of the medulla, appears to be the primary site of action of emetic drugs and if this region of the brain is destroyed these drugs no longer cause vomiting. Though the natural stimulus for vomiting is the presence of irritating substances in the stomach, the same effects can be produced by strong enough stimulation of almost any kind; overstimulation of the labyrinth (as occurs in motion-sickness), or of the sensory nerves from the heart or other viscera, and strong emotion, may all cause vomiting.

Many compounds cause vomiting by a central action but they are not used for this action. They include the cardiac glycosides, the veratrum alkaloids, anti-tumour drugs, apomorphine, and related compounds. If it is necessary to produce vomiting in a person in order to eject toxic substances from the stomach, the most simple methods are to give the patient a salt solution to drink or to place a finger in his oesophagus.

Reflex vomiting is caused by irritation of the gastro-intestinal tract and is abolished by destruction of the chemoreceptive trigger zone. Drugs which cause reflex vomiting when taken by mouth include copper sulphate, zinc sulphate, and mercuric chloride. When vomiting is due to irritation of the gastric mucosa it may cure itself by the removal of the irritant, but local methods to protect the mucous membrane are also sometimes effective. The neutralization of excess acid with alkalis may stop vomiting, particularly if it is associated with acidosis.

Many drugs with antihistamine actions act also as anti-emetics perhaps by virtue of their atropine-like action and their sedative effects.

Chlorpromazine is a potent anti-emetic and prevents vomiting caused by drugs, pregnancy, and inner ear disease. It has no effect in the prevention of motion-sickness.

DRUG WHICH RELIEVE MOTION-SICKNESS

The number of remedies for motion-sickness is legion, and none of them cure all cases, since some people are sea-sick by suggestion, some by stimulation of the labyrinth, some by stimulation of sensory nerves in the abdominal viscera, and some by other causes.

The agents which are most effective against motion-sickness often share with atropine the property of antagonizing the actions of muscarine on peripheral tissues and it is possible they act by paralysing cholinergic systems in the CNS.

The most effective drug in the treatment of motion-sickness is **hyoscine.** This is now widely used. It is taken before motion-sickness is likely to be encountered and its effects last 6 or 7 hours. High doses produce extremely unpleasant side-effects. Compounds of this type will also protect against vomiting induced by drugs.

Promethazine is effective against motion-sickness and vomiting induced by drugs. It is an antihistamine with atropine-like properties and may cause side-effects, including a dry mouth and blurred vision.

Other compounds used in the treatment or prevention of motion-sickness include:

> **Antazoline** (*Histostab, Antistin*), **chlorcyclizine** (*Di-paralene, Derazil, Histantin*), **dimenhydrinate** (*Dramamine*), **diphenhydramine** (*Benadryl*).

The last two compounds are particularly effective and useful anti-emetics.

BILE

The bile is continuously excreted by the liver and collected in the gall-bladder, where it is concentrated about ten times. Bile contains bile salts which are emulsifying agents and aid the absorption of fats and fat-soluble vitamins in the intestine. It also contains bile pigments which come from haemoglobin, inorganic salts, water, mucin, cholesterol, and lecithin. It may contain many other substances in small quantities, including many drugs which are excreted in this way.

The bile salts are reabsorbed from the intestine, so that they may circulate and be used again. In their absence, fats are not emulsified and are only poorly absorbed. When food is present in the duodenum the gall-bladder contracts and empties its contents down the bile-duct. This contraction is partly under nervous control and is partly due to circulating hormones. Stimulation of the vagus or the administration of drugs with muscarinic actions causes contraction of the gall-bladder and relaxation of the sphincter of Oddi at the lower end of the bile-duct.

A complicated train of events is involved in the hormonal control of bile secretion. The presence of fats in the duodenum causes the liberation of **cholecystokinin,** which causes a contraction of the gall-bladder. This throws the bile salts into the duodenum where they stimulate the liberation of **secretin,** which causes not only pancreatic secretion but also bile secretion in the liver, so that the gall-bladder is refilled. There are thus several ways in which drugs may act as cholagogues (choleretics) to increase the flow of bile.

The most effective choleretics are the bile salts themselves and they may be used to flush out the biliary ducts to remove small gall-stones or infections. They may occasionally be used to aid digestion. Preparations which contain the bile salts are: extract of ox bile, **sodium tauroglycocholate,** and **bilein** and all these may be used as choleretics. **Dehydrocholic acid** produces a watery bile and is used to treat flatulence and abdominal discomfort due to gall-bladder disease. It is also used to treat inflammatory conditions of the biliary system but is not used in the presence of obstructive jaundice.

PURGATIVES

The intestine makes movements of various kinds. Rhythmic contractions of the longitudinal muscles are called pendulum movements and they pull the mucous membrane back and forwards over the food. Rhythmic movements of the circular muscles cause segmentation which mixes the food. The progression of food down the intestine is not increased by either of these movements and is entirely due to peristalsis. This is controlled by Auerbach's plexus, which causes the circular muscle to relax below the food and contract above it and so force the intestinal contents along.

Peristalsis is increased by the presence of bulky substance in the intestine which excites sensory receptors in the mucous membrane.

All these movements are increased by stimulation of the vagus or the administration of eserine or drugs with muscarine-like actions, and these effects are antagonized by atropine. Sympathetic stimulation and the administration of adrenaline have the opposite effect. The response of the ileocolic sphincter to both nerve stimulation and drugs is the opposite of the rest of the intestine.

The purgative group of drugs include a very large number of compounds which act in a number of different ways. They all cause defaecation and are in wide use, often unnecessarily, in all parts of the world. Terms which are used synonymously with purgative include laxative, cathartic, purge, drastic evacuant, and aperient and, although they may suggest different degrees of purgative action, they all mean the same thing in the end.

Depending largely on the dose used, a purgative may have a gentle action and well-formed stools will be produced. In larger doses, badly formed stools will be produced, and in still larger doses the stools will be watery.

The purgatives act either by a bulk effect, by lubrication, or by irritation.

Bulk purgatives

The presence of bulky substances in the intestine provides the normal stimulus for peristalsis by stretching the wall of the intestine.

Fruit and vegetables contain cellulose which is not normally digested, and this acts as roughage and increases intestinal mobility. **Bran,** which is often taken as a cereal, contains a large proportion of insoluble fibres and prunes, in addition to providing cellulose and fibre, also contain **diphenylisatin** which is a stimulant purgative.

Numerous substances act as bulk purgatives because they are not absorbed through the intestinal wall but swell by the absorption of fluid.

Agar is a dried extract of Japanese seaweed and consists largely of an insoluble carbohydrate, which swells up with water to form a jelly. If flakes of it are taken by the mouth they swell up in the alimentary canal and increase peristalsis. It is not normally used as a purgative alone because large quantities have to be ingested to be effective.

Magnesium sulphate is isotonic in 3·5 per cent solution and is a commonly used, bitter-tasting purgative. The bitter taste is usually disguised with a variety of additives. Both magnesium and sulphate ions are only very slightly absorbed and other salts containing them make effective purgatives. These include **sodium sulphate, heavy magnesium oxide,** and **heavy magnesium carbonate** and the corresponding light salts.

Tartrates and phosphates are both only partly absorbed from the intestine and may act as mild saline purgatives.

Lubricant purgatives

Liquid paraffin (mineral oil) is an inert, oily liquid consisting of a mixture of aliphatic hydrocarbons that is used as a mild laxative. It acts as a lubricant and increases the bulk and softness of the faeces. In reasonable doses it is useful in the treatment of chronic constipation and for patients with haemorrhoids and heart disease who should avoid straining at stool.

It is liable to leak past the anal sphincter and large doses may delay the absorption of carotene, calcium, phosphates, and vitamins D and K.

Dioctyl sodium sulphosuccinate is a wetting agent and is used to soften the stools. It appears to have little effect on intestinal mobility. It has not yet been fully tested but may be useful for patients who must avoid straining at stool.

Enemas

The bulk effect of about one pint of warm soapy water causes rectal distention with stimulation of muscle activity in the rectum and colon and so promotes defaecation.

Irritant purgatives

These compounds have a local irritant or stimulant action on the intestinal wall and so excite Auerbach's plexus and cause peristalsis. They may act at any part of the intestinal tract and are commonly used when a patient is being treated with drugs that cause constipation and after food poisoning or the administration of anthelminthics.

Bisacodyl was developed as a result of studies of compounds structurally related to the purgative, phenolphthalein. The purgative action of bisacodyl resembles that of

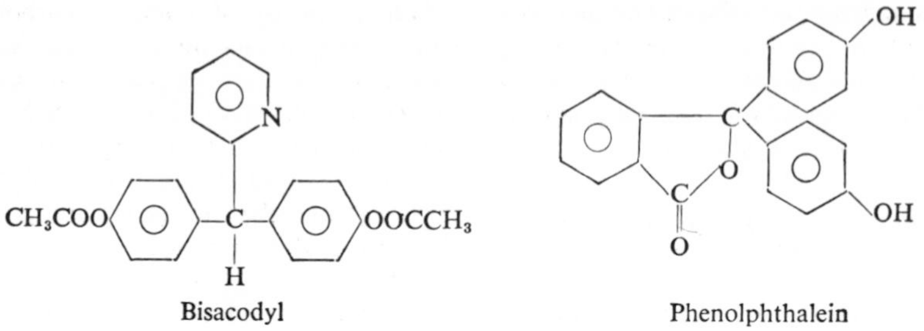

Bisacodyl

Phenolphthalein

Fig. 12.1. The structures of bisacodyl and phenolphthalein.

other irritant purgatives but it is more active on the large bowel than on the small intestine. Unlike other irritant purgatives, it can be given rectally as well as by oral administration.

This compound is sometimes known as a 'contact purgative' because it acts directly on sensory nerve endings in the mucosa to stimulate peristalsis. This effect can be blocked by the topical application of cocaine.

Mercurous chloride (calomel) has a prolonged irritant action on the intestinal mucosa and was once used as a purgative. Although mercurous chloride itself is almost insoluble and is therefore not absorbed, a proportion of the mercurous salt may be converted to the mercuric form. Mercuric ions are absorbed and may cause mercury poisoning.

Castor oil is a triglyceride consisting of glycerides of ricinoleic acid and isoricinoleic acid. It is expressed from the seeds of the castor-oil plant of tropical Africa.

The oil itself is soothing and is used as eye-drops to protect the eyes from irritation, but in the small intestine it is hydrolysed by lipase to produce ricinoleic acid which stimulates the small intestine. If bile is deficient the oil is not properly emulsified, so that the lipase cannot hydrolyse it and there is no purgation. Castor oil is safe and it is useful in acute constipation but its use may be followed by a period of constipation. It is used to rid the bowel of irritants and infections.

Phenolphthalein is colourless in acids and goes red in alkalis. Its purgative action was discovered as the result of the proposal that it should be added to adulterated wines so that they could be identified by adding alkali to them. Phenolphthalein does not act directly on the small intestine, its effect is due to an action on the colon, which is followed by reflex stimulation of peristaltic activity in the small intestine. The drug is absorbed in the small intestine but some is then secreted into the bile and the colon. This, and its indirect stimulant action, makes its effect slow to appear and prolonged in duration.

Since it is active in small doses, an overdose is easily taken and harm may be done when the compound is distributed in laxative chocolate or in chewing gum form among irresponsible people. It produces diarrhoea and some individuals are unusually susceptible to its action.

Anthracene purgatives

Aloes, cascara, rhubarb, and **senna** are popular drugs for treating chronic constipation. They are classed together because they contain the anthracene group, usually combined with two atoms of oxygen to form anthraquinone, and with other groups to form emodine. In the crude drug the anthracene group is also combined with sugars to form glycosides. These glycosides are themselves inactive but the active emodine is liberated in the body.

Anthracene purgatives act after a comparatively long latent period (about 10 hours). This is because, like phenolphthalein, they do not act directly on the small intestine. They are absorbed in the small intestine and their active principle is re-secreted in the bile and the colon. **Emodine,** the active principle, then acts directly on the colon and the reflexes arising from this stimulus cause reflex stimulation of the small intestine. The active substances are partly converted in the body to chrysophanic acid, which is very similar to emodine in chemical structure.

PROTECTIVES, DEMULCENTS, AND ASTRINGENTS

Protectives are used in medicine to remove undesirable substances from the intestine and also when gases or poisons have been produced in the intestine itself and are causing flatulence and diarrhoea. Protectives act as adsorbents and are used in a form in which they have a large surface area. Adsorbents are not specific in their action and they may adsorb enzymes and nutrients as well as noxious substances. Activated charcoal is an extremely efficient adsorbent of gases and substances in solution. It is used in the form of a powder or as lozenges in the treatment of food poisoning and diarrhoea.

Kaolin is a natural aluminium silicate with great absorptive power. It is practically insoluble and when taken by the mouth it protects the gut by covering it. Its value in the treatment of diarrhoea may be partly due to this mechanical action, but is mainly due to the absorption of toxins.

Other protectives include **magnesium trisilicate, kieselguhr, fuller's earth, zinc oxide, chalk,** and **starch.**

A demulcent is a colloidal solution of a high molecular weight gum or protein, the molecules of which are adsorbed on surfaces where they form a thin, but fairly consistent, protective film.

They are used in the form of mouth washes and gargles, and as pastilles and lozenges to treat inflamed surfaces of the mouth and throat. They are also used to protect inflamed regions of the gastro-intestinal tract.

Gums consist of complex carbohydrates which yield sugars on hydrolysis with acid: colloidal solutions of gums in water are known as mucilages. **Tragacanth** and **acacia** are gums used for making emulsions and suspensions, and as a basis for pills. Demulcents include **glycerin, propylene glycol,** and the **polyethylene glycols.**

Astringents are compounds which precipitate proteins, and this effect can easily be demonstrated by adding the astringent to a protein solution in a test-tube. They are applied locally to mucous membranes and the skin where their actions are confined to the surface layers. They form a protective layer of precipitated protein and inhibit exudations and the secretion of mucous glands. The membrane looks pale and the word astringent (drawn together) denotes the fact that it has a puckered appearance. In this intestine they tend to check diarrhoea and cause constipation. Many of the heavy metals are astringents. Aluminium, copper, zinc, iron, and lead are all applied as astringents to the skin or used as mouth washes and gargles. Substances of vegetable origin containing tannin possess astringent properties. Tannic acid, which is liberated from these preparations, produces water-insoluble protein precipitates which can be dissolved in acids or alkalis with the reformation of the tannic acid.

Preparations containing **tannic acid** have limited therapeutic uses but, in combination with silver nitrate, they have been used externally for the treatment of burns and skin ulcers. Tannic acid also precipitates alkaloids and heavy metals and has found a limited use in cases of poisoning by these substances. Other forms of treatment for burns and poisoning are usually preferred because they are more effective and precipitated tannates may be absorbed to cause general toxic effects.

FURTHER READING

Brody, M. and Bachrach, W. H. (1959). Antacids I. Comparative biochemical and economical considerations, *Amer. J. dig. Dis.* **4,** 435.

Gregory, R. A. (1965). Secretory mechanisms of the gastrointestinal tract, *Ann. Rev. Physiol.* **27,** 395.

James, A. H. (1957). *The physiology of gastric digestion*, London.

Wang, S. C. (1965). Emetic and antiemetic drugs, in *Physiological pharmacology*, ed. Root, W. S., and Hoffman, F. G., Vol. 2, p. 256, New York.

13

VITAMINS

THE vitamins are organic compounds which must be supplied in the diet or injected into the body in order to maintain health. Essential amino acids, which are required in larger quantities are not usually called vitamins, but the daily dose separating vitamins from other dietary essentials has not been defined and the exact boundaries of this chapter depend upon convention. Vitamins are classified as water or fat soluble.

THE WATER-SOLUBLE VITAMINS

[see Table 13.1 and Fig. 13.1]

Vitamin C (ascorbic acid)

This is a white crystalline solid related to the hexoses. The natural active isomer rotates polarized light to the right, but it is called L-ascorbic acid because it is related to other sugars which are L-isomers.

Vitamin C is a strong reducing agent and is rapidly oxidized by oxygen, especially in alkaline solutions or in the presence of traces of copper. It is easily destroyed by cooking and by an enzyme present in plant tissue.

The first product of oxidation is dehydroascorbic acid and this compound contains all the biological activity of the vitamins and will cure scurvy. Further oxidation is irreversible and abolishes biological activity.

Ascorbic acid is readily absorbed from the intestine and is stored in various tissues, particularly the liver, adrenals, pituitary, and the corpus luteum.

Large doses of vitamin C produce no observable effects in the normal individual but in the vitamin C-deficient person there is immediate alleviation of the deficiency symptoms.

It is likely that ascorbic and dehydroascorbic acid play a part in cellular respiration. Ascorbic acid can be oxidized by cytochrome oxidase in the presence of cytochrome c while dehydroascorbic acid can be reduced by glutathione. Ascorbic acid can serve as a hydrogen donor in respiratory systems and may help to maintain —SH activated enzymes in their reduced forms.

Ascorbic acid is concerned in carbohydrate metabolism and deficient animals tend to be hyperglycaemic and to have a diminished glucose tolerance.

A lack of ascorbic acid causes scurvy in man, monkeys, and guinea-pigs, but other animals such as dogs and rats do not get scurvy because their intestinal bacteria can synthesize ascorbic acid. The fundamental lesion caused by a lack of ascorbic acid is that the intercellular cement is weakened because the collagen fibres, normally embedded in it, disappear. Scurvy develops slowly and is associated with weakness and a general appearance of illness. The strength of the capillaries is diminished and haemorrhages occur all over the body and particularly in the skin, gums, periosteum, joints, and intestine. The patient often becomes anaemic due to the presence of numerous small haemorrhages and blood losses into the gastro-intestinal tract and urine. There are characteristic changes in the teeth and the bones become weakened. During infections more ascorbic acid is used by the body and, unless the intake is large, the stores become depleted. Wounds heal slowly or not at all and the scars lack strength. Minor degrees of vitamin C deficiency are common, though outright scurvy only occurs when the diet is markedly

Table 13.1. The water-soluble vitamins

Vitamin	Other name	Approx. daily requirement (adult)	Main natural source	Deficiency disease	Therapeutic use
C	Ascorbic acid	70–75 mg	Fruit, vegetables, potatoes, rose hips, etc.	Scurvy	Prevention and treatment of scurvy
P	Rutin, Citrin	..	Fruit, vegetables, potatoes, rose hips, etc.	None in man	Treatment of purpura (?)
B_1	Aneurine, Thiamin	1·6 mg	Yeast, wheat germ, pork fat, rye bread	Beriberi	Thiamine deficiency and some kinds of neuritis
B_2	Riboflavine Lactoflavin	1·8 mg	Yeast, liver, meat extract, human milk, beef	Ariboflavinosis	Riboflavine deficiency
B_6	Pyridoxine, Adermine	1·5 mg	Yeast, potatoes, liver	Rare in man	Pyridoxine deficiency
Nicotinamide	Niacin, Nicotinic acid	20 mg	Meat extract, yeast, liver bread	Pellagra	Treatment of pellagra
Pantothenic acid	..	10 mg	Yeast, liver	Unknown in man	No established use
Folic acid	..	50 μg	Yeast, liver, vegetables	Megaloblastic anaemia, sprue	Folic acid deficiency
B_{12}	Cobalamin, Cyanocobalamin	10 μg	Liver	Pernicious anaemia	Cobalamin deficiency
H	Biotin	..	Yeast, chocolate, intestinal bacterial flora	Rare in man	No established use
Choline	..	250–600 mg	Eggs, meat, cereal, milk, etc.	Fatty liver (?)	Some forms of liver disease (?)

deficient in fresh fruit and vegetables. Milk is not a good source of ascorbic acid, and if it is boiled it loses its activity, so that infants should always be given orange juice or some such other supplement.

Ascorbic acid has been used to treat various diseases in which haemorrhages are particularly likely to occur. The fact that the body tends to become unsaturated during fevers has led to its administration in various infections.

Vitamin P (citrin, rutin, hesperidin)

The existence of vitamin P was suggested when it was found that crude extracts of ascorbic acid were more effective than the pure substance in prolonging the lives of scorbutic animals. Several substances share the biological action of vitamin P in reducing capillary permeability and all are related to flavone. Substances called vitamin P are sometimes also known as flavonoids.

Vitamin P has not been chemically identified but rutin has the same biological properties and its structure is shown in Fig. 13.1.

Little, if any, vitamin P is absorbed from the gastro-intestinal tract and experiments designed to show an antiscorbutic action for this vitamin require its parenteral injection. For this reason there is some doubt as to whether vitamin P should be considered a natural vitamin.

The substances included under the term 'vitamin P' have a direct constrictor action on capillaries and reduce their fragility and permeability.

The status of vitamin P as a natural vitamin is not well established and deficiency symptoms have not been demonstrated but it has been used widely for a variety of therapeutic

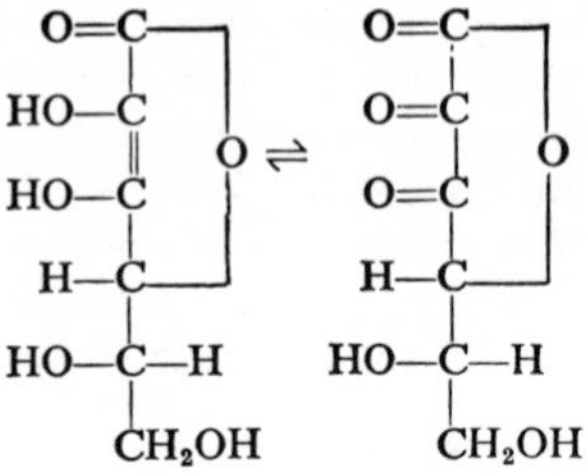

Ascorbic acid ⇌ Dehydroascorbic acid

Vitamin C

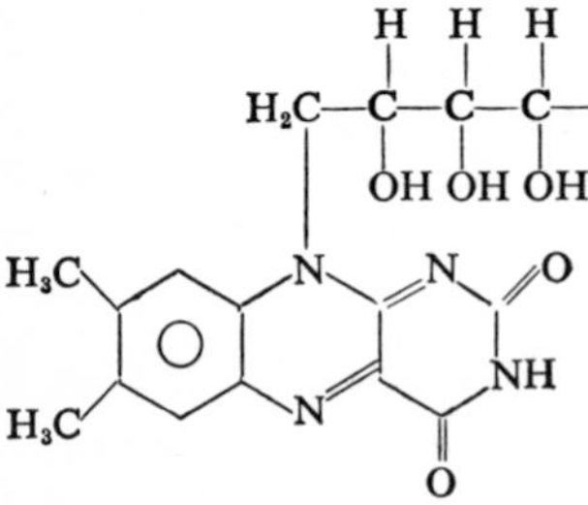

Riboflavine

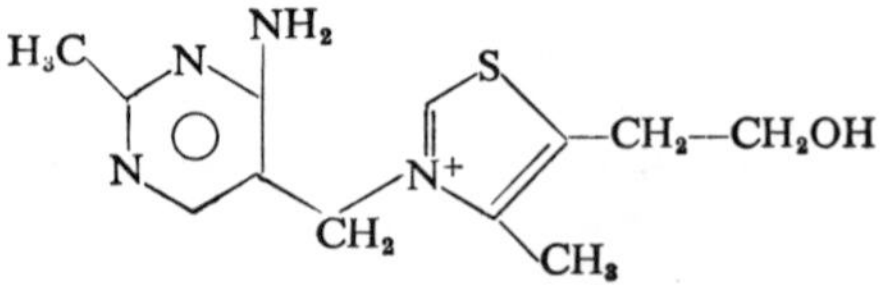

Vitamin B_1

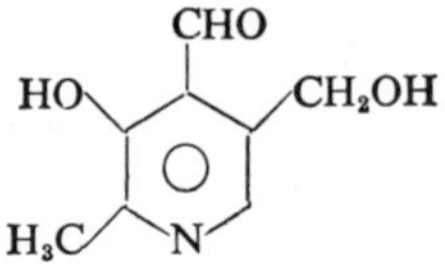

Pyridoxal

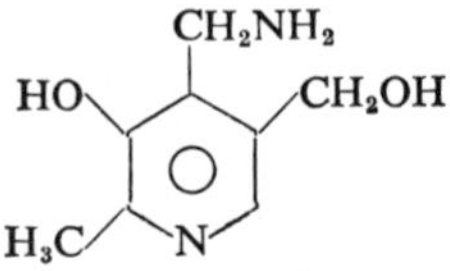

Pyridoxamine

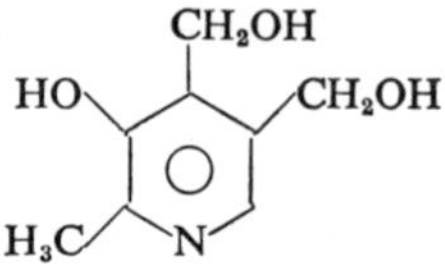

Pyridoxine

Vitamin B_6

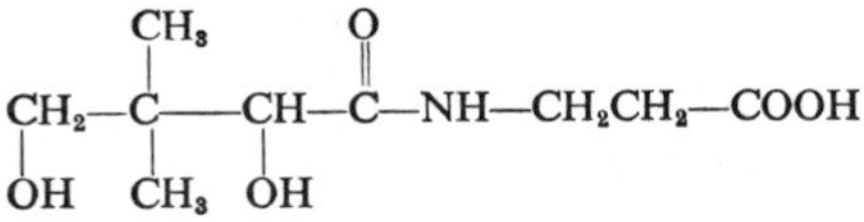

$CH_2(OH)$—$C(CH_3)_2$—$CH(OH)$—CO—NH—CH_2CH_2—$COOH$

Pantothenic acid

Pteridine | PABA | Glutamic acid

Pteroic acid

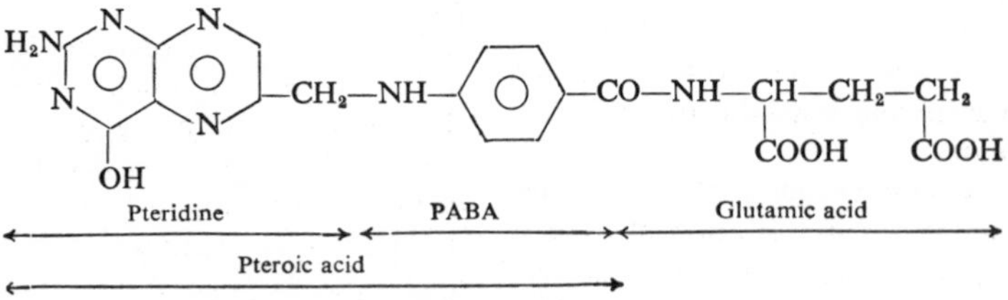

Folic acid

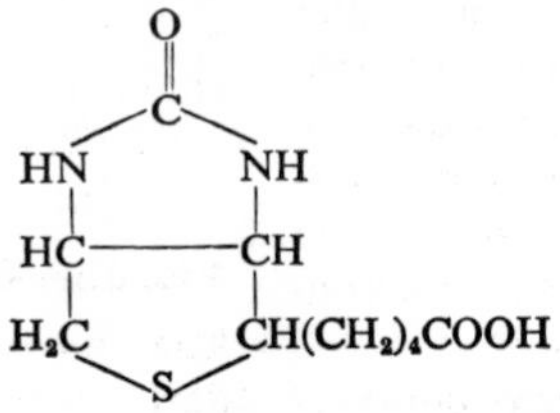

Vitamin H

Fig. 13.1. The structures of the water-soluble vitamins.

reasons. It is usually given orally even though it is probably not absorbed by this route. It has been chiefly used to treat diseases where there is capillary bleeding and increased capillary fragility, i.e. allergic states and diabetes mellitus.

THE VITAMIN B COMPLEX

The vitamins in this group comprise a large number of chemically different compounds with a variety of actions. They are commonly grouped under one heading because they are all water soluble and may be extracted from liver and yeast.

The substances forming the vitamin B complex are **aneurine** (thiamin, vitamin B_1), **riboflavine** (vitamin B_2), **pyridoxine** (vitamin B_6), **nicotinic acid, pantothenic acid, cyanocobalamin** (vitamin B_{12}), **folic acid, biotin** (vitamin H), and **choline.**

Vitamin B_1 (aneurine, thiamin)

Vitamin B_1 is more stable than ascorbic acid, but less stable than the other vitamins. In neutral solutions a little less than half of it is destroyed in 4 hours at 100° C. Certain bacteria can synthesize vitamin B_1 and they may occur in the intestine and protect an animal from deficiency diseases.

The vitamin contains a pyrimidine ring and a thiazole ring and is active in the body as the coenzyme thiamin pyrophosphate. The formation of this coenzyme requires the presence of adenosine triphosphate. Antimetabolites to thiamin have been synthesized and these include **neopyrithiamin** (pyrithiamin) and **oxythiamin.**

Thiamin pyrophosphate is the coenzyme necessary for the decarboxylation of pyruvic and α-keto-glutaric acids and is therefore important in carbohydrate metabolism. Animals fed on a thiamin-deficient diet suffer from deficiency of this coenzyme so that pyruvic acid accumulates, and this causes an accumulation of lactic acid, since lactic acid is normally converted to pyruvic acid. Both acids accumulate, and abnormally high concentrations are found in the blood.

The accumulation of lactic acid deranges the earlier phases of carbohydrate metabolism, and the animal is unable to tolerate normal quantities of carbohydrate in the diet. The fact that a carbohydrate-rich diet was liable to accentuate beriberi has been known for a long time, but the detailed explanation of this effect has only become evident fairly recently.

Thiamin deficiency eventually leads to the condition known as beriberi. Beriberi was one of the first deficiency diseases to be recognized and, although it can now be easily diagnosed and treated, it is still widespread in some parts of the Far East.

The symptoms of this deficiency disease include polyneuritis, cardiac failure, and reduced growth.

Thiamin is used therapeutically in the treatment of beriberi, and various kinds of neuritis, including alcoholic neuritis and neuritis of pregancy, both of which may actually be due to a lack of this vitamin.

Vitamin B_2 (riboflavine)

Riboflavine consists of an orange–yellow pigment, lumiflavin, combined with ribose. It can be made synthetically, and is fairly stable, but is destroyed by alkali or by light, in which it gives off a bright green fluorescence.

Riboflavine acts in the body in the form of riboflavine phosphate or flavine adenine dinucleotide. These coenzymes act as hydrogen carriers between pyridine nucleotides and cytochrome systems and play an important part in metabolism.

Rats fed on a riboflavine-deficient diet do not grow, and eventually develop inflammation of the skin, and cataracts. Deficiency in man causes pallor followed by inflammation of the tongue (glossitis) and skin (seborrhoeic dermatitis). The cornea becomes vascularized, apparently because it is normally dependent on riboflavine for its metabolism. Riboflavine is also necessary for the growth of certain kinds of bacteria.

Riboflavine is used therapeutically only for the correction of deficiency disease.

Vitamine B_6 (pyridoxine)

Like nicotinic acid, pyridoxine is a simple derivative of pyridine. It can be estimated chemically and is present in yeast, wheat germ, liver, muscle, and various vegetables.

Pyridoxine is only one of three forms in which vitamin B_6 can exist naturally, the other forms are pyridoxal and pyridoxamine. The active forms of the vitamin are pyridoxal phosphate and pyridoxamine phosphate whose formation is catalysed by pyridoxal kinase. An important role for pyridoxine is as a coenzyme for decarboxylases.

Isonicotinic acid hydrazide (isoniazid) antagonizes the pyridoxal kinase reaction and so has an anti-vitamin-B_6 action by blocking the formation of the active form of the vitamin.

Lack of pyridoxine in the diet of rats makes their extremities red, swollen, and oedematous. This condition was once thought to be identical with pellagra, and was known as rat pellagra. It is said that this is worse in cold weather and is analogous to chilblains. Prolonged deficiency may cause anaemia and fits.

Pyridoxine may be given to people receiving isoniazid in order to prevent peripheral neuritis. It is not certain whether man can become pyridoxine-deficient but this vitamin usually given if there is any deficiency of B complex vitamins.

Nicotinamide (niacin, nicotinic acid)

Nicotonic acid has a more simple molecule than other vitamins, and can easily be synthesized. Its presence in yeast was discovered in 1912, but its function as a vitamin was not known until 1938. Its amide **(nicotinamide)** has the same action.

In the body nicotinic acid is converted to diphosphopyridine nucleotide (NAD) or to triphosphopyridine nucleotide (NADP) and these compounds have an important role as coenzymes for many proteins involved in tissue respiration. Nicotonic acid but not nicotinamide has a direct action on blood vessels causing vasodilatation.

A deficiency of nicotinic acid in the diet produces pellagra, a disease which still occurs among poorly nourished populations in Egypt, the southern states of North America, and other countries in the same latitude. The classical signs of the disease are dermatitis, diarrhoea, and dementia. The most obvious changes are in the skin, which becomes particularly susceptible to sunburn, so that all exposed parts become inflamed and blistered. The nervous symptoms include disturbances of the brain, the spinal cord, and the peripheral nerves.

Most of these symptoms are the result of a deficiency of nicotinic acid and the disease is particularly liable to occur among alcoholics, partly because alcoholics do not usually choose their food carefully, and possibly also because they lose the power of absorbing nicotinic acid.

Nicotinic acid and nicotinamide are used in the treatment of pellagra. High doses may be needed initially and nicotinic acid, in these doses, may cause vasodilatation with flushing and itching of the skin.

Pantothenic acid

Pantothenic acid is converted to coenzyme A in the body and is active in this form. Pantothenic acid was first recognized as the factor whose absence was responsible for a form of dermatitis in chickens. The effects of deficiency in rats are a loss of weight, grey hair, inflammation of the nose with a red discharge containing porphyrin, and haemorrhages and atrophy in the adrenals. It is essential for the growth of yeast and some bacteria.

Coenzyme A is essential in metabolism as a coenzyme for many enzyme-catalysed reactions involving the transfer of acyl groups.

There is no accepted therapeutic use for pantothenic acid.

Folic acid (pteroylmonoglutamic acid)

Folic acid got its name from the fact that it is commonly present in green leaves. It appeared first as vitamin M and then as vitamin B_c, vitamins which were necessary for the health of monkeys and chickens respectively.

Studies of the nutritional requirements of *Lactobacillus casei* led to the isolation of folic acid in 1945. It contains 2-NH_2-4-OH-pteridine, para-aminobenzoic acid, and glutamic acid (see Fig. 14.2). Natural folic acid is found conjugated with several molecules of glutamate attached to it in peptide linkages.

Folic acid is converted in the body to dihydrofolate and tetrahydrofolate by folate reductase and these compounds accept a transferable one-carbon group which plays an important part in the synthesis of purine rings and some amino acids. If there is a shortage of purine compounds this means there is a shortage of materials from which nucleic acid is made, and it is therefore not surprising that the production of new cells may depend on the presence of folic acid.

Vitamin B_{12} (cyanocobalamin)

Liver extracts do not contain enough folic acid to account for all their therapeutic effects in megaloblastic anaemia. Fractions had been prepared which were more active, in smaller doses than folic acid, and which cured lesions of the spinal cord on which folic acid had no effect. These fractions were further purified in Britain but a comparatively quick microbiological assay was developed in America and vitamin B_{12} was isolated there in 1948, just before it was isolated in Britain. The original vitamin B_{12} is known as cyanocobalamin. Other cobalamins, with groups other than cyanide, are known, but can easily be converted to cyanocobalamin which is the one generally available.

Cyanocobalamin is a complex porphyrin-like ring structure called cobamide with a co-ordinate cobalt atom (see Fig. 14.1). Cyanocobalamin is concerned in the biosynthesis of the methyl groups of thymidine and methionine and, through these, most of the *N*-methyl, *S*-methyl, and *O*-methyl groups of naturally occurring compounds. It is thus associated, at least indirectly, with every known metabolic system.

It is essential for normal growth, haematopoiesis, and for the production of epithelial cells and the maintenance of myelin in the nervous system.

Its action on the blood-forming elements and the results of deficiency are described in Chapter 14.

Vitamin H (biotin)

Biotin acts as a coenzyme for several enzyme-catalysed carboxylation reactions and therefore plays an important role in CO_2 fixation.

The effects of deficiency include loss of weight and hair, exfoliative dermatitis, hyperkeratosis, and spasticity. This condition is rare in man, but a striking case has been described. An Italian labourer had a passion for raw eggs, and ate about ten a day. Raw egg white contains a protein known as avidin which combines with biotin and prevents its absorption. His blood biotin fell and he had dermatitis. The administration of biotin reversed this condition.

Choline

Choline cannot be classed as a true vitamin because it is present in the body in much larger amounts than are usually associated with vitamins and because no co-factor concerned in enzymic reactions and containing choline has been found.

Choline has qualitatively similar pharmacological actions to acetylcholine but is very much less potent. It is involved in fat metabolism and is important as a methyl donor in intermediary metabolism. It is also a precursor for acetylcholine.

In order to produce a choline-deficient animal it is necessary to deprive it, not only of choline, but also of methionine. This is because choline can be synthesized from phosphatidylethanolamine with methionine acting as a methyl donor.

As a result of choline deficiency the fat content of the liver increase and hepatic cirrhosis may result. It seems unlikely that this ever happens in man and no effects of choline deficiency have been observed on cholinergic mechanisms.

Choline and methionine have sometimes been used in the treatment of liver disease.

FAT-SOLUBLE VITAMINS

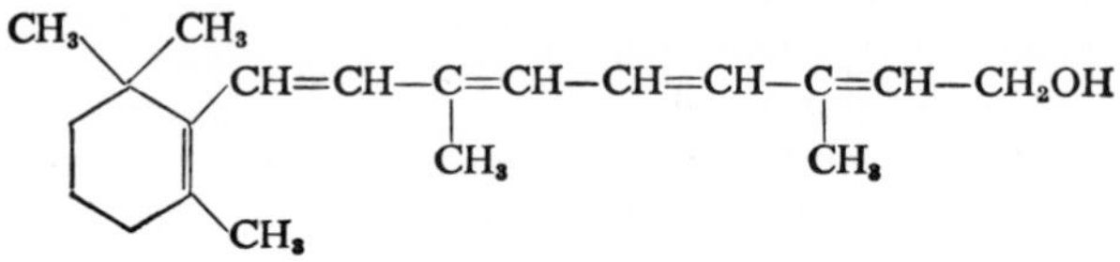

CH_3 CH_3 $CH{=}CH{-}C{=}CH{-}CH{=}CH{-}C{=}CH{-}CH_2OH$ CH_3 CH_3 CH_3

Vitamin **A**

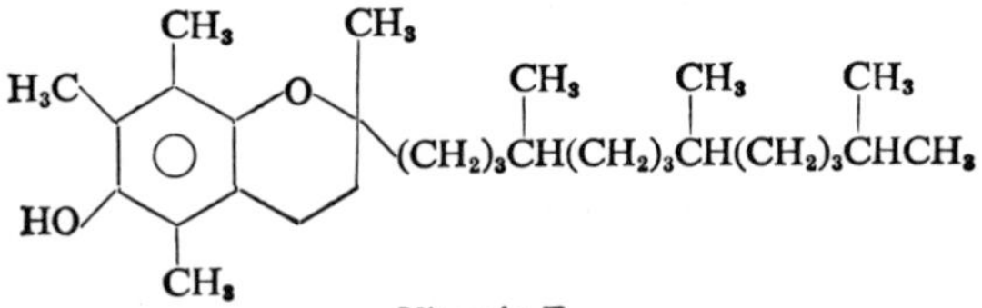

CH_3 CH_3 H_3C O CH_3 CH_3 CH_3 $(CH_2)_3CH(CH_2)_3CH(CH_2)_3CHCH_3$ HO CH_3

Vitamin E

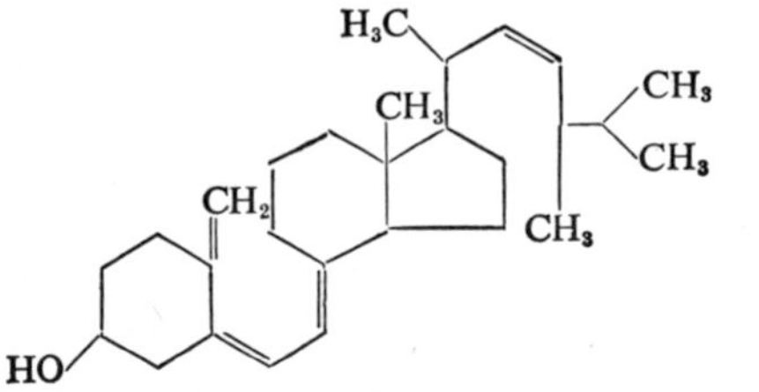

H_3C CH_3 CH_3 CH_3 CH_2 CH_3 HO

Vitamin D_2

CH_3 CH_3 CH_3 CH_3 CH_2 HO

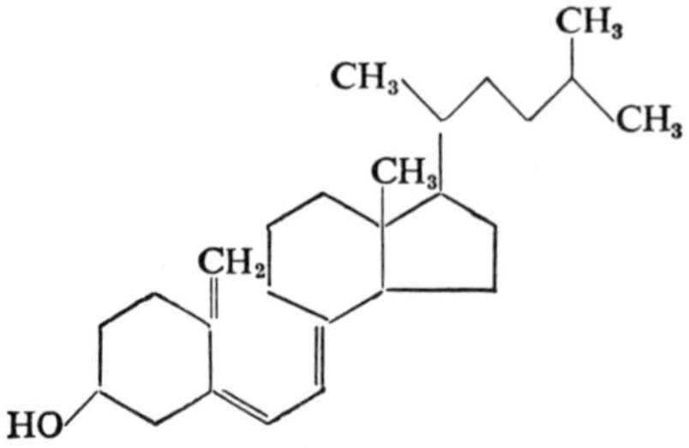

Vitamin D_3 (cholecalciferol)

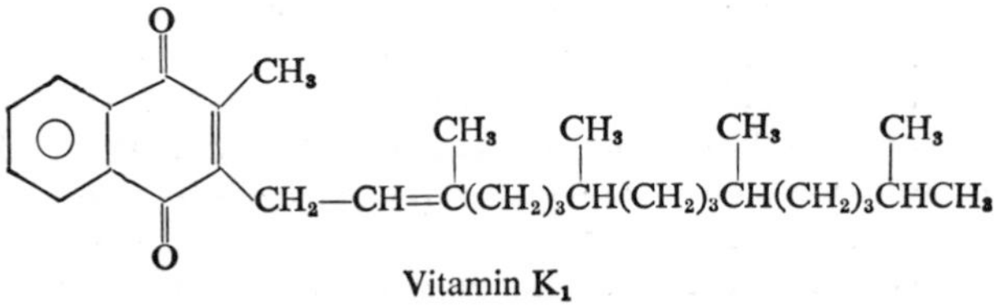

O CH_3 CH_3 CH_3 CH_3 CH_3 $CH_2{-}CH{=}C(CH_2)_3CH(CH_2)_3CH(CH_2)_3CHCH_3$ O

Vitamin K_1

O CH_3 O

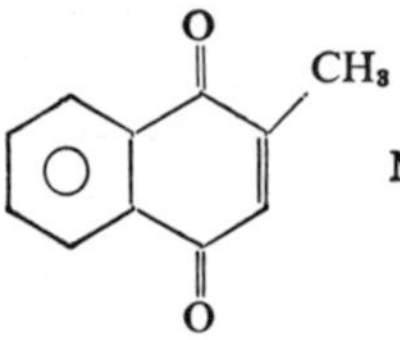

Menaphthone (menadione)

Fig. 13.2. The structures of fat-soluble vitamins.

Vitamin A

Vitamin A is a long-chain alcohol with five double bonds and is obtained from fish-liver oils. If two such molecules are joined together by a double bond with the elimination of two molecules of water at the place where the hydroxyl group is, the result is β-carotene. Carotenes form the red pigment in carrots; they are converted by the body to vitamin A, each molecule of carotene forming one molecule of vitamin A.

Vitamin A is fairly stable at temperatures up to 120° C in the absence of oxygen, but it is oxidized by aeration even at room temperature and is destroyed by light. Neither vitamin A nor carotene is destroyed by ordinary cooking.

Vitamin A is well absorbed through the wall of the gastro-intestinal tract, and only if an amount exceeding the daily requirement is ingested does any appear in the faeces. Since the vitamin is fat soluble, its absorption will be related to lipid absorption and in cases of disordered fat absorption it may be necessary to use water-miscible solutions of the vitamin.

Vitamin A plays an essential role in the function of the retina, in the maintenance of epithelial cells, and probably in the synthesis of glucocorticoids. There is also evidence that it may be a growth-promoting factor.

Deficiency of vitamin A reduces vision in dim light because adaptation of the retinal rods to poor illumination is affected. The chemical concerned with dim light vision is rhodopsin which is a combination of a protein, opsin, and a prosthetic group, retinene (11-*cis*-vitamin A aldehyde). During the synthesis of rhodopsin, *cis*-vitamin A is converted into *cis*-retinene and this then combines with opsin to form rhodopsin. The action of light on rhodopsin converts the retinene part of the molecule into the *trans*-isomer, *trans*-retinene (Fig. 13.3).

The *trans*-retinene then dissociates from the opsin and nerve impulses are generated.

The *trans*-retinene can be reconverted to rhodopsin, via *cis*-retinene, or may be reduced to *trans*-vitamin A and then back to vitamin A.

In vitamin A deficiency the retinal rhodopsin concentration falls because it can no longer be synthesized in adequate amounts.

The failure to dark-adapt as a result of vitamin A deficiency is quickly overcome by administering the vitamin.

Reserves of the vitamin in the tissues are usually sufficiently large to prevent deficiency except in cases of disordered fat absorption.

Because vitamin A deficiency, when it does occur, leads to epithelial lesions and infections, the vitamin is sometimes given to combat infections but this use is unjustified. The only legimate use of vitamin A is to treat a deficiency of this vitamin. It may be given as **cod-liver oil** or as **halibut-liver oil.**

Vitamin D (cholecalciferol)

The term vitamin D refers to vitamin D_3 (cholecalciferol) which is the only vitamin D to occur naturally in man. It is present in halibut and cod-liver oil and is produced in the skin by the action of sunlight on the sterol 7-dehydrocholestrol.

The exposure of certain inactive food substances or cholesterol and other steroids to

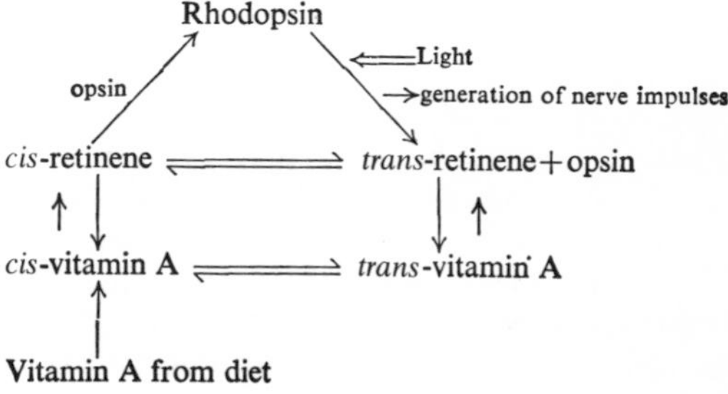

Fig. 13.3. The rhodopsin cycle.

sunlight or artificial ultraviolet light produces compounds which have as a common property the ability to prevent rickets. These compounds have the same ring structure as cholesterol and include vitamin D_2 (ergocalciferol, calciferol). Vitamins D_1 and D_2 do not differ greatly in their antirickitic potencies when given orally to man.

These substances are soluble in fats and fats solvents, are reasonably stable, and are not destroyed by ordinary cooking procedures.

Vitamin D is essential for the proper absorption of calcium and phosphorus from the intestine into the blood and it is likely that it acts by stimulating the synthesis of calcium-binding protein which may be involved in the absorption of this ion. An adequate level of calcium absorption is essential for the formation of bone and the proper functioning of nerves and muscles and for the coagulation of blood. Abnormal levels of calcium in the body may cause malfunction of these systems and so signify a possible deficiency of vitamin D. In rickets the calcification of bone is deficient. Dogs and humans get rickets when they lack vitamin D and this is normally a disease of the young. Osteomalacia is a similar disease, due to similar causes, occurring in adults and particularly in pregnant women, who are more susceptible than others because they lose calcium and phosphorous to the foetus.

The signs of vitamin D deficiency are:

(1) The bones are deficient in calcium and phosphorus, soft and liable to bend, so that the person becomes bow-legged or knock-kneed, and the thorax and pelvis are deformed.
(2) The teeth are badly formed and liable to become diseased.
(3) If the blood calcium falls very low, tetany is produced, and this may occur among children with rickets.
(4) The parathyroids become overactive to maintain the blood calcium by liberating calcium from the bones; this tends to make the rickets worse.

Hypervitaminosis D is not uncommon. It occurs in any person who receives excess of the vitamin, often during the treatment of vitamin D deficiency.

The level of calcium and phosphate in the blood is dependent on the circulating level of vitamin D, but an important role in the absorption of these ions is also played by the parathyroid hormone. If the levels of vitamin D fall there is a fall in circulating calcium and a compensatory rise in the output of parathyroid hormone. This hormone raises the plasma calcium and phosphate at the expense of bone which becomes demineralized and excretion through the kidneys, particularly of phosphate, is increased.

The part played by vitamin D is further complicated because it is itself required in order to maintain full parathyroid activity.

Vitamin E (tocopherol)

There are several active tocopherols, known collectively as vitamin E. They are fat-soluble alcohols, which have been synthesized, and are associated with reproductive processes. Vitamin E is unstable in rancid fats, being easily oxidized but stable to ordinary cooking. It is stored in the body, and signs of deficiency take many months to develop. An important chemical property of vitamin E is that it is an anti-oxidant and forms reversible oxidation–reduction systems.

Vitamin E is absorbed through the gastrointestinal tract in the same way as other fat-soluble vitamins. It is stored in the tissues and the body can be supplied from these stores for a long period. For this reason a vitamin E deficiency can only be obtained by the prolonged ingestion of a vitamin E-deficient diet.

Despite numerous investigations into the action of vitamin E in the body, the subject is still controversial. Even animals whose tissues contain no vitamin E are able to reproduce normally and bear normal offspring.

It may be that vitamin E merely mimics and supplements a naturally occurring coenzyme with similar properties. Where vitamin E acts as an anti-oxidant it is likely that other, unrelated anti-oxidants can take over its role during periods of deficiency.

Vitamin K

Vitamin K is essential for the synthesis in the body of several factors concerned with the clotting of blood. Animals which are deficient in vitamin K tend to bleed easily and this has been shown to be due to a fall in the circulating level of prothrombin.

Vitamin K is fat soluble and consists of at least two naturally occurring substances (vitamins K_1 and K_2), both of which are derivatives of naphthoquinone. More simple substances which contain this group, e.g. **menaphthone** (menadione), have the same effect as the natural vitamins and are slightly more water soluble.

Vitamins K_1 and K_2 are only absorbed from the gastro-intestinal tract if bile salts are present. A deficiency of the vitamins may arise when bile is held back in obstructive jaundice. Other conditions which reduce its absorption include ulcerative colitis, sprue, or large doses of liquid paraffin. Menaphthone is absorbed in the absence of bile salts and enters the blood directly, unlike the natural vitamin K which is absorbed via the lymphatic system.

Vitamin K in the intestines is partially derived from the food and is partly formed by intestinal flora. When rats are raised under sterile conditions, without vitamin K in their diet and without bacteria in their intestines, haemorrhages occur but they disappear in a few days if the normal intestinal flora is allowed to develop.

There appears to be no significant storage of vitamin K in the body.

Vitamin K is concerned in the synthesis of prothrombin and factors VII, IX, and X in the liver and this is described in detail in Chapter 14.

FURTHER READING

Diem, K. (ed) (1962). Vitamins. In *Documenta Geigy, Scientific Tables*, p. 449. Geigy Pharmaceuticals, Manchester.

Harris, J. L. (1955). *Vitamins in theory and practice*, Cambridge.

Marks, J. (1968). *The vitamins in health and disease.* Churchill, London.

Sebrell, W. H., and Harris, R. S. (1954) *The vitamins: chemistry, physiology, pathology*, New York.

Weissbach, H., and Dickerman, H. (1955). Biochemical role of vitamin B_{12}, *Physiol. Rev.* **45,** 80.

14

BLOOD

RED blood cells are formed in the bone marrow from stem cells which divide and give rise to more mature cells which show two prominent changes as they mature, the acquisition of the iron-containing respiratory pigment haemoglobin and the dissolution and disappearance of the nucleus so that the mature cell when released into the circulation is a biconcave disk of about 7·5 μm diameter and containing 33 per cent haemoglobin (0·1 per cent iron). The cells survive in the circulation for some 120 days before degenerating and being removed from the circulation, the released pigment is metabolized, the iron set free, and returned to the stores. This means that a little less than 1 per cent of the circulating red cells are being replaced daily. The circulating red cell mass is controlled by homeostatic processes probably mediated by both central nervous and renal mechanisms that control the secretion of a glycoprotein, erythropoietin, which stimulates red cell production. Normal red cell formation depends also on an adequate supply of iron and of the coenzymes, coenzyme B_{12} and tetrahydrofolate which are necessary for nucleotide synthesis.

The total iron pool of the body is composed of that in the red cell mass (2·5 g), tissue iron (myoglobin, haemenzymes, etc. 0·3 g), that in iron stores (1 g), and the small amount circulating in the plasma (4 mg). The iron stores are mainly in the form of ferritin, a complex of ferric iron with a protein apoferritin found mostly in the liver, spleen, and bone marrow. Iron is transported in the plasma in ferric form in another complex with a special plasma protein transferrin, so that virtually no free iron is normally present, indeed whereas the plasma iron concentration is about 1·2 mg/l the binding capacity of the transferrin present is about 3·2 mg/l so that the plasma is capable of accepting a further 2 mg/l of iron (a total of 10 mg iron) without its binding capacity being saturated. Since 1/120 of the red cells are being broken down and newly formed each day the amount of iron required each day is about 20 mg but nearly all of this is recycled from the stores and the normal amount absorbed from the diet is only about 1 mg a day, this being balanced by excretion in the urine and by the gut.

Because such a small proportion of the iron is obtained from dietary intake extra losses of iron are very important. These are especially so in women who lose iron in menstruation, pregnancy, and lactation and are therefore much more susceptible to iron deficiency than males. The effects of dietary deficiency of iron take a long while to develop—if there were no iron at all in the diet and the loss remained at 1 mg a day it would take 3 years to drain the iron stores. Iron loss can occur much more rapidly with acute or chronic blood loss, thus the loss of 1 litre of blood is equivalent to the loss of 0·5 g iron, or half the reserve. In chronic iron deficiency the red cells are reduced in numbers and they are small and deficient in haemoglobin content. On administration of iron in adequate amounts rapid restoration can occur at rates of up to 15 g haemoglobin (50 mg Fe) per day.

Iron is not very well absorbed from food, the overall absorption being about 5–10 per cent and may be lower owing to natural chelators such as phytate in the diet. Inorganic iron salts administered orally are well absorbed (20–30 per cent) when given in small amounts but the fraction absorbed decreases as the total amount is increased. In iron deficiency absorption is considerably improved but it is still not clear why this should be so.

ORAL IRON PREPARATIONS

The most commonly used are **ferrous sulphate, ferrous gluconate, ferrous fumarate,** and **ferric ammonium citrate.** In severe iron deficiency the amounts given must be quite large, i.e. of the order of 100–300 mg a day with lesser amounts in milder cases. All these preparations are liable to cause such gastrointestinal disturbances as epigastric pain, colic, and diarrhoea and these side actions may make it impossible to give adequate doses by mouth. Serious toxicity is rare in adults but it is not uncommon and highly dangerous in children, who are attracted by iron tablets which are sugar coated and brightly coloured. Iron toxicity demands energetic treatment including sequestration of the iron by the chelator desferrioxamine given by lavage and intravenously and supportive therapy must be given to deal with the accompanying shock. Desferrioxamine is a hydroxypeptide isolated from *Streptomyces pilosus*, each molecule of which can bind one molecule of trivalent iron.

In patients who are unable to tolerate oral iron preparations, iron may be given by intramuscular injection as the non-ionic complexes **iron sorbitol** and **iron dextran.** Iron dextran and iron dextrin may be given intravenously. The amount of iron given by these routes is commonly 20–50 mg. Since this exceeds the plasma iron binding capacity there is considerable risk of systemic toxicity. There may be anaphylactic-like effects with dizziness, tachycardia, sweating, nausea and vomiting, and circulatory collapse. Moreover, delayed allergic type responses may also occur. Because of the unpleasantness and danger of these responses parenteral iron should be restricted to those who really need it, i.e. those really intolerant of oral iron and those who are refractory to oral preparations.

MACROCYTIC ANAEMIAS

When there is a dietary deficiency of **cobalamins** or **folates** the erythrocytes are decreased in numbers but increased in size and some nucleated cells may escape into the circulation. The defect appears to be one of nucleic acid synthesis which retards cell division. Both of these substances form coenzymes concerned in the transfer of one carbon unit in the biosynthesis of purines and pyrimidines. The effects of deficiency are not confined to the bone marrow, effects also being seen on epithelia in the gut, skin, and hair. Cobalamins are also necessary for the survival of neurones in the CNS and in deficiency a characteristic syndrome, subacute combined degeneration, develops.

The role of cobalamins in erythrocyte development stems from the discovery by Minot and Murphy that liver had a curative effect in pernicious anaemia (the commonest form of macrocytic anaemia in temperate climates) and the finding by Castle that there was no dietary deficiency *per se* but a failure

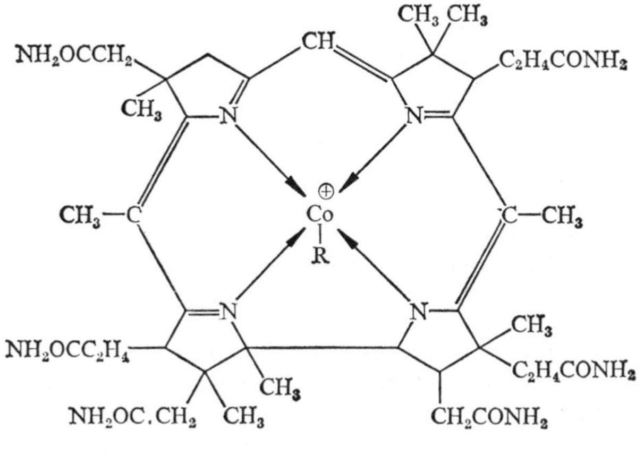

Fig. 14.1. Cobalamin (vitamin B_{12}).

to absorb a dietary factor due to the lack of the absorption promoting factor, 'intrinsic factor', a mucoprotein secreted by the gastrointestinal epithelium. Purification eventually led to isolation and characterization of cyanocobalamin. This was greatly aided by the finding that the liver factor was a growth factor for some bacteria such as *Lactobacillus lactis.* The vitamin is red in colour, and it was noticed that cultures of *Streptomyces* var. gave pink-coloured culture fluids which were found to be rich in cobalamins. This is now the source of the material used therapeutically.

Cobalamins are not synthesized by animals, which are therefore dependent on dietary sources; deficiency can occur from inadequate intake but is much more frequently due to gastro-intestinal disturbances interfering with absorption (see Chapter 13). The estimated daily requirement is about 10 μg. In normal individuals cyanocobalamin is rapidly and efficiently absorbed (>50 per cent) and is stored in the tissues, notably in the liver, which may contain about 1 mg/kg wet weight.

Colbalamin has a very complicated chemical structure based on a ring structure closely related to the porphyrins with a cobalt atom held in co-ordinate linkage at its centre. The cobalt also may bind an additional group of which the most important are cyanide in **cyanocobalamin,** hydroxyl in **hydroxocobalamin,** and deoxyadenosine in the biochemically active form **coenzyme B_{12}**.

The former two are used therapeutically and differ mainly in their duration of effect. Excess cyanocobalamin is rapidly excreted in the urine because the plasma binding capacity for cyanocobalamin is low so that after giving large doses most is unbound to plasma protein, is filtered in the glomerulus, and cleared rapidly. On the other hand, hydroxocobalamin is bound to a greater extent and is rather more slowly excreted. The therapeutic advantage is debatable.

Since cobalamins are readily available and reasonably cheap, massive doses may be given at infrequent intervals. In treating pernicious anaemia, for instance, it is common to give 1 mg twice weekly by intramuscular injection until the blood picture is normal and then the same dose once a month. Oral absorption in the enterogenic anaemias is too irregular and uncertain to be relied upon.

Folic acid

Folic acid is another dietary factor necessary for normal erythrocyte formation but its deficiency does not lead to subacute combined degeneration of the spinal cord. It is available in many foods including green vegetables and deficiency is due either to a poor diet, which is the usual reason in tropical areas (tropical sprue), or to deficient absorption (non-tropical sprue, coeliac disease) frequently associated with intolerance to the protein gluten present in wheat flour (see Chapter 13).

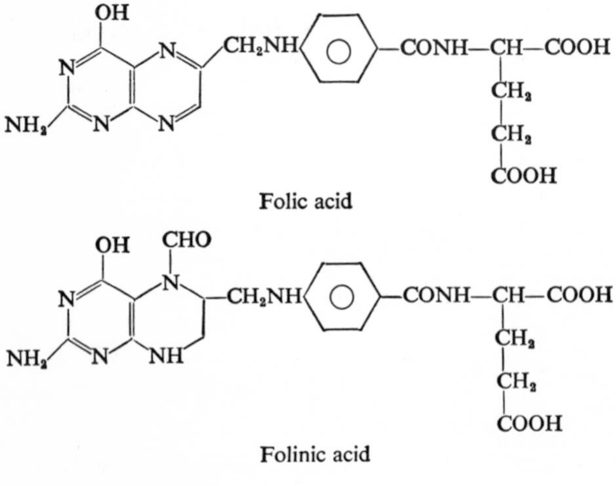

Folic acid

Folinic acid

Fig. 14.2. The structures of folic acid and folinic acid.

Utilization of folic acid may be defective during chronic administration of anti-epileptic drugs such as phenobarbitone and phenytoin.

Folic acid itself is not the active coenzyme of one carbon transfer but must first be reduced to tetrahydrofolic acid by the enzyme folic reductase. Like the cobalamins, folic acid is efficiently stored so that only small amounts of administered doses are lost by excretion. In the treatment of true dietary deficiency satisfactory responses occur with as little as 25 μg a day although usually 1–5 mg is given. In coeliac disease larger doses are necessary to compensate for the poor absorption and usually 10–30 mg are given. An effective folic acid deficiency is produced by the antifolic drugs which are specific inhibitors of the enzyme folic reductase (see Chapter 19). In this case reversal of the untoward effects cannot be achieved with folic acid but requires a tetrahydrofolate such as folinic acid (N^5-formyltetrahydrofolinic acid).

POLYCYTHAEMIA VERA

In this condition the number of red cells produced is greater than normal due to a low-grade neoplastic change in the erythropoietic cells. The excess cells can be removed by **acetylphenylhydrazine** which causes haemolysis but this is rather dangerous. Alternatively cell production may be depressed with radioactive phosphorus, but the simplest procedure is to carry out periodic bleeding; while this reduces the cell volume directly it would in itself have only transient effects, but if the bleeding is sufficient to deplete the iron stores and this is combined with moderate restriction of dietary iron intake, the red cell mass becomes dependent on availability of iron and the red cell count remains low for long periods.

BLOOD COAGULATION

Blood coagulation involves a very complicated series of reactions ending in the conversion of the soluble plasma protein fibrinogen into a polymerized meshwork of the insoluble derivative fibrin.

The process can be initiated either in shed blood, or in the body by tissue factors, in both cases leading to the generation of factors called thromboplastins which react with prothrombin in the presence of Ca^{2+} to form thrombin (Table 14.1).

Thrombin is a peptidase which splits off a peptide fragment fibrinopeptide from fibrinogen, leaving fibrin which then polymerizes to produce the clot.

Blood is kept fluid in the circulation by antagonists which either inhibit the steps referred to above or are able to remove or destroy the small amounts of active materials being produced. When activation of the system occurs a positive feedback ('autocatalytic') reaction develops.

Heparin

Heparin is a natural anticoagulant found in many tissues (first isolated from the liver and hence the name). It is especially concentrated in the mast cells which are basophil cells found in tissues and blood. With certain basic dyes, such as toluidine blue, the granules in these cells alter the colour of the dye from blue to purple. This metachromatic reaction is characteristic of heparinoids. Heparin has been extracted from tissues and purified; it is a polymer containing the repeating unit

Table 14.1. Blood clotting factors

	Blood thrombo-plastin	Tissue thrombo-plastin
Ca^2	+	+
Factor V	+	+
Factor VII	−	+
Factor VIII	+	−
Factor IX	+	−
Platelet factors	+	−
Tissue factors	−	+

$$\text{Prothrombin} \xrightarrow[\text{Ca}^{2+}]{\text{Thromboplastin}} \text{Thrombin}$$

$$\text{Fibrinogen} \xrightarrow{\text{(Thrombin)}} \textit{Fibrin}$$

O,N,sulphato-glycosamino-glucuronate. Heparins extracted from different tissues and by different processes differ in their degree of polymerization and sulphation. Concentrations of heparin must still be specified in Units related to an international standard (~120 Units/mg).

Heparin prevents the coagulation of blood when added *in vitro* as well as when administered systemically; the mechanism is complex, it certainly inhibits the effects of thrombin on fibrinogen provided that a co-factor is present, but it also has effects on various stages of thromboplastin generation. While clotting time is prolonged by heparin, bleeding time is little affected and the risk of haemorrhage is not great. A further interesting effect of heparin is to cause the clearing of turbid lipaemic serum by activation of the enzyme lipoprotein lipase. The physiological role of heparin is uncertain. Heparin is inactive when given orally in part due to its polyanionic character and in part to instability in the gastric juice. Injected subcutaneously or intramuscularly absorption is irregular probably due to tissue binding and local tenderness and induration may develop. It is, therefore, usually given intravenously, intermittently, or by infusion. The effects of a single intravenous injection are brief, the half-time being of the order of 0·5–2 hours. This is not due to rapid excretion since only traces are found in the urine, but due to rapid metabolism in the liver by desulphation and depolymerization.

Heparin readily forms compounds with bases. It has already been noted that toluidine blue reacts forming a molecular complex, this is inactive as an anticoagulant. A similar complex is formed by the basic polymer hexadimethrine. Proteins also form complexes with heparin that are especially strong if the protein is rich in the basic amino acids arginine and lysine. An example is the low molecular weight nuclear protein protamine. Both protamine (as the sulphate salt) and hexadimethrine can be used to reverse heparin actions *in vivo* and approximately 1 mg of either will neutralize the effects of 1 mg heparin. They both have anticoagulant effects themselves and overdosage must be avoided. In addition, they are both liable to produce hypotension, bradycardia, flushing, etc., perhaps by releasing histamine and other vascularly active autocoids.

Heparin itself is of low toxicity and is an excellent anticoagulant whose use is largely restricted by the inconvenience of the intravenous route, the short duration of action, and high cost. Synthetic sulphated polysaccharides have been shown to be active but up to the present have shown undesirable toxicity.

The most important use of heparin is in cardiovascular surgery, in keeping blood fluid for heart–lung machines, and for brief post-operative periods to prevent mural thrombi developing at sites of surgical injury. It is also necessary in plasma dialysis (artificial kidney machines).

It is widely used in acute thrombotic disease such as cardiac infarction, pulmonary embolism, and venous thrombosis as a stopgap until longer-term anticoagulant therapy can become effective.

The coumarin group

The action of this group was discovered during the investigation of a haemorrhagic disease affecting cattle fed on improperly cured sweet clover. It was found that the active agent was 3,3-methylene-bis (4-hydroxycoumarin) which was given the trivial name of **dicoumarol.** Dicoumarol has no action on blood clotting *in vitro* nor does it have any immediate effect when given *in vivo* but following its administration there is a gradual decline in the concentration of both prothrombin and some of the thromboplastin components notably Factors VII, VIII, and IX; the most important of these is Factor VII. The maximum effect is produced in 1–2 days. The slowness of the effect is related to the usual turnover of these proteins. The evidence is strongly in favour of dicoumarol acting by depressing the synthesis of these proteins in the liver, so that their levels in the plasma decline as the circulating proteins are catabolized. The effects of dicoumarol can be antagonized by vitamin K in what appears to be a competitive manner. Indeed, a similar pattern of defective coagulation appears in vitamin K deficiency. Consideration of the chemical structure of vitamin K and the dicoumarol group suggests that these are structural analogues. It is not known what role vitamin K plays in the synthesis of these proteins, although vitamin K appears to be related to the important quinone coenzymes called ubiquinones which are concerned with hydrogen transfer. Dicoumarol itself has draw-backs as a therapeutic agent mainly due to its poor and irregular absorption. Many analogues have been preparted, some of which, **warfarin, phenindione,** and **nicoumalone (acenocoumarol)** are most used. Warfarin acquired its name in a curious way. Rats are very susceptible to this group of drugs and die from haemorrhage if the dose is large enough. This led to their introduction as rat poisons and the most widely used was called warfarin. Later it was found that warfarin was a very satisfactory anticoagulant for clinical use.

The toxicity of the dicoumarol group is low and is mainly attributable to overdose leading to haemorrhage particularly from mucous membranes and the genito-urinary tract. Because the effects of the drugs of this group are rather long lasting, when rapid reversal of the effect on blood clotting is required, this can be achieved by intravenous vitamin K as a water-soluble derivative such as **menadiol diphosphate.** Although the clotting factors begin to rise in concentration almost immediately, a significant effect as far as stopping haemorrhage is concerned may take several hours, and if the haemorrhage is serious it may be wise to supply the missing factors by a transfusion of fresh blood or fresh frozen plasma. The usage of phenindione is decreasing because sensitivity reactions involving a rash, leukopenia, and fever are not uncommon.

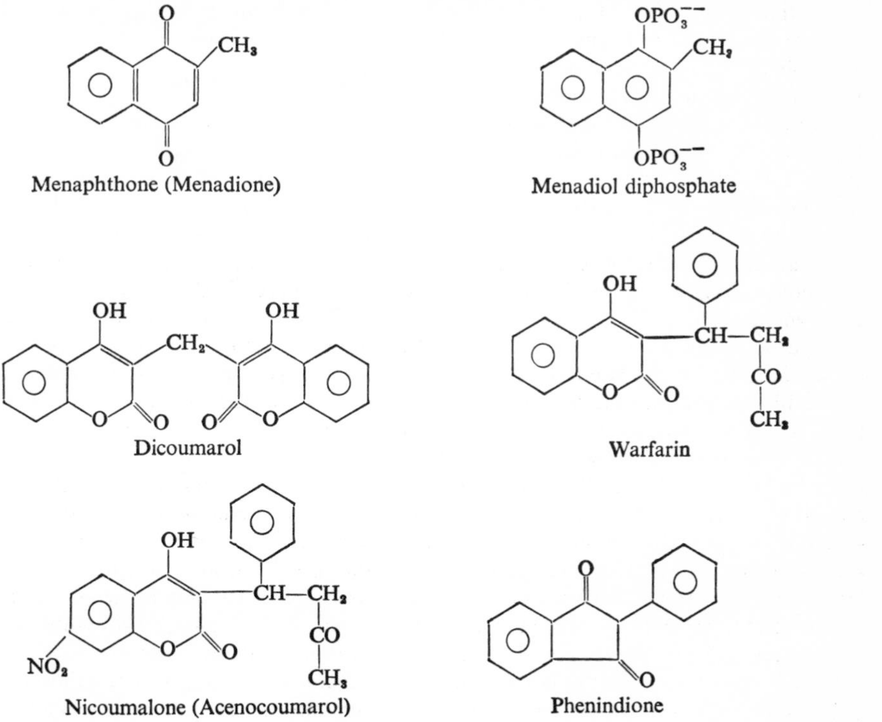

O
CH_3
O
Menaphthone (Menadione)

OPO_3^{--}
CH_3
OPO_3^{--}
Menadiol diphosphate

OH
CH_2
OH
O
O
O
O
Dicoumarol

OH
CH—CH_2
CO
CH_3
O
O
Warfarin

OH
CH—CH_2
CO
CH_3
NO_2
O
O
Nicoumalone (Acenocoumarol)

O
O
Phenindione

Fig. 14.3.

The long-term use of dicoumarol-type anticoagulants in thrombotic disease is a hotly debated issue at present. It is very difficult to establish that such therapy reduces the long-term risks of further thrombotic incidents. However, there is fairly general agreement that the short-term mortality is reduced, almost certainly due to a reduction in deep vein thrombosis which is a frequent accompaniment of confining elderly people to bed.

FURTHER READING

Bothwell, T. H. and Finch, C. A. (1962) *Iron metabolism*, Boston.

Douglas, A. S. (1962) *Anticoagulant therapy*, Oxford.

Ellenbogen, L. and Highley, D. (1963). Intrinsic factor, *Vitam. and Horm.* **21,** 1.

Engelberg, H. (1963). *Heparin*, Springfield, Ill.

Friedkin, M. (1963). Enzymatic aspects of folic acid, *Ann. Rev. Biochem.* **32,** 185.

Girdwood, R. (1960). Folic acid, its analogs and antagonists, *Advanc. clin. Chem.* **3,** 235.

Gross, F. (ed.) (1964). *Iron metabolism*, Berlin.

Ingram, G. I. C. (1961). Anticoagulant therapy, *Pharmacol. Rev.* **13,** 279.

Mollin, D. (ed.) (1971). *Haemopoietic agents*, Oxford.

O'Brien, J. S. (1962). The role of folate coenzymes in cellular division, *Cancer Res.* **22,** 267.

Smith, E. L. (1960). *Vitamin B_{12}*, London.

15

HORMONES

THE word 'hormone' was introduced by Starling in 1905 to denote 'chemical messengers' and was applied to substances liberated by special glands of internal secretion and which were carried in the blood to produce effects in other parts of the body.

Hormones may be used therapeutically in conditions of hormone deficiency or to affect physiological functions. Drugs may be used to increase or reduce the release of hormones and to antagonize the actions of individual hormones.

The hormones themselves may act at one or more sites, including cell membranes, enzyme systems, subcellular structures, or on nucleic acids, but although most of the hormones were isolated in a pure form between 1920 and 1935, it is still impossible to decide their precise mechanism of action. For many years it was thought that they worked by activating enzymes, a view which was supported by the knowledge that vitamins were a part of coenzymes, but this hypothesis has not yet been fully substantiated.

A more recent suggestion is that hormones may act by regulating the activity of certain genes. The evidence for this type of action has been obtained using the metamorphosis hormone **(ecdysone)** of insects. This is a steroid hormone which can be shown to influence the giant chromosomes in the salivary glands of midge larvae. The injection of ecdysone into mature larvae causes 'puffing' at one or two gene loci. These puffs contain and synthesize RNA and this RNA is assumed to act as messenger-RNA, the first transcript of the genetic message. The puff is thought to be the region in which genetic information is read and transferred to the cytoplasm to direct the synthesis of proteins.

There is also good evidence that ecdysone is able to cause enzyme induction. When ecdysone is injected into *Calliphora* larvae there follows a darkening of the cuticle due to the incorporation of a tyrosine metabolite, *N*-acetyl-dopamine. This substance is produced from DOPA by decarboxylation and the decarboxylating enzyme is induced by ecdysone. Inhibitors of RNA and protein synthesis prevent this synthesis.

Mammalian cells lack giant chromosomes so it is not possible to observe directly the action of a hormone on genetic material but several indirect pieces of evidence strongly suggest that this does occur.

Hydrocortisone (p. 173) appears to be a potent inducer of several enzymes, mainly those which are concerned with gluconeogenesis from amino acids and this action could account for the physiological effect of hydrocortisone on carbohydrate metabolism.

Further evidence suggests that other hormones act in this way. Enhanced RNA synthesis has been demonstrated in the testosterone-treated rat, and growth hormone, oestrogens, and thyroxine seem to act in a similar manner. The effects of oestrogens can be blocked by actinomycin and puromycin which are inhibitors of RNA and protein synthesis. If messenger-RNA mediates hormone action then the action of hormones should be reproduced by injecting the appropriate messenger. This has been done by isolating messenger-RNA from the uterus of oestrogen-treated castrated rats and injecting it into the uterus of ovariectomized rats. This procedure produces clear oestrogenic effects.

It is unlikely that all hormones act in this way. Insulin, for instance, acts primarily on cell permeability as does the antidiuretic hormone. It is also unlikely that hormones with a very rapid action can work by what is, from its very nature, a slow process.

THE PITUITARY GLAND

Although the pituitary gland is not essential for life, the hypophysectomized animal is far from normal. The gland is divided into two major hormone-producing parts, the anterior lobe (adenohypophysis) and the posterior lobe (neurohypophysis). The anterior lobe secretes hormones which regulate the growth of body tissues and the activity of the other endocrine glands. The posterior lobe secretes the antidiuretic hormone and oxytocin.

THE ANTERIOR LOBE

Hormones secreted by the anterior lobe include the growth hormone and the trophic hormones, thyrotrophin (TSH), corticotrophin (ACTH), and the gonadotrophins. The latter group consist of the follicle-stimulating hormone (FSH), the luteinizing hormone (LH), and prolactin.

Most of these substances produce their effects on the body through other endocrine glands and removal of the pituitary causes atrophy of the sex glands, the thyroid, and the adrenals: the injection of anterior lobe extracts has the opposite effect. In adults, suppression of anterior lobe secretion may be fatal as in Simmonds' disease but more often the suppression is not complete.

Releasing factors

Control of anterior lobe secretions is exerted, to a large extent, by feedback mechanisms involving an action of circulating hormones on the hypothalamus. A vascular plexus connects the hypothalamus and the anterior pituitary; this acts as a portal system and transports hormones released in the hypothalamus and which control anterior pituitary secretions. These hormones are known as releasing factors (or pituitary stimulating and inhibiting hormones) and they allow the central nervous system to exert a fine control over pituitary function.

Several releasing-factor hormones have been isolated and synthesized and they all appear to be small polypeptides.

Thyrotrophin releasing factor (TRF) stimulates the release of thyrotrophin (TSH). It may also cause the release of prolactin and is active when given orally or intravenously. The hormone has been identified as pyroglutamylhistidylprolinamide.

Luteinizing hormone releasing factor (LRF) causes the release of both luteinizing hormone (LH) and follicle-stimulating hormone (FSH) and has been shown to be a decapeptide.

Corticotrophin releasing factor (CRF) is thought to release corticotrophin after haemorrhage and other stimuli. Other releasing factors produced in the hypothalamus include prolactin releasing factor (PSF) and prolactin release-inhibiting factor (PIF), growth hormone releasing factor (GRF) and growth hormone release-inhibiting factor (GIF), and melanocyte stimulating hormone (MSH).

Thyrotrophin (TSH)

TSH is a glycoprotein which acts on the thyroid causing hyperplasia of the cells and the secretion of thyroxine. The mechanism by which TSH stimulates thyroid secretion is unknown despite many studies on the chemical and enzymatic changes that are produced in the gland or in tissue slices.

The control of TSH secretion is largely regulated by the amount of thyroxine circulating in the blood and if thyroxine is injected into the blood stream, then TSH secretion is reduced by this negative feedback mechanism. Any reduction in circulating thyroxine leads to increased TSH secretion and thence to increased thyroid activity. TSH is not used therapeutically but it may be used in the evaluation of thyroid function in conjunction with radioactive iodine.

Long-acting thyroid stimulator

This substance appears in the blood of patients suffering from hyperthyroidism and, when injected into animals, it causes prolonged stimulation of thyroid function. It appears to be a gamma globulin and is probably not liberated from the pituitary.

Exophthalmos-producing substance

Pituitary extracts injected into animals cause protrusion of the eyeballs. The nature of the substance responsible for this effect has not been determined.

Growth hormone

Over-production of growth hormone is sometimes associated with an eosinophil adenoma of the anterior pituitary. If it occurs before the epiphyses have united it produces a giant. If it occurs later it produces acromegaly.

If an animal is deprived of its pituitary when young it does not grow, but remains a dwarf. The condition can be prevented by the injection of growth hormone, large and continued doses of which produce giants.

Growth hormone acts directly on all cells and causes a rapid growth of bones, associated with a rise of alkaline phosphatase and inorganic phosphate in the plasma. The amount of protein and water in the organs increases, and the amount of fat generally falls. Nitrogen is retained by the body and there is an increased blood glucose level.

This hormone is species specific and because supplies of human growth hormone are severely limited it is only used to treat a small number of cases of dwarfism.

The growth hormone releasing factor, which is produced in the hypothalamus, has recently been isolated and found to be a small acidic peptide with only fifteen amino acid residues. It should be relatively simple to synthesize this compound and it may prove invaluable in the treatment of dwarfism and similar growth disorders.

Corticotrophin (adrenocorticotrophic hormone, ACTH)

Corticotrophin is an anterior pituitary hormone whose chemical structure is known. The hormone from pig, ox, and sheep pituitary contains thirty-nine amino-acid residues and if one amino acid from the NH_2-terminal of the molecule is lost then all biological activity disappears. ACTH stimulates the adrenal cortex to secrete cortisol, corticosterone, and a number of weakly androgenic substances. The gland increases in weight, loses ascorbic acid and cholesterol, and undergoes histological changes, mainly in the zona fasiculata.

The most important therapeutic use of ACTH is as a diagnostic agent in studies of disorders of the anterior pituitary and adrenal cortex, i.e. Addison's disease, but it may also be used in the early stages of some inflammatory diseases, and to increase the output of corticoids in children. An injection of ACTH will result in a reduced excretion of sodium, perhaps leading to oedema, and loss by excretion of potassium, nitrogen, uric acid, and 17-keto-steroids. Blood sugar levels will be raised and there may be a fall in circulating red blood cells.

The release of ACTH is under the influence of the nervous system and the negative feedback effect of circulating corticosteroids. ACTH is released under various conditions of stress including haemorrhage, burning, cold, and after a large injection of almost any drug. Emotional stress is an extremely effective stimulus for the release of ACTH.

Gonadotrophins

The anterior pituitary releases three gonadotrophic hormones which affect the ovary: (1) the follicle-stimulating hormone (FSH); (2) the luteinizing hormone (LH); and (3) prolactin.

FSH stimulates the tissues which form the ova and follicles in the female and LH then causes maturation of the follicle, ovulation, and the formation of the corpus luteum. Prolactin maintains the secretory activity of the corpus luteum. These gonadotrophins initiate puberty and regulate the menstrual cycle in females. Prolactin also initiates the production of milk after parturition.

In the male, FSH stimulates the tissues which produce spermatozoa. LH stimulates the interstitial cells of the testes to secrete androgens which causes enlargement of the prostate and seminal vesicles.

The placenta secretes chorionic gonadotrophin which acts like a mixture of the luteinizing hormone and prolactin. It can be extracted from the urine of pregnant women and is used therapeutically.

The gonadotrophins are used mainly for the treatment of infertility and cryptorchism. They are particularly useful for the induction of ovulation in women who are infertile because of ovarian malfunction, even crude extracts of gonadotrophins often producing ovulation. The main complications encountered have been excessive ovarian enlargement and multiple pregnancies. By the careful adjustment of dosage, the number of cases of multiple pregnancies has now been markedly reduced.

Melanophore-stimulating hormone

This hormone is released from the intermediate tissue of the pituitary gland. The nature of its action in mammals is not clear but in patients with certain endocrine disorders who show pigmentation chanbes, an alteration in the circulating level of this compound in the blood may be detected.

This hormone has a marked action in causing darkening of the skin of amphibia through the dispersal of the dark pigment granules of the melanophores.

THE POSTERIOR LOBE
(Neurohypophysis)

Extracts of the posterior lobe of the pituitary contain two hormones, the antidiuretic hormone (vasopressin, pitressin) and oxytocin.

The former acts primarily on the kidneys and is described on p. 188. The latter hormone causes contraction of the uterus and is particularly effective during the later stages of pregnancy and for a few days after parturition.

THE THYROID

Thyroxine and triiodothyronine are the active principles of the thyroid gland (Fig. 15.1), they are both iodine-containing amino acids. Thyroxine was isolated and chemically identified some time before the existence of a second thyroid component was suspected but in 1948 the isolation and synthesis of the second, and more active principle, triiodothyronine, occurred.

The synthesis of thyroid hormone has been studied in considerable detail because most disturbances of thyroid function arise from abnormalities in the synthesis.

Synthesis in the gland takes place in several stages: (1) iodine uptake by the gland; (2) oxidation of iodine and the iodination of tyrosyl groups; (3) formation of thyroxine and triiodothyronine from iodotyrosines; and (4) release of thyroxine and triiodothyronine.

Iodine is taken up from the blood by the thyroid gland and concentrated 20–100 times. This uptake mechanism is an active membrane process and may be inhibited by thiocyanate, perchlorate, or by cardiac glycoisdes. Once in the gland, the iodine is oxidized and incorporated into the tyrosyl groups of thyroglobulin.

It is this stage in the synthesis which is blocked by antithyroid drugs. These agents produce an enlarged, goitrous thyroid and numerous compounds are now known which have this action and are known to act by inhibition of the synthesis of thyroid hormone.

The antithyroid drugs fall into four groups: (1) the thioamides, i.e. thiourea; (2) aniline derivatives, i.e. sulphonamides; (3) polyhydric phenols, i.e. resorcinol; and (4) miscellaneous compounds.

The structures of some of the compounds which have been used as antithyroid drugs are shown in Fig. 15.2.

These antithyroid drugs have an almost immediate effect, when there is no reserve of thyroxine, because they act at the first stage of iodine incorporation by the gland. The iodine is still concentrated in the gland but these drugs prevent its incorporation into

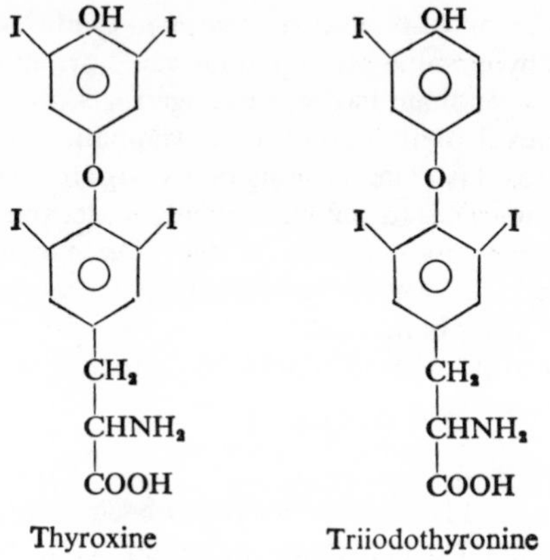

Thyroxine Triiodothyronine

Fig. 15.1. The thyroid hormones.

the organic form perhaps by antagonizing the oxidation of iodine which is brought about by peroxidase. It is also possible that they inhibit the synthesis of the thyroid hormone by blocking the coupling of iodotyrosines to form iodothyronines but firm evidence on this is difficult to obtain.

In the normal person, whose thyroid contains much thyroxine, thiouracil has no effect on the metabolism for several months, but in hyperthyroidism there is usually little thyroxine in the gland, and the drug is quickly effective.

While the initial high doses of thiouracil or related compounds are being given, toxic effects may occur, including rashes, fever, oedema, swelling of the lymph glands, and conjunctivitis. The most serious effects are the disappearance of white cells and platelets from the blood; treatment must therefore be controlled with blood counts and stopped if necessary.

The most commonly used antithyroid preparations of this type are **carbimazole** (*Neo-Mercazole*), **propylthiouracil, methylthiouracil** (*Methiacil, Thimecil*), **methimazole** (*Tapazole*). The drug of choice is probably carbimazole.

The synthesis of thyroid hormone continues with oxidation of the iodine by a peroxidase, and the inactive compounds moniodotyrosine and diiodotyrosine are formed. The next stage of the synthesis, in which two molecules of diiodotyrosine are coupled, produces the active hormone thyroxine. Triiodothyronine, which is also active, is formed at the same time. These active compounds are synthesized and stored as parts of the molecule of thyroglobulin and

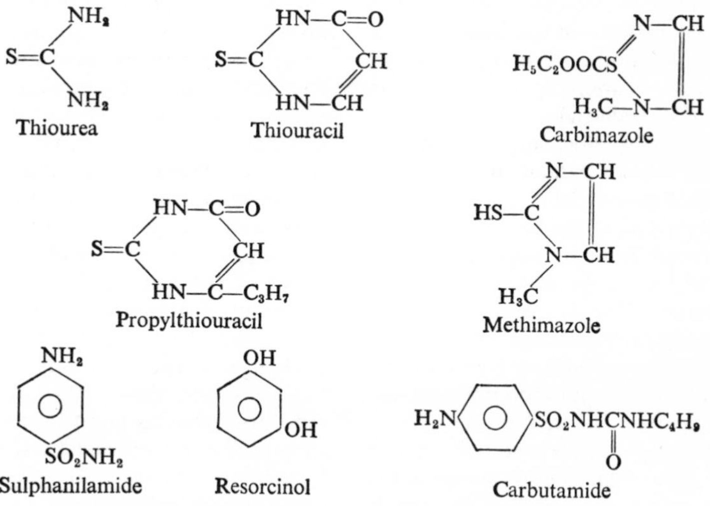

Fig. 15.2. The structures of some antithyroid drugs.

are released from the gland as free amino acids. Proteases must be concerned in this release process and, as would be expected, moniodotyrosine and diiodotyrosine are liberated as well but they are not secreted into the blood. Instead, they are broken down enzymatically and the iodine, liberated in the form of iodide, is reincorporated into protein.

Thyroxine in the blood is bound to proteins called 'thyroid binding proteins' and this binding can be competitively antagonized by substances which are chemically similar to thyroxine or by a variety of other substances including aspirin and diphenylhydantoin. When this antagonism occurs the thyroxine levels in the blood fall but secretion by the gland is unchanged.

Increased thyroxine binding occurs in pregnancy and this is brought about by circulating oestrogens.

The thyroid hormones act directly on cells and stimulate metabolic activity. The actual changes in the oxygen consumption of cells in different parts of the body vary widely after thyroxine. The testes, for instance, are hardly affected but the oxygen consumption of the heart may double. The thyroid also controls growth and hypothyroid humans do not grow up but become cretins. Because of these various effects it is unlikely that thyroxine acts on a single cellular mechanism. One possible mechanism of action was suggested by the observation that minute amounts of the thyroxine caused a swelling of fragmented mitochondria. If the hormone was altering the permeability of the mitochondrial membrane then it could also be regulating the energy output of the cell.

Alternatively, thyroxine may act by increasing protein synthesis and certainly, in rats given thyroxine, there is an increase in the incorporation of amino acids into tissues when their oxygen consumption rises. Tissues like the testes, where the oxygen consumption does not rise, do not incorporate amino acids in the presence of thyroxine.

The finding that the presence of puromycin, which reduces amino acid incorporation, reduces the effect of thyroxine on oxygen consumption, suggests that this results from an action of thyroxine on protein synthesis.

Thyroxine is slowly eliminated from the body and so has a prolonged action and removal of the liver slows elimination even more. The liver conjugates thyroxine with glucuronic and sulphuric acids and excretes these compounds in the bile. These conjugates are hydrolysed in the intestine and the free compounds are reabsorbed so that they return to the liver and the process is repeated.

THYROID DEFICIENCY

Thyroid deficiency causes myxoedema (Gull's disease), in which the skin is dry, the hair loose, the body cold, the pulse is slow, and mental functions are impaired. The metabolic rate falls and a mucoid substance accumulates in the subcutis giving the patient a puffy appearance (myxoedema). Cholesterol accumulates in the blood. Failure of the thyroid early in life produces a cretin, who, in addition to the above symptoms, fails to grow either mentally or physically.

The cure of myxoedema by the administration of thyroid was the first, and one of the most dramatic, triumphs of hormone therapy.

Various reports of the effects of grafting thyroids in thyroidectomized animals were published in 1890, and the next year G. R. Murray successfully treated myxoedema with crude extracts of sheep thyroids. Providing the right dose of thyroid hormone is taken, a patient with myxoedema can look forward to a perfectly normal and full life. Thyroxine and triiodothyronine are also used for this treatment.

Normal secretion by the thyroid requires an adequate intake of iodine and when this is lacking in the diet the thyroxine levels in the blood fall, thyrotrophin is secreted in excess, and the thyroid enlarges. The enlarged gland is about ten times more efficient in concentrating iodine than the normal gland so hypothyroidism does not usually result from an iodine-deficient diet. This condition is known as simple or non-toxic goitre and is treated by adding iodine to the diet, often in combination with salt.

THYROID HYPERACTIVITY

An excessive increase in thyroid secretion often leads to striking changes. The most typical symptoms are staring eyes, often with protrusion of the eyeballs, and a rise in metabolic rate. There is an increase in an nitrogen excretion in the urine, the reserves of carbohydrate disappear from the liver, fats from the fat deposits, and cholesterol from the blood. The excretion of water and of calcium in the urine is increased. All these factors lead to a general loss of weight, but the increase in the work of the heart, lungs, liver, kidneys, and adrenals leads to an increase in the weights of these organs. The excitability of the sympathetic receptors is increased, and this is associated with an increase in the pulse rate and a disturbance of the cardiac rhythm.

Thyroxine produces all these effects in the normal, whole animal. In exophthalmic goitre (Graves' disease, Basedow's disease) or in cases of secreting adenomas, the thyroid becomes overactive and the patient shows all the symptoms of an overdose of thyroid hormone.

DRUGS WHICH INHIBIT THYROID FUNCTION

Inhibitors of thyroid function, apart from the antithyroid drugs which interfere with synthesis, may be classified as follows: (1) ionic inhibitors that block the uptake of iodine by the gland; (2) iodide which suppresses the secretion of thyroxine in hyperthyroidism; and (3) radioactive iodine which impairs thyroid function by radiation damage.

Ionic inhibitors

These substances affect the power of the thyroid to accumulate iodine. The active agents are anions and in some way resemble iodide ions.

Thiocyanate and perchlorate. Thiocyanate is not concentrated in the gland but inhibits the uptake of iodide and has a weak inhibitory action on iodide binding. Perchlorate is concentrated in the gland and is excreted unchanged in the urine.

Iodide

This is the oldest treatment for hyperthyroidism. If iodide is given to patients with exophthalmic goitre, it causes a temporary cure with disappearance of the symptoms of hyperthyroidism. This is probably because thyroxine is retained in the gland instead of being released into the blood. The beneficial effects usually reach a maximum in 10–14 days and the symptoms then recur in spite of the continuance of the treatment, and though the cure is not permanent, it still serves a useful function in preparing hyperthyroid patients for the operation of thyroidectomy, because it reduces the size and vascularity of the gland.

Often it is used for this purpose after previous treatment with antithyroid drugs.

Radioactive iodine

This is prepared as sodium iodide (^{131}I) and is used for the study of thyroid function and in the management of hyperthyroidism.

^{131}I emits gamma and beta rays and is rapidly taken up by the thyroid, where the radiation will destroy the tissue of the gland, It is not easy to judge the correct dose to destroy just sufficient thyroid tissue, but nevertheless this treatment is often regarded as the one of choice for the management of hyperthyroidism.

Tracer studies with ^{131}I have been widely applied to disorders of the thyroid gland. The uptake of iodine can help the diagnosis of hyperthyroidism and myxoedema and the response of the thyroid to TSH and antithyroid drugs can be judged. Since the thyroid accumulates iodine the position of the gland and its size can be estimated with radiation-detecting equipment after the administration of ^{131}I.

THE PARATHYROIDS

The normal function of the parathyroids is to keep the blood calcium level constant. Removal of the parathyroids causes death with tetany due to a fall in the concentration of calcium ions.

The chemistry of the hormone is not yet fully understood. Bovine parathyroid hormone consists of 76 to 83 separate amino acid residues, at least 33 of these residues being necessary for the hormone to have biological activity.

The hormone acts to regulate the blood calcium by several means: (1) it promotes absorption of calcium from the gastrointestinal tract; (2) it mobilizes the calcium in bone; and (3) it increases renal capacity for calcium reabsorption and regulates the excretion of the ion in the faeces, sweat, and milk. The most important of these effects is that of bone calcium regulation.

Parathyroid injection is used therapeutically only for the early control of the tetany associated with hypoparathyroidism. The hormone acts slowly so calcium is normally given intravenously to obtain immediate relief. The hormone must be used with extreme care in order that hypercalciuria or hypercalcaemia are not produced. Once the tetany is brought under control its recurrence may be prevented by instituting a careful diet and by treating with vitamin D (p. 151).

Calcitonin (thyrocalcitonin)

This hormone produces opposite effects to those of the parathyroid hormone, causing a decrease in plasma calcium concentrations. Calcitonin is probably produced in the parafollicular cells of the thyroid gland and it is a single-chain polypeptide containing 32 amino acids and containing an S–S link. The hormone has been synthesized and can be detected in the blood using radioimmunological methods.

Calcitonin acts principally on bone where it decreases calcium release and may enhance calcium incorporation. This results in reduced calcium plasma levels which may be further reduced by increased renal excretion.

The secretion of calcitonin is stimulated by a rise in plasma calcium levels.

Calcitonin is used therapeutically in patients with Paget's disease of the bone which is due to an accelerated bone resorption rate and is often associated with prolonged periods of pain. Calcitonin may produce dramatic relief of the bone pain when simpler methods have failed and, in mild cases of the disease, it can induce biochemical evidence of remission.

THE PANCREAS

INSULIN

Insulin is secreted by the β cells of the islets of Langerhans in the pancreas and is used in the treatment of diabetes mellitus. It plays an important part in the regulation of blood sugar levels and its relation to other regulative factors is shown in Fig. 15.3.

In 1926, four years after active extracts of insulin were obtained from the pancreas, crystalline insulin was isolated and an investigation into its structure became possible. It has a molecular weight of about 5700 and is made up of two parallel amino acid chains of thirty and twenty-one amino acids crosslinked by disulphide bonds of cystine residues. There are species differences in the structure of insulin which are usually confined to three amino acids in one of the chains. The sequence of amino acids in the chains was worked out by Sanger in 1960 and insulin was synthesized for the first time in 1964 by Katsoyannis.

The diabetic is characterized by marked changes in all phases of carbohydrate, protein, and fat metabolism. The rise in blood sugar level is a result of the decreased utilization of glucose and also the increased production of glucose. Storage of glucose as glycogen is reduced and glucose production from non-carbohydrate sources, especially

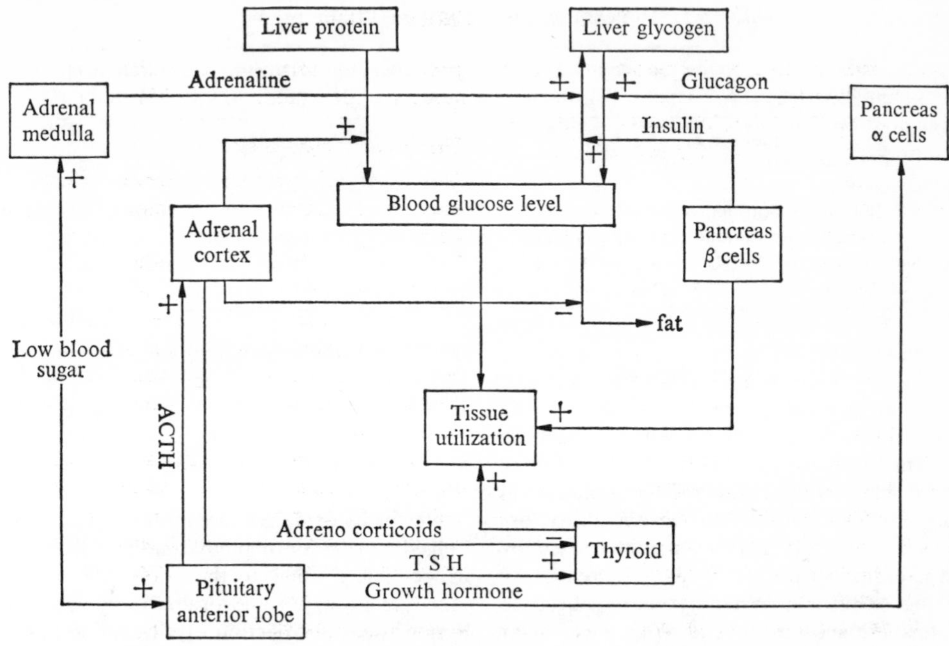

Fig. 15.3. The factors controlling blood sugar levels.
+ potentiation of effect or secretion.
− inhibition of effect or secretion.

fat, is increased. Until 1949 it was believed that insulin acted on the sugar metabolizing systems within the cell but it is now known that its primary action is on the cell membrane itself, and glucose is not utilized because it cannot penetrate the cell at the normal rate. If insulin is provided, the glucose can again cross the membrane and be metabolized. This theory of the action of insulin explains why glucose is not deposited as glycogen and why the rate of glucose oxidation is reduced. There is also strong evidence that insulin has a part in regulating glycogen synthesis by an independent action on the enzyme system involved. It is still not certain whether the impairments in fat and protein synthesis in diabetes are secondary effects of changes in carbohydrate metabolism or whether they directly require the presence of insulin. Insulin has been shown to stimulate the incorporation of amino acids into rat diaphragm bathed in a glucose-free medium so, at least as far as protein synthesis is concerned, insulin must be exerting a direct effect.

When circulating insulin is deficient or not fully effective, symptoms of diabetes mellitus will occur. These include hyperglycaemia, glycosuria, thirst, and alterations in weight. The causes of insulin lack or insufficiency may be: (1) lack of insulin secretion due to absence, degeneration, or poisoning of the islet cells; (2) tissue insensitivity to insulin; (3) excess of insulin antagonists, i.e. adrencortical hormones, pituitary hormones, glucagon, and insulin auto-immunity; and (4) depressed insulin release or transport.

The diabetic, without treatment, utilizes less glucose than the normal person, and there is an increased formation of new sugar. The storage of sugar is depressed and all these factors tend to increase the blood sugar level so that glycosuria may be present when the renal threshold is exceeded. The

Table 15.1. The characteristics of some insulin preparations

Insulin type	Time of onset (h)	Duration of action (h)
Soluble (frequent injections required)	1	6–8
Globin zinc (rarely used)	1–2	12–18
Isophane	1–2	18–20
Zinc suspension, lente	1–2	20–24
Zinc suspension (amorphous), semilente	1–2	12–16
Zinc suspension (crystalline), ultralente	4–6	24–30
Protamine	4–6	24–30

metabolism of fat increases to compensate for the decreased sugar metabolism, and this leads to the loss of body fat and to the formation of ketone bodies, which poison the patient, increase his respiration, and may make him unconscious and eventually kill him. Diabetic coma is not always easily distinguishable from hypoglycaemia caused by an overdose of insulin: it may be treated by giving sugar and insulin together, because both these substances tend to increase sugar metabolism and so relieve the fat metabolism and decrease the formation of ketone bodies. The disease is treated by reducing hyperglycaemia and ketonuria and the maintenance of body weight. Obesity, which is often present, may be reduced by a low-calorie diet and the pancreas may be stimulated to produce more insulin by drug therapy. Alternatively, the insulin deficiency may be remedied by giving insulin in a suitable form or the tissue uptake of sugar may be increased by a synthetic drug.

Hypoglycaemia may occur in a diabetic patient treated with insulin or a synthetic hypoglycaemic agent, due to unpredictable changes in the insulin requirement or the failure to eat properly or because of an insulin overdose. Hypoglycaemia will also result from over-secretion of the islet cells as happens in some types of pancreatic tumours. The symptoms of hypoglycaemia are often heralded by a feeling of hunger or nausea, sometimes accompanied by bradycardia and mild hypotension. There is usually a feeling of apprehension and sweating, faintness, and yawning may occur. The slow heart rate is replaced by a fast rate as adrenaline is released into the circulation and if the hypoglycaemia becomes severe, coma and death may result.

Most of these symptoms may be attributed to the effect of low blood sugar on the CNS, which relies exclusively on glucose as a substrate for its oxidative metabolism and a prolonged period of hypoglycaemia will cause irreversible damage to the brain. The symptoms are promptly and dramatically relieved by glucose. An injection of adrenaline has a similar effect by releasing sugar from the liver.

Absorption

Insulin is generally injected subcutaneously. Intravenous injections are less effective but quicker in their action. Administration by the mouth is ineffective because insulin is destroyed by the gastric juice. A number of attempts have been made to prolong the action of subcutaneous doses, so as to avoid frequent injection (Table 15.1). One successful method is that of Hagedorn, who found that in neutral solutions insulin combines with simple proteins known as protamines to form a precipitate. If a suspension of this precipitate is injected it breaks up slowly in the tissue where it is injected, and produces prolonged effects. If a small quantity of zinc is also added the effect is even more prolonged, and protamine zinc insulin is widely used in the treatment of diabetes. Insulin zinc suspensions (lente insulins) which contain no protein other than insulin have the advantage that hypersensitivity reactions are rare and a single daily injection gives a smooth control of blood sugar for 24 hours.

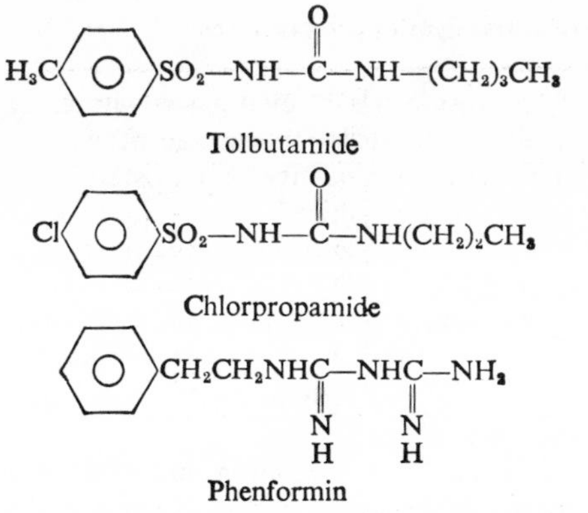

$$H_3C\langle\bigcirc\rangle SO_2{-}NH{-}\overset{\overset{\displaystyle O}{\|}}{C}{-}NH{-}(CH_2)_3CH_3$$

Tolbutamide

$$Cl\langle\bigcirc\rangle SO_2{-}NH{-}\overset{\overset{\displaystyle O}{\|}}{C}{-}NH(CH_2)_2CH_3$$

Chlorpropamide

$$\langle\bigcirc\rangle CH_2CH_2NH\underset{\underset{\displaystyle NH}{\|}}{C}{-}NH\underset{\underset{\displaystyle NH}{\|}}{C}{-}NH_2$$

Phenformin

Fig. 15.4. The structures of some oral hypoglycaemic agents.

ORAL HYPOGLYCAEMIC AGENTS

The management of diabetes mellitus was made very much easier with the introduction of orally effective hypoglycaemic drugs. There are two major types of oral hypoglycaemic agents, the sulphonylureas and the biguanides (Fig. 15.4).

Sulphonylureas

Tolbutamide (*Orinase*) and **chlorpropamide.** These compounds are arylsulphonylureas with substitutions on the benzene and urea groups. Their hypoglycaemic action is probably mediated by stimulation of insulin release from the islet cells of the pancreas.

Both substances are readily absorbed through the intestinal wall; tolbutamide appears in the blood 30 minutes after ingestion and is bound to plasma proteins and has a plasma half-life of about 5 hours. Chlorpropamide is also bound to plasma proteins and, unlike tolbutamide, it is excreted unchanged.

The drugs should be used with great care in patients with a history of liver disease. Toxic reactions include allergic rashes, gastro-intestinal and haematological disturbances.

Biguanides

Phenformin (*D.B.I.*, *Dibotin*). Phenformin does not stimulate the secretion of insulin by the pancreas and hypoglycaemia is not induced in normal subjects by this drug. The mechanism of action is unknown but it may prevent the degradation of insulin or reduce the effectiveness of an insulin antagonist. The latter possibility would explain why phenformin has a hypoglycaemic action only in diabetic patients. The drug is well absorbed from the gastro-intestinal tract and its effects last from 6 to 15 hours. It is used in the treatment of diabetes which presents for the first time in the mature patient and may be used in combination with the sulphonylureas or with insulin. The usefulness of the latter combination of drugs is still a matter of debate and is still undergoing clinical trial.

GLUCAGON

When commercial preparations of insulin are administered there is a brief period of hyperglycaemia before the prolonged hypoglycaemic effect begins. This, and subsequent experimental observations, suggested the existence of a discrete hyperglycaemic factor in the preparations and this was named glucagon. Glucagon has now been isolated and chemically purified and is a peptide containing twenty-nine amino acids.

Glucagon is present in the pancreas and is probably secreted by the α cells. The administration of glucagon depletes liver glycogen and the glycogenolytic action of glucagon is not, unlike that of adrenaline, blocked by anti-adrenergic drugs.

It seems unlikely that glucagon plays an important physiological role but it is used to counteract insulin-induced hypoglycaemia.

THE ADRENAL STEROIDS

Under the influence of adrenocorticotrophic hormone, the cortex of the adrenal gland is stimulated to synthesize a number of separate steroid hormones from cholesterol. The adrenal cortex is essential to life and if it is removed death occurs within a few days.

Under-activity of the adrenal cortex leads to Addison's disease and over-activity produces Cushing's disease or the adrenogenital syndrome. The secretion of the cortex is controlled by the adrenocorticotrophic hormone (p. 163) so the symptoms of adrenocortical abnormality may be secondary to disease of the pituitary.

About forty-three crystalline steroids have been isolated from the adrenal cortex but only seven of these are active in the body. They are usually classified into two groups, the mineralocorticoids and the glucocorticoids. The mineralocorticoids control salt and water balance by acting on the renal tubules to cause the retention of sodium, chloride, and water. The glucocorticoids accelerate the formation of glucose from protein (gluconeogenesis) (see p. 169) and have only slight effects on salt and water balance. The glucocorticoids also inhibit antibody formation and tissue responses to inflammation.

Two features, common to all these steroids, appear essential for biological activity, an $\alpha\beta$ unsaturated carbonyl group in ring A at C_3 and a two carbon side chain on ring D with a ketone group at C_{20} (see Fig. 15.5). Differences in activity between these compounds are related to the presence or absence of an α-hydroxyl group at C_{17} and of a ketonic or β-hydroxyl group at C_{11}. The absence of an oxygen atom at C_{11} makes the compound effective in causing sodium retention. When an oxygen atom is present at C_{11} the compound is moderately potent with respect to both electrolyte and carbohydrate activity. When both an oxygen atom at C_{11} and a hydroxyl group at C_{17} are present, the compound has strong carbohydrate regulating activity and has anti-inflammatory actions but little electrolyte regulating activity. For these reasons the term 11-oxycorticoids refers to glucocorticoids and 11-deoxycorticoids refers to the mineralocorticoids. Aldosterone does not fit into this classification.

The adrenal cortex also synthesizes oestrogens, androgens, and progesterone but their importance under normal conditions is not certain. The action of these hormones is described on p. 175.

BIOSYNTHESIS OF ADRENAL STEROIDS

By perfusing the adrenal gland with carbon-labelled cholesterol and acetate it was found that some radioactive corticosteroid hormones were produced and it was concluded that cholesterol and acetate can act as precursors.

Cholesterol appears to be the main precursor and the first stage of synthesis involves a cleavage of six carbon atoms in the cholesterol side chain to yield a C_{21} product, pregnenolone. Progesterone is then formed by an $\alpha\beta$ unsaturated 3-ketone oxidation and then a number of hydroxylating enzymes catalyse hydroxylations stepwise at C_{11}, C_{17}, and C_{21}.

Of the seven active steroids which are secreted into the blood, only three are secreted in physiologically significant amounts; they are corticosterone, hydrocortisone (cortisol), and aldosterone.

Synthesis of the steroid hormones may be inhibited by drugs which affect the hydroxylation reactions. The most important of these drugs are metyrapone and amphenone B (Fig. 15.7).

Table 15.2. The adrenocorticoids

Mineralocorticoids (11-deoxy)	
11-deoxycorticosterone (DOCA) (deoxycortone acetate, desozycorticosterone acetate)	High sodium retention, slight carbohydrate activity
17-hydroxy-11deoxycorticosterone	Only slight activity
18-aldocorticosterone (aldosterone)	High sodium retention
Glucocorticoids (11-oxy)	
11-dehydrocorticosterone	Moderate sodium and carbohydrate activity
Corticosterone	Moderate sodium and carbohydrate activity
11-dehydro-17-hydroxycorticosterone (cortisone acetate)	Weak sodium retention, strong carbohydrate and anti-inflammatory activity
17-hydroxycorticosterone (cortisol, hydrocortisone)	Weak sodium retention, strong carbohydrate and anti-inflammatory activity

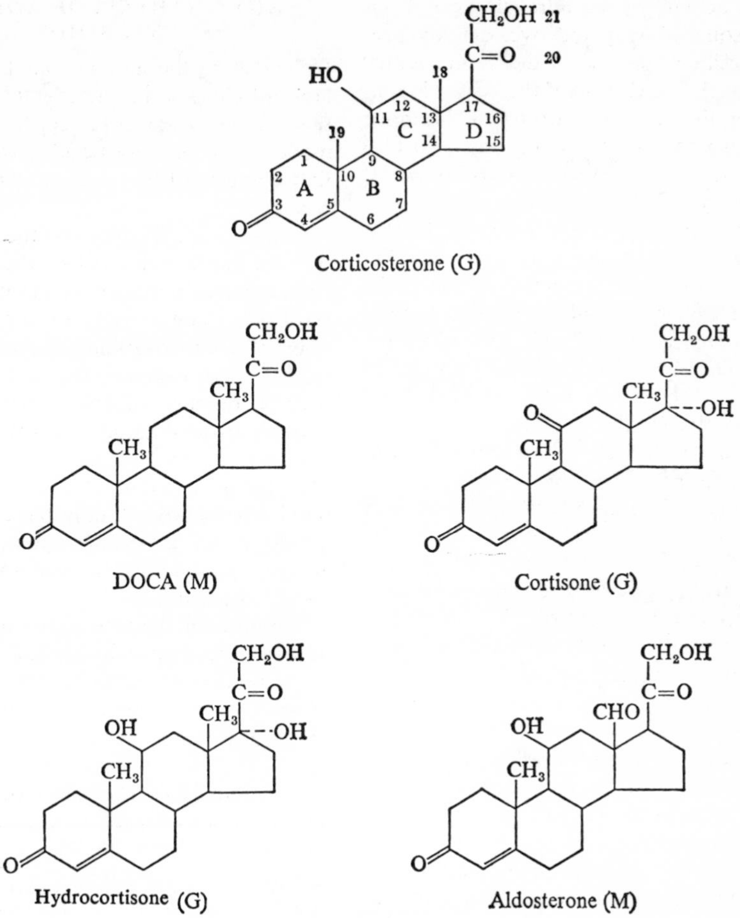

Corticosterone (G)

DOCA (M)

Cortisone (G)

Hydrocortisone (G)

Aldosterone (M)

Fig. 15.5. Structural formulae of the five most physiologically active steroids. M, mineralocorticoids; G, glucocorticoids.

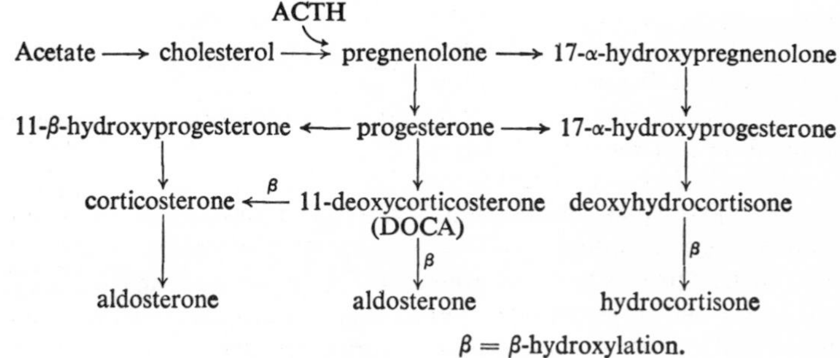

Fig. 15.6. The biosynthesis of adrenal steroid hormones and the point of action of ACTH and β-hydroxylation.

Amphenone B

Metyrapone

Fig. 15.7. The structures of drugs which inhibit the biosynthesis of steroid hormones.

Metyrapone and amphenone B

These compounds suppress the synthesis of aldosterone, corticosterone, and hydrocortisone by inhibiting β-hydroxylase which catalyses the β-hydroxylation of DOCA and deoxyhydrocortisone.

When circulating hydrocortisone levels are reduced in this way there is an increased output of DOCA and deoxyhydrocortisone and so, after giving these drugs, there is a fall in the blood levels of hydrocortisone and a rise in 17-hydroxycorticosteroids. The urinary 17-hydroxycorticosteroids and 17-ketosteroids rise and aldosterone falls. Metyrapone is used as a test for hypothalmic-pituitary function. After the drug is administered the urinary 17-hydroxycorticosteroids and 17-ketosteroids are measured. If ACTH release is low then the urinary levels of these compounds will not rise.

Spironolactone

The actions of the mineralocorticoids can be specifically inhibited by certain compounds. Various steroid lactones, e.g. spironolactone, act by competitive displacement of steroids such as aldosterone from redeptor sites in the distal renal tubule. This effect is described in Chapter 16.

CONTROL OF CORTICOSTEROID SECRETION

With the exception of aldosterone, the secretion of these hormones is largely under the control of ACTH. The factors affecting ACTH release have been described on p. 163.

The control of aldosterone secretion is an extremely complex subject and is still a matter for debate. A wide variety of conditions have been associated with an increased aldosterone secretion including: (1) low sodium diet; (2) high potassium diet; (3) decreased extracellular volume; (2) haemorrhage; and (5) emotional stimuli.

It does seem certain that aldosterone secretion is relatively independent of control by the anterior pituitary and it seems more likely that a trophic hormone, known as angiotensin II, is mainly responsible for increased production of aldosterone by the adrenal cortex.

Angiotensin II is an octapeptide which is formed from the decapeptide angiotensin I in the plasma. Angiotensin I is derived from plasma globulin when the enzyme renin is present. Renin is produced by the kidney and the stimuli for its production include a reduced arterial pressure and probably changes in circulating electrolyte levels (see Chapter 16). It is possible that angiotensin II also exerts some regulatory influence over the secretion of hydrocortisone.

ACTIONS

The corticosteroids have a great variety of actions in the body; they affect the metabolism of fats, carbohydrates, proteins, and purines; they influence the functions of the cardiovascular system, the kidneys, muscle, and the nervous system; they also help the body overcome conditions of stress.

The corticosteroids increase gluconeogenesis, oppose the action of insulin, and cause hyperglycaemia. Glucose is formed from amino acids released in tissue breakdown and fat is mobilized, often producing ketosis. The adrenalectomized animal is hypersensitive to insulin as is a patient with

Addison's disease. Administration of large doses of cortisol over a long period, or cortical hypersecretion as occurs in Cushing's disease, produces metabolic changes which are, in general, the opposite of those occurring in adrenocortical insufficiency.

The regulation of electrolyte and water balance is probably the most important role of the adrenocortical hormones. When secretion is deficient there is sodium loss, hypercalcaemia, reduction of extracellular fluid volume, and the cells take in water. When there is hypersecretion there is sodium gain, hypocalcaemia, and an increase in extracellular fluid volume.

Alterations in electrolyte and water balance caused by adrenal insufficiency will lead to disturbances in the cardiovascular system. The most important changes will be a fall in blood volume and consequent increase in blood viscosity. A lack of adrenocortical hormones also reduces the efficiency of the myocardium and patients with Addison's disease often have small hearts. Hypertension is a common symptom of adrenocorticoid hypersecretion; this is mainly due to the mineralocorticoids and is a common symptom in Cushing's diesease.

Hydrocortisone and various synthetic analogues are able to inhibit the development of local inflammation. The mechanism of this effect is not known but may be due to an action of the steroids on the metabolism of the cells involved in the inflammatory process. Steroids are often used locally for a variety of skin complaints and for arthritis.

Corticosteroids act beneficially in some diseases in which hypersensitivity is important. The corticosteroids do not inhibit antibody production in man, nor is the interaction of antigen and antibody, or the release of histamine from sensitive cells affected. It seems reasonable to conclude that the adrenocorticosteroids do not influence the immune reactions that lead to cell injury, but rather reduce the inflammatory reactions of the cell to injury.

Table 15.3 summarizes the characteristics of some of the corticosteroids which are used clinically. The structural formulae of some of the more important synthetic compounds are shown in Fig. 15.8.

SIDE-EFFECTS

Prolonged use of adrenal steroids may lead to a Cushing-type syndrome due to:

1. The retention of electrolytes and water. The symptoms include 'moon face', weight gain, oedema, raised blood pressure, and heart failure.
2. Metabolic disturbances. The symptoms include those associated with diabetes.
3. Sexual changes including abnormal hairiness and menstrual disturbances. These changes occur with very low doses but are usually reversible.

Treatment with corticosteroids may suppress the secretion of corticotrophin and so lead to atrophy of the adrenal cortex. Sudden withdrawal of the steroid treatment may then produce acute adrenal insufficiency.

Other side-effects that may occur with prolonged usage include a susceptibility to infection, peptic ulceration, muscle weakness, osteoporosis, increased coagulability of the blood, and psychoses. This last complication is not uncommon and may be dangerous and take the form of manic depression or schizophrenia. These side-effects can usually be eliminated by a careful reduction in steroid dose.

THE SEX HORMONES

The sex hormones are all steroids and are formed mainly in the interstitial cells of testes in the male and in the corpus luteum and placenta of the female.

The natural sex hormones are the oestrogens, progesterones, and the male hormones, the androgens, and they have a variety of important functions.

Table 15.3. The characteristics of some clinically useful natural and synthetic corticosteroids

Compound	Alternative name	Origin	Relative sodium retaining potency	Relative carbohydrate regulating potency	Relative anti-inflammatory potency	Main therapeutic use	Usual route of administration
Glucocorticoids							
Hydrocortisone	Cortisol	Adrenal cortex	1	1	1	Acute allergic states; Skin disease	Topical, oral, I.V.
Cortisone acetate	Cortisone	Adrenal cortex	1	0·6	0·6	Adrenal insufficiency	Oral
Prednisolone	Deltahydro-cortisone	Synthetic	<1	3	4	Rheumatoid arthritis	Oral, topical injection
Prednisone	Deltahydro-cortisone	Synthetic	<1	3	3·5	General use	Oral
Methylprednisolone	Medrol	Synthetic	0	5	5	Skin disease	Oral
Triamcinolone	Kenacort	Synthetic	<1	4	3	General use except in adrenal insufficiency	Topical, I.M.
Paramethasone acetate	Haldrone	Synthetic	0	8	10	Anti-inflammatory	Oral
Betamethasone	Celestone	Synthetic	0	?	25	Anti-inflammatory	Oral
Mineralocorticoids							
Deoxycortone acetate; Desoxycorti-costerone acetate	DOCA	Adrenal cortex	100	0	0	Adrenal insufficiency	Implant, injection
Fludrocortisone acetate	Alflorone	Synthetic	125	10	10	Adrenal insufficiency and skin disease	Topical, oral
Aldosterone	Aldocorten	Adrenal cortex	3,000	0·3	?	None	—

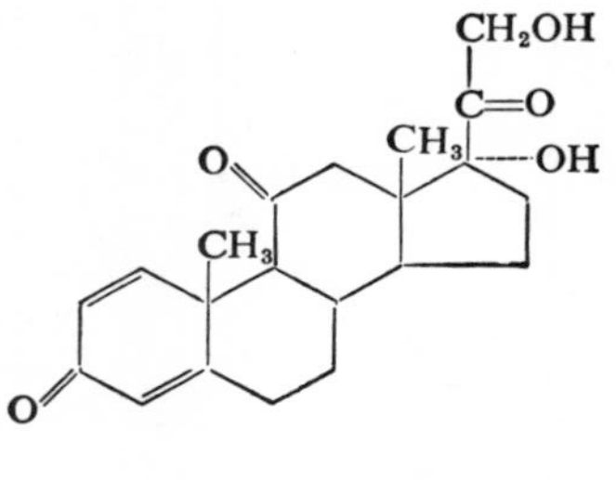

Prednisone

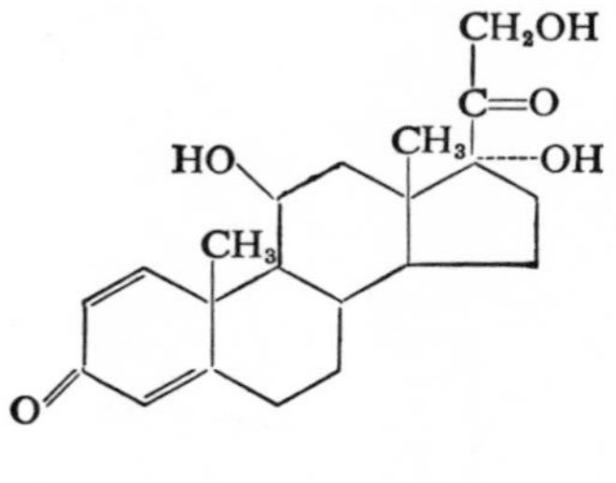

Prednisolone

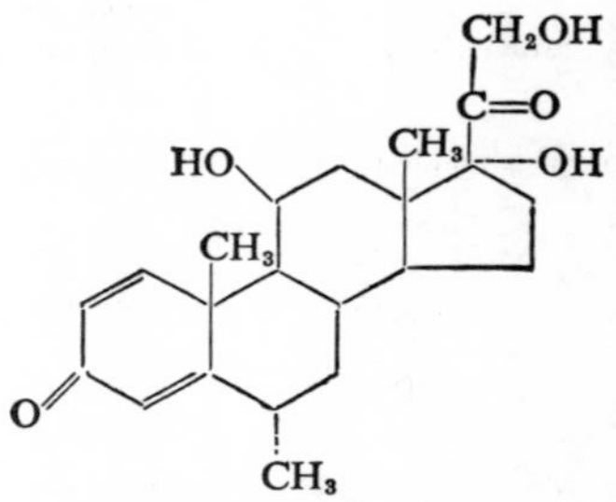

Methylprednisolone

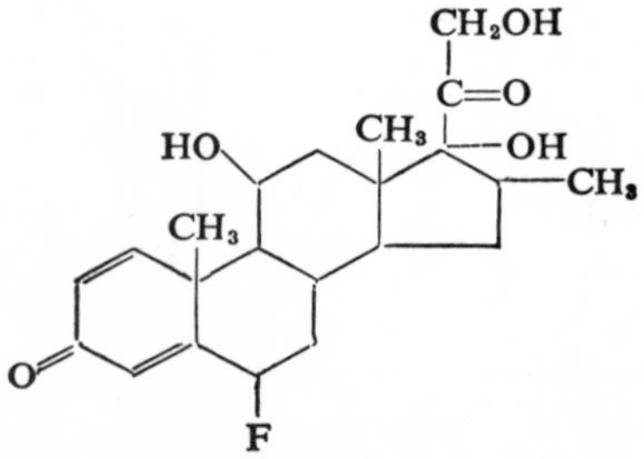

Paramethasone

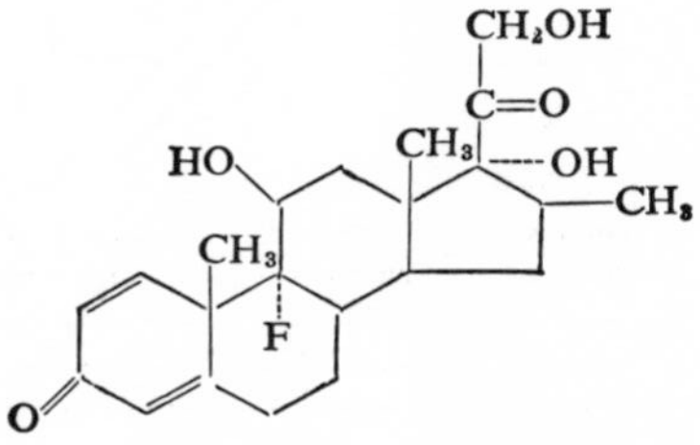

Betamethasone

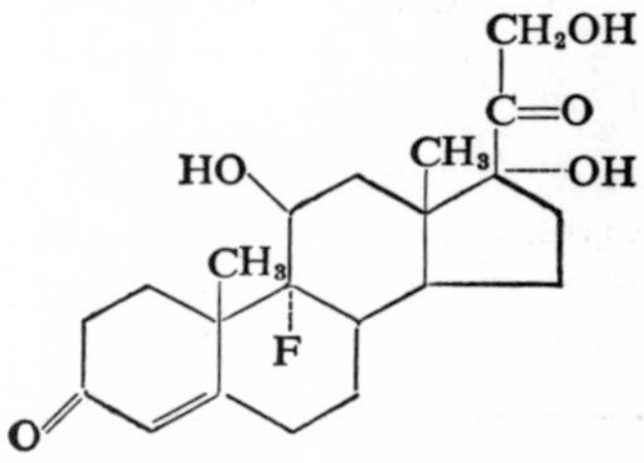

Fludrocortisone

Fig. 15.8. The structures of some synthetic steroids.

THE OESTROGENS

The oestrogens are female sex hormones responsible for the development and maintenance of accessory sex organs and secondary sexual characteristics in the female.

They increase the motor activity of the uterus and increase the size of the mammary glands and induce oestrus. They cause proliferation of the endometrium (Fig. 15.9) and menstruation occurs when they are withdrawn.

The ovary secretes three oestrogenic compounds, oestradiol, oestriol, and oestrone. These compounds are also secreted in small amounts from the adrenal cortex, the testes, and the placenta. Oestradiol is the most potent oestrogen secreted by the ovary and it is readily oxidized in the body to oestrone which can then be hydrated to oestriol. These changes occur mainly in the liver and all three compounds are excreted in the urine as glucuronides and sulphates. In pregnancy the oestrogens originate from the placenta and the urine of pregnant women is rich in natural oestrogens.

Oestrogens are used to correct deficiency states. Probably the most common disorder of this type is the syndrome occurring at menopause when oestrogens are no longer secreted. The syndrome is characterized by hot flushes, weakness, and psychological disturbances and the administration of oestrogens usually secures some relief.

If menstruation ceases for more than 3 months in the absence of pregnancy or disease, a condition of amenorrhoea is said to exist. The normal cycle may be induced to begin again by the careful use of oestrogens and progesterones.

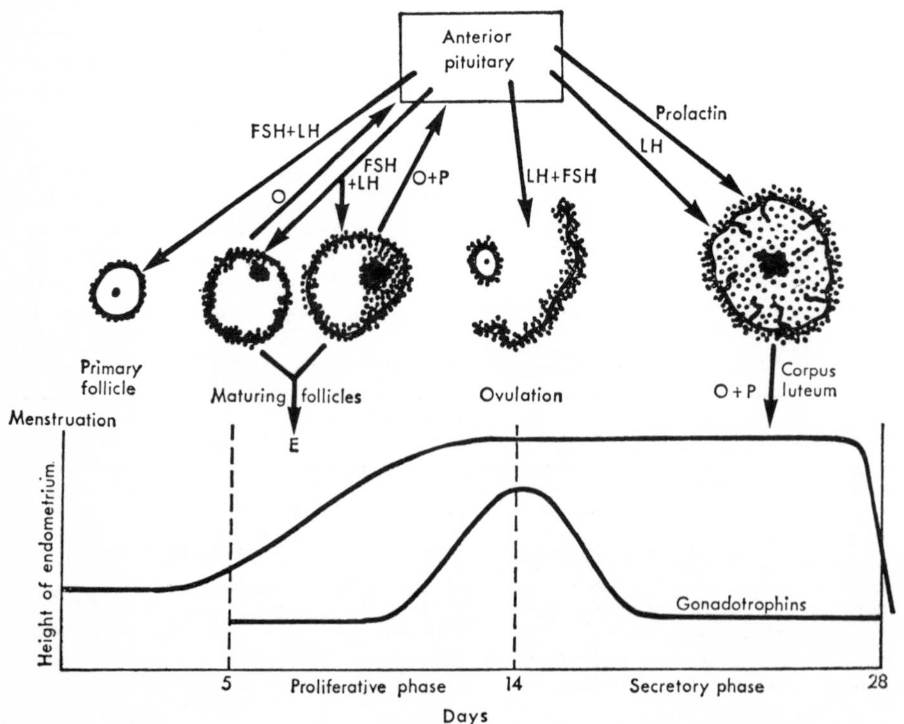

Fig. 15.9. The relationship between the anterior pituitary, ovary, and uterus during the menstrual cycle. O, oestrogen; P, progesterone; LH, luteinizing hormone; FSH, follicle-stimulating hormone.

The progress of carcinoma of the breast and prostate may be inhibited by the use of oestrogens because both these tissues are dependent upon a balance of sex hormones for their growth and function. Oestrogens suppress the growth of the prostate by antagonizing testosterone and inhibiting gonadotrophin which would stimulate the production of testosterone. The mammary gland is not affected by the administration of male sex hormones but testosterone, in combination with cytotoxic or antimetabolite drugs and the removal of other endocrine glands, may influence the course of the disease.

The most common side-effect of oestrogen therapy is nasuea, rather similar to the 'morning sickness' of pregnancy. There may also be anorexia, vomiting, and diarrhoea. These symptoms usually disappear as treatment continues.

THE INDIVIDUAL NATURAL AND SYNTHETIC OESTROGENS

Many preparations of naturally occurring and synthetic sex hormones are used therapeutically but the responses produced by all of them are very similar so the choice of drug is often determined by the convience to the patient. Oral administration is nearly always preferred.

These compounds may all be used for the following complaints: disorders of the menstrual cycle, menopausal symptoms, senile vaginitis, pruritus vulvae, and cervicitis. A few of the oestrogen-type hormones which have found a place in therapeutics are listed in Table 15.4 and their structures shown in Figs. 15.10 and 15.11.

ANTI-OESTROGENS

Progesterones and androgens may be considered as anti-oestrogens and their properties are discussed in relation to oral contraception on p. 180.

Two important anti-oestrogens have recently been discovered. They are related to chlorotrianisene and are called **ethamoxytriphetol** (MER–25) and **clomiphene** (MRL–41).

Chlorotrianisene, which is weakly oestrogenic, was found to give no enlargement of the pituitary in rats even when given in high doses. Oestradiol normally causes pronounced enlargement of the pituitary and this effect may also be reduced with chlorotrianisene. The chemically related compound ethamoxytriphetol has no oestrogenic activity but is strongly anti-oestrogenic and it inhibits naturally released oestrogens as well as stilboestrol and chlorotrianisene. The action of this compound in man has not been fully investigated.

Clomiphene interferes with the release of gonadotrophins from the pituitary, has no

Table 15.4. Some clinically useful compounds with oestrogen-like activity

Compound	Origin	Usual route of administration	Comments
Oestriol	Natural	i.m.	
Oestradiol	Natural	i.m.	
Ethinyloestradiol (Ethinyl Estradiol)	Synthetic	Oral	Very potent
Mestranol	Synthetic	Oral	Very potent
Stilboestrol (Diethylstilboestrol)	Synthetic	Oral	
Dienoestrol	Synthetic	Oral	
Chlorotrianisene	Synthetic	Oral	Stored in adipose tissue, prolonged weak action.
Methallenoestril	Synthetic	Oral	Potent; little withdrawal bleeding.

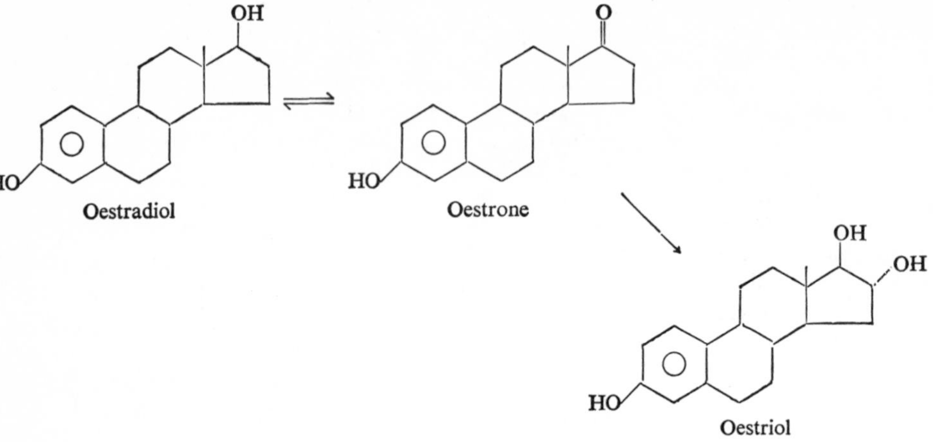

Oestradiol ⇌ Oestrone → Oestriol

Fig. 15.10. The interconversion of the oestrogen hormones.

oestrogenic activity and moderate anti-oestrogen potency. Small doses stop the oestrous cycle of normal rats and cause a reduction in the size of the ovaries. Given to humans, this compound causes an enlargement of the ovaries and it has been used in the treatment of infertility.

PROGESTERONES

Progesterone is the naturally occurring progestational hormone and it is secreted by the corpus luteum which is formed in the uterus after ovulation, half-way through the menstrual cycle. Progesterone causes proliferation of the endometrium and the inhibition of its secretion initiates menstruation.

The hormone also reduces the excitability of the uterine muscles and causes the embedding of a fertilized ovum and the development of the placenta and alveolar proliferation in the mammary gland. Progesterone secretion also inhibits ovulation.

Progesterone is only active when given by injection but a number of synthetic compounds have now been discovered which can be given orally.

The compounds that are used therapeutically can be divided into two classes, the progesterone derivatives and the compounds related to 19-norsteroids (Table 15.5). Orally active progesterones are used for a number of gynaecological disorders. A common disorder which may be treated is functional uterine bleeding. In this condition there are prolonged and irregular periods of bleeding, probably due to the irregular production of oestrogens with interruption by the secretion of progesterone. Progesterones are specific in alleviating this condition and they are usually most effective when administered with oestrogens.

ORAL CONTRACEPTIVES

Mechanism of action

Under the influence of progesterone secreted by the corpus luteum, the oestrogen-dominated uterus is able to receive a fertilized ovum and pregnancy will be maintained. During this time the circulating levels of oestrogens and progesterones are high and they act on the anterior pituitary to inhibit the release of gonadotrophins and so stop further ovulation occurring.

The administration of an oestrogen or a progesterone or both will inhibit ovulation and therefore pregnancy.

The mechanism of this effect is probably that oestrogens stop the secretion of FSH from the pituitary and the presence of progesterone prevents the release of LH.

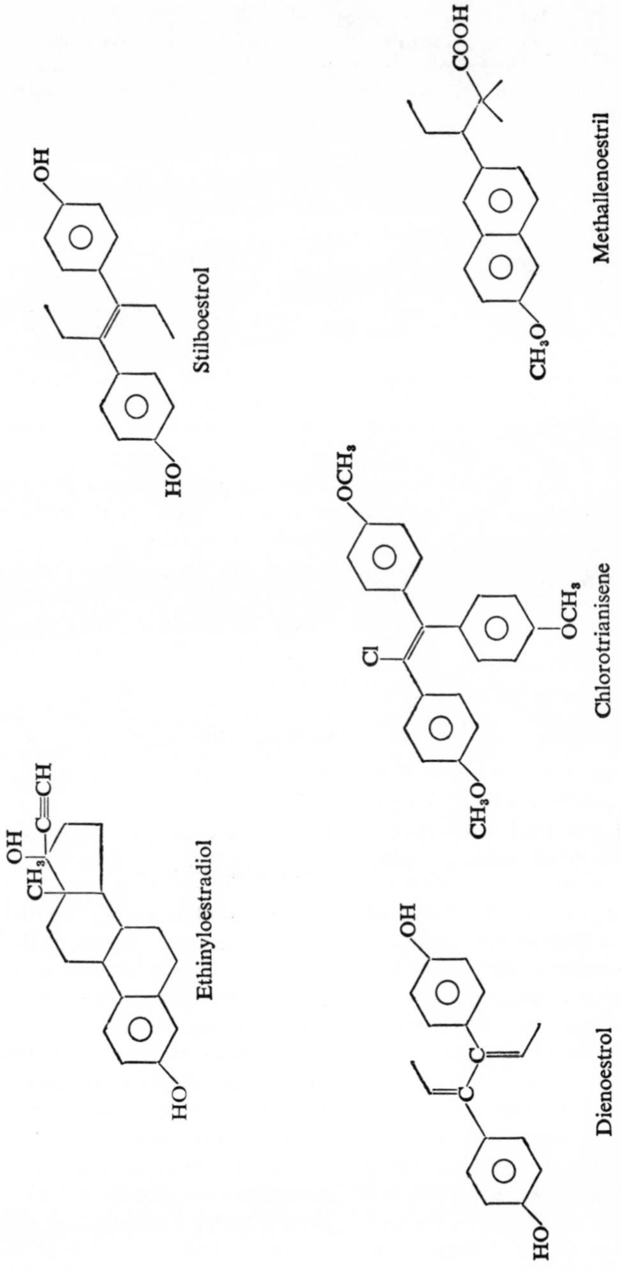

Ethinyloestradiol

Stilboestrol

Chlorotrianisene

Dienoestrol

Methallenoestril

Fig. 15.11. The structures of some clinically useful oestrogens.

Table 15.5. Compounds with mainly progesterone-like activity

Compound	Method of administration	Progesterone activity	Androgen activity	Therapeutic use
Progesterone Injection only	Injection only	high		Habitual abortion, amenorrhoea, uterine bleeding, dysmenorrhoea
Ethisterone	Oral	Delayed, prolonged	+	
Megestrol	Oral	High		Oral contraception
Medroxyprogesterone acetate	Oral	High		
Dydrogesterone	Oral			
Chlormadinone	Oral	Very high		Anti-oestrogen, contraception
Norethisterone	Oral	High, prolonged	+	Contraception
Norethynodrel	Oral	Oestrogen and progesterone activity		Contraception

Ovulation can therefore be prevented either by stopping the stimulus to ovulation or by preventing follicle growth and either of the steroids will effectively do this. In theory, therefore, either an oestrogen or a progesterone should alone be sufficient to prevent ovulation. In practice the two steroids are usually combined, the oestrogen inhibiting ovulation and the progesterone being mainly responsible for ensuring that withdrawal bleeding will be of short duration and prompt.

Oral contraceptives (the pill) are available as combined or sequential formulations of oestrogen and progesterone or of progesterone alone. The daily administration of a progesterone in combination with a small amount of oestrogen from the fifth to the twenty-fifth day of the menstrual cycle will prevent conception. Alternatively, the sequential method can be used in which oestrogen is given daily for fifteen or sixteen days of the cycle, followed by a progesterone-oestrogen combination for five days. Two to four days after completing this treatment, withdrawal bleeding occurs and the next cycle of treatment is started on the fifth day after the beginning of the bleeding.

Some oral contraceptive formulations carry progesterone only and these are taken daily without interruption. Progesterone makes the cervical mucus thick during the whole cycle and thus prevents the passage of sperm and hinders implantation of the ovum. Although this type of contraceptive is not as effective as the combination types, the absence of oestrogen reduces the risk of thrombosis and possible undesirable effects on metabolism.

Because the contraceptive compounds can be taken orally, and because fertility is not impaired and conception can occur normally when the drug is discontinued, it is likely that oral contraceptive techniques will become increasingly popular. There are still obvious improvements to be made to this type of contraception such as the elimination and assessment of side-effects and the production of compounds with long-lasting actions. This latter property now seems a real possibility and there are reports of slow-release contraceptive compounds which can be implanted subcutaneously and remain effective for many years.

There is also the possibility that post-coital contraceptives may be developed. One class of compounds that might prove useful here

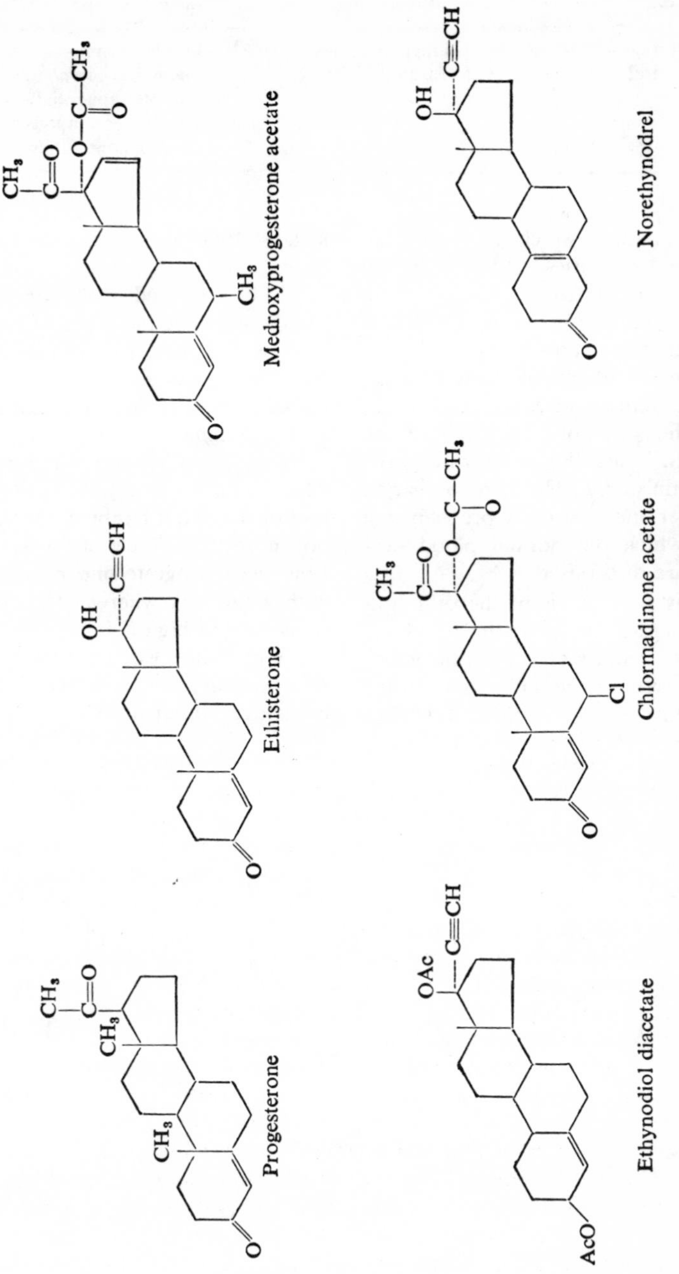

Progesterone

Ethisterone

Medroxyprogesterone acetate

Ethynodiol diacetate

Chlormadinone acetate

Norethynodrel

Fig. 15.12. The structures of some compounds with progesterone activity.

Table 15.6. The composition, name and type of some oral contraceptives

Progesterone	Oestrogen	Name and type
Norethisterone	Ethinyloestradiol	*Anovler*, combined
Norethynodrel	Mestranol	*Conovid*, combined
	Mestranol	*Ovanon*, sequential
Ethynodiol diacetate		*Femulen*, continuous
Norethisterone		*Noriday*, continuous

are the prostaglandins, which have been applied as vaginal pessaries and will inhibit implantation in the uterus.

There are a number of minor side-effects associated with the majority of oral contraceptives. These side-effects include occasional nausea, vomiting, dizziness, and weight gain. These effects do not usually persist and they can be attributed almost entirely to the oestrogen administered. They are similar to symptoms experienced in early pregnancy, a condition in which the normal blood oestrogen levels are also raised.

More serious side effects of the oral contraceptives are rare but there have been a large number of reports of venous thromboembolisms occurring in young women using the pill. Extensive epidemiological studies suggest that deep vein thrombosis and pulmonary embolism occur more often than would be expected by chance in women taking the pill. The incidence of cerebral thrombosis is also greater in women taking the pill, but these risks have to be set against the risks involved in other types of contraception and in pregnancy itself.

In order to minimize the risks, most of which seem to be due to the oestrogen content of the pill, it has been recommended that not more than 50 μg of this steroid be used. Low dose progesterone pills are associated with a low risk whereas sequential preparations carry a high risk.

There is no evidence that oral contraceptives increase the incidence of cancer of the breast, cervix, or uterus.

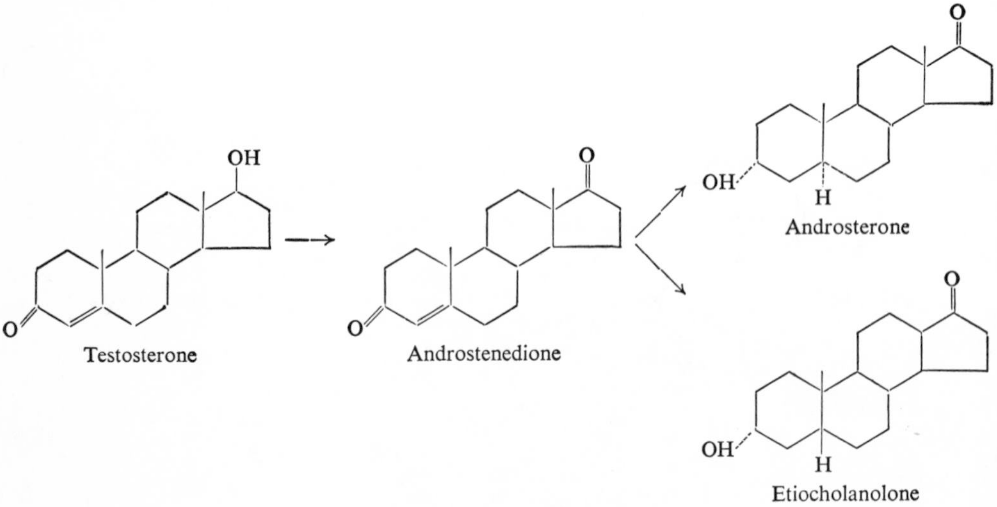

Fig. 15.13. The degradation of testosterone.

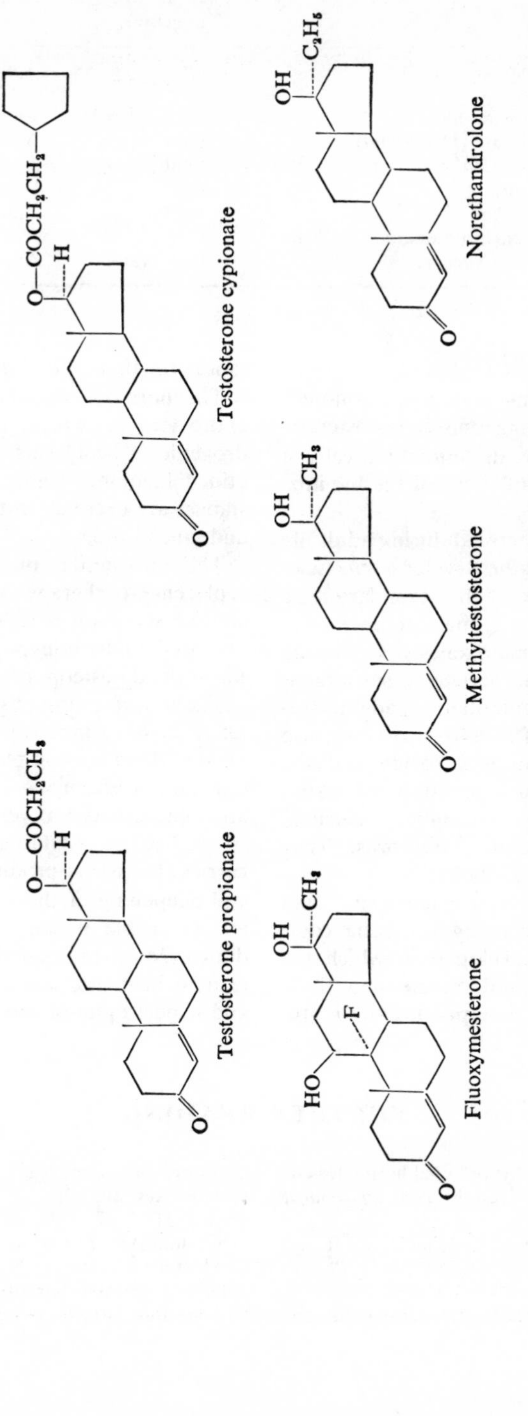
O—COCH$_2$CH$_3$
H
Testosterone propionate
O—COCH$_2$CH$_2$
H
Testosterone cypionate
OH
CH$_3$
F
HO
Fluoxymesterone
OH
CH$_3$
Methyltestosterone
OH
C$_2$H$_5$
Norethandrolone
O

Fig. 15.14. The structures of some compounds with androgen-like properties.

Table 15.7. Individual androgen compounds

Compound	Route of injection	Main use
Testerone propionate injection (*Androteston*)	i.m.	Androgen
Testerone cypionate injection	i.m.	Androgen
Testerone enanthate (*Delatestryl*)	i.m.	Androgen
Fluoxymesterone (*Halotestin*)	Oral	Androgen
Methyltestosterone	Oral	Weak androgen
Testosterone implants	Implantation	Androgen
Nandrolone phenylpropionate (*Durabolin*)	i.m.	Anabolic
Norethandrolone (*Nilevar*)	i.m., oral	Anabolic

ANDROGENS

The androgens are the male sex hormones. The naturally occurring one is testosterone and this is secreted by the interstitial cells of the testes under the influence of the luteinizing hormone.

It is continuously secreted during adult life and is responsible for the development, function, and maintenance of the secondary male sexual characteristics, the male accessory sex organs, and for spermatogenesis. Castration causes atrophy of the accessory sex organs but this may be prevented by the administration of androgens. The androgens are also secreted from the adrenal cortex and the ovaries and they cause retention of water, nitrogen, potassium, sodium, calcium, chloride, sulphate, and phosphorus. They also increase protein anabolism.

Testosterone has both androgenic and anabolic activity but many synthetic compounds have been developed in which the anabolic properties predominate and these have proved useful therapeutically to promote growth and the formation of new tissue.

The hormone is degraded in the liver to androsterone, which is only weakly androgenic, and its inactive isomer, etiocholanolone (Fig. 15.13). These substances are excreted in the urine as sulphates and glucuronides.

The most important use of androgens is in replacement therapy when normal testosterone secretion is reduced or absent. They are used to treat hypogonadism, hypopituitarism, and oesteoporosis.

The use of androgens as anabolic agents is likely to have important applications but at present there are complications, including the difficulty of producing an androgen with high anabolic activity but very low androgenic activity. The use of androgens in women always carries the risk of producing masculinization. and deepening of the voice but these effects are reversible if the drug is quickly withdrawn. More prolonged administration may lead to baldness, acne, excessive body hair, and hypertrophy of the clitoris.

FURTHER READING

Berde, B. (1968). Neurohypophysial hormones and similar polypeptides *Handb. exp. Pharmacol.* Vol. 23.

Bush, I. E. (1962). Chemical and biological factors in the activity of adrenocortical steroids, *Pharmacol. Rev.* **14,** 317.

Copp, D. H. (1964). Parathyroids, calcitonin and control of plasma calcium, *Recent Progr. Hormone Res.* **20,** 59.

Dixon, H. B. F. (1964). Chemsitry of pituitary hormones, in *The hormones*, Vol. 5, New York.

Guillemin, R. (1964). Hypothalamic factors releasing pituitary hormones, *Recent Progr. Hormone Res.* **20,** 89.

Karlson, P. and Sekeris, C. E. (1966). Biochemical mechanisms of hormone action, *Acta endocr.* (*Kbh.*) **53,** 505.

Laragh, J. H. and Kelly, W. G. (1964). Aldosterone: its biochemistry and physiology, in *Advances in metabolic disorders*, New York.

Matsuzaki, F. and Raben, M. S. (1965). Growth hormones, *Ann. Rev. Pharmacol.* **5,** 137.

Metz, R. and Best, C. H. (1960). Insulin and glucagon, *Practitioner*, **185,** 593.

Rall, J. E., Robbins, J., and Lewallen, C. G. (1964). The thyroid, in *The hormones*, Vol. 5, New York.

Schally, A. V., Artimora, A., and Kaston, A. J. (1973). Hypothalamic regulating hormones. *Science*, N. Y. **179,** 341.

Schwyzer, R. (1964). Chemistry and metabolic action of non-steroid hormones, *Ann. Rev. Biochem.* **3,** 259.

Young, F. G. (1960). Insulin, *Brit. med. Bull.* **16,** 175.

16

RENAL PHARMACOLOGY

THE kidneys are responsible for maintaining the water and electrolyte composition of the whole body and particularly the blood plasma. They do this not by a simple filtering action but by performing work in the regulation of concentration gradients and for this they consume as much oxygen, weight for weight, as does the heart.

NORMAL FUNCTIONS OF THE KIDNEY

The functions of the kidney include the maintenance of the blood osmotic pressure (chiefly by excretion of variable amounts of water), and the excretion of the waste products of nitrogenous metabolism and inorganic and organic constituents of the food which are not required in the body. The kidneys also maintain the alkali reserve of the blood by excreting excess non-volatile acids and by the formation of ammonia to neutralize excess acid.

These complex tasks are carried out in the kidneys by more than one million similar units, each unit being called a nephron. The nephron consists of a glomerulus, proximal convoluted tubule, loop of Henle, distal convoluted tubule, and collecting duct. The loop of Henle is divided into a thick descending limb, a thin descending and ascending segment and a thick ascending limb.

Proximal tubule

Blood is filtered into the glomerulus by hydrostatic pressure at about 120 ml per minute. About 60–80 per cent of this filtrate is reabsorbed isosmotically in the proximal tubule and sodium is reabsorbed by an active process. Reabsorption at this site is influenced by several factors. It has been shown that extracellular fluid volume can alter the reabsorption of sodium in the proximal tubule and there is evidence for the existence of a natriuretic hormone released in response to expansion of the extracellular fluid volume and which reduces sodium reabsorption.

Ascending limb of Henle's loop

The remaining filtrate becomes increasingly hypertonic as it travels into the descending loop of Henle, into the medulla of the kidney, and the tip of the loop. As it travels up the ascending limb, about 25 per cent of the remaining sodium is reabsorbed. This mechanism is concerned with the countercurrent multiplier system responsible for maintaining the medullary osmotic gradient. This gradient ranges from 300 milliosmols at the cortico-medullary junction to 1500–3000 milliosmols at the tip of the renal papilla. Sodium absorption in the ascending limb is passive on both the thin and thick segments where it follows the active reabsorption of chloride ions. Sodium reabsorption continues in the cortical part of the ascending limb and this results in a hypotonic solution passing on the distal tubule.

The distal tubule

As the filtrate passes through the distal tubule sodium is reabsorbed in exchange for potassium and hydrogen ions. This mechanism is regulated by aldosterone and accounts for reabsorption of up to 5 per cent of the filtered load of sodium.

The collecting duct

Here the filtrate is hypotonic but it may be modified in its passage through the medulla by antidiuretic hormone (ADH). When this hormone is present the walls of the duct are permeable to water and fluid is lost to the hypertonic medulla because of the osmotic

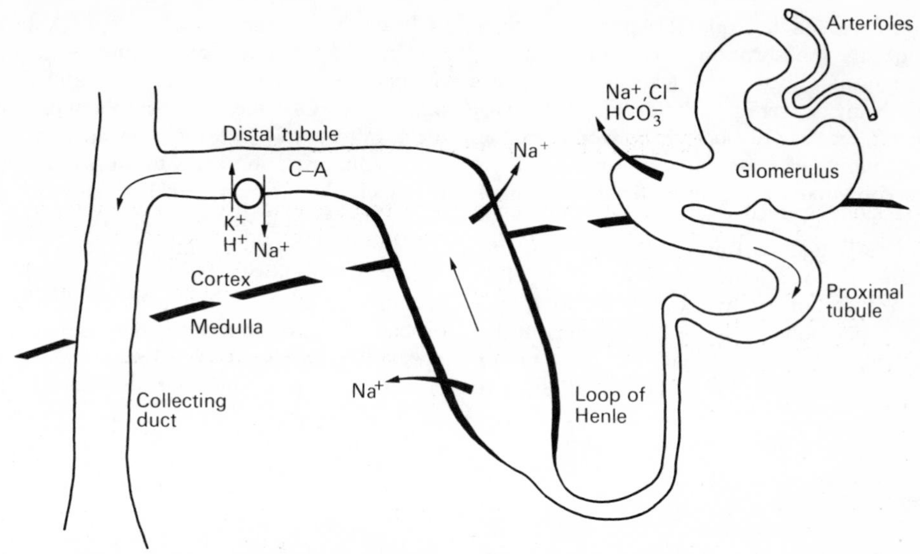

Fig. 16.1. The nephron with sites of major ion exchange.

gradient; thus a concentrated urine is excreted. When ADH is not present, only a small amount of water passes to the medulla and, because the collecting duct can reabsorb sodium, a dilute urine is produced.

The action of drugs which affect the kidney will now be considered against this background of normal function.

ACTION OF DRUGS

Organic mercurials

Inorganic mercury compounds have been known to have diuretic properties for several centuries, the discovery of this action being coincidental to their use as antisyphilitics. Their use is very limited owing to excessive toxicity. The first organic mercurial diuretic was discovered in a similar way during the clinical trial of the compound for its antisyphilitic action. It was, however, much more potent than inorganic mercury compounds and of low toxicity. Several organic mercurials have come into general use as diuretics and their structures are shown in Fig. 16.2.

The major action of the organic mercurials

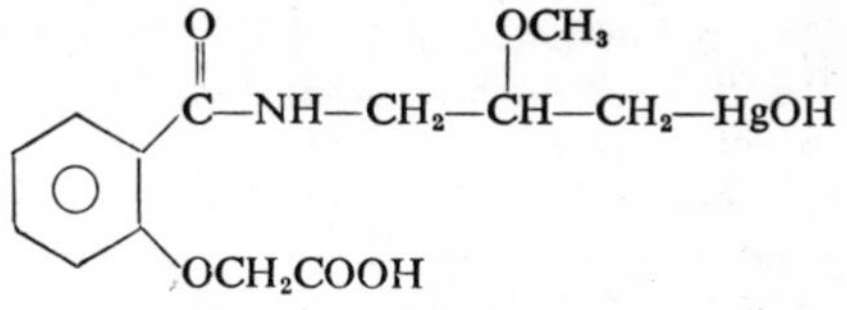

$C_6H_4(OCH_2COOH)$–C(=O)–NH–CH_2–CH(OCH_3)–CH_2–HgOH

Mersalyl

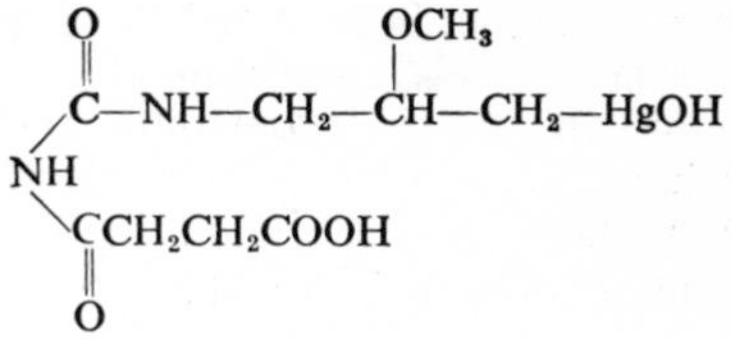

$HOOCCH_2CH_2$C(=O)–NH–C(=O)–NH–CH_2–CH(OCH_3)–CH_2–HgOH

Meralluride

cyclopentane ring [C(=O)–NH–CH_2–CH(OCH_3)–CH_2–HgOH; CH_3, CH_3; CH_3, COOH]

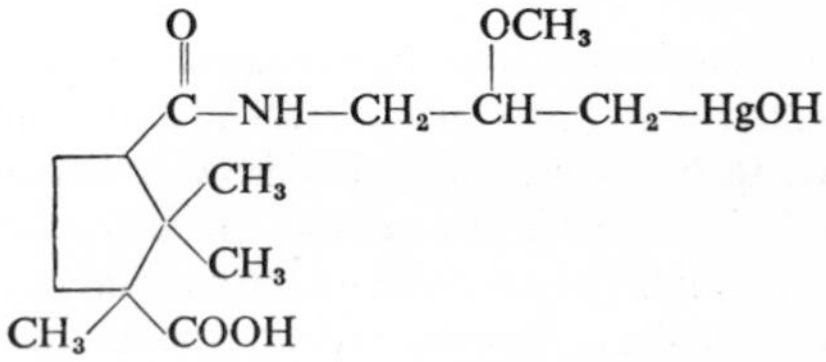

Mercurophylline

Fig. 16.2. The structures of organic mercurials.

is on the ascending loop of Henle where they reduce the reabsorption of sodium and hence of anions and water and lead to much more fluid being delivered to the distal tubule. The greater amount of sodium delivered to the distal tubule increases the reabsorption there and consequently increases the excretion of hydrions. However, the net effect is to cause a diuresis and natriuresis. A moderate increase in potassium loss also occurs. The extra excretion of hydrions leads to a systemic metabolic alkalosis. Characteristically the response to mercurials develops rather slowly and this has led to the hypothesis that the organic mercurial is not directly diuretic but slowly liberates divalent mercuric ions in the tubules which are the actual diuretic agent.

The pH dependence of their action is of practical importance as with repeated doses the mercurials become less effective. This is due to the alkalosis referred to above and the diuretic action may be restored by correction of the alkalosis with acidifying salts such as ammonium chloride.

The main use of the mercurials is in oedema due to cardiac failure in which they are highly effective. They are also used in ascites due to cirrhosis of the liver and portal obstruction and occasionally in renal oedema. When the glomerular filtration rate is low and tubule function is impaired the action of the mercurials is generally poor.

Carbonic anhydrase inhibitors

When carbonic anhydrase is inhibited the supply of hydrions to the distal cation exchange process is reduced, a smaller amount of hydrions are secreted, and despite a compensatory increase in potassium secretion the total amount of cation leaving the tubule cell is reduced and in consequence the amount of sodium that can be reabsorbed is reduced. Although this is mainly an action on the distal tubule there is some evidence that a similar action is produced elsewhere in the nephron. A secondary effect of the decreased hydrion secretion is a reduced conversion of bicarbonate to carbonic acid and hence reduced bicarbonate reabsorption. A large number of aromatic and heterocyclic sulphonamides are potent carbonic anhydrase inhibitors. Of these **acetazolamide** and **dichlorphenamide** are those in current use. Their administration leads to a brisk diuresis in which the urine is alkaline and rich in bicarbonate and potassium. A systemic acidosis and hypokalaemia result. The response to successive doses of these drugs becomes reduced as the acidosis develops, probably because in acidosis the formation of hydrions uncatalysed by carbonic anhydrase occurs at a rate sufficient to operate the cation exchange process at an adequate level. Both acetazolamide and dichlorphenamide are effective given orally but are little used as diuretics alone; they may, however, be used in conjunction with mercurials and are of special value in pulmonary heart disease owing to their effects on the alkalosis present in this condition.

Acetazolamide reduces intra-ocular tension by interfering with the secretion of aqueous humour and may be used in the treatment of glaucoma. It may also reduce the frequency of attacks in petit mal and grand mal epilepsy. Toxic effects are infrequent.

Thiazides

The carbonic anhydrase inhibitors are all sulphonamides with the amide group unsubstituted. In the search for better drugs of this group the benzthiadiazines were synthesized and found to be diuretics with a different type of action. The derivative first introduced and still the most widely used is **chlorothiazide,** although **hydrochlorothiazide** and **bendrofluazide** (*Bendroflumethiazide*) (Fig. 16.3) are also used and are more potent. Because of the possession of the sulphonamide group the thiazide are carbonic anhydrase inhibitors and so have in a mild degree the action of this group but having in addition a powerful depressant action on distal tubular reabsorption, and may be said to combine the actions of mercurials and carbonic anhydrase inhibitors. They are powerful orally acting diuretics producing an

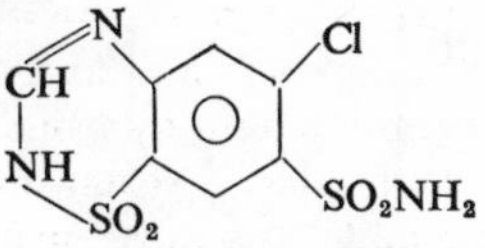

Chlorothiazide

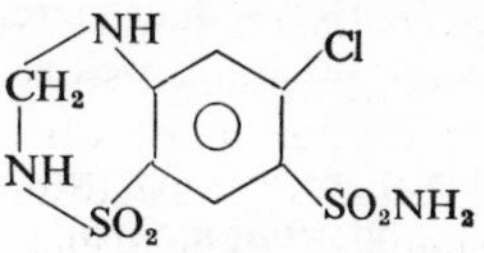

Hydrochlorothiazide

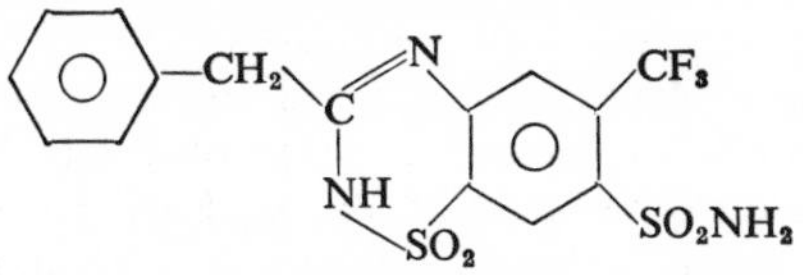

Bendrofluazide

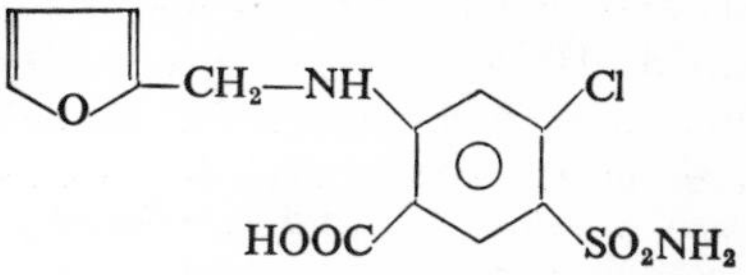

Frusemide

Fig. 16.3

alkaline urine and potassium loss with hypokalaemia. For this reason they are combined with potassium salts since hypokalaemia is to be guarded against in treating cardiac conditions because of its potentiation of the cardiac actions of the cardiac glycosides.

The thiazides are in wide use as effective diuretics in cardiac disease. They also exert useful mild antihypertensive action. A curious action of thiazides is to *reduce* the diuresis in diabetes insipidus. There is no satisfactory explanation of this action.

Clinical toxicity of the thiazides is infrequent but they tend to cause hyperglycaemia and may precipate diabetes mellitus. They cause hyperuricaemia by interfering with uric acid excretion and may cause acute attacks of gout in those predisposed to the condition.

Frusemide (Fig. 16.3)

Frusemide is related to the thiazides and produces a similar pattern of electrolyte loss. It is, however, more rapid in action and more potent in the sense that it can produce a greater peak effect than thiazides. It is useful when very rapid effects are needed as in acute heart failure and pulmonary oedema. It should be pointed out here, however, that although power and speed in a diuretic are pharmacologically dramatic, the production of a torrent of urine can be embarrassing to the patient and may lead to an undesirable contraction of the plasma and extracellular fluid space, accompanied by hypotension.

Ethacrynic acid (Fig. 16.4)

Ethacrynic acid is a diuretic of novel structure with a highly reactive ethylene (boxed in the formula). This group reacts with sulphydryl groups like many other olefins (e.g. maleic anhydride) to form adducts. It is probable that it exerts its action by reacting with sulphydryl groups in the kidney tubules associated with the active transport mechanism for sodium. Since this is basically the mode of action postulated for mercurials it is not surprising that these two diuretics tend not to be additive, nor that their general pattern of action is similar. Ethacrynic acid, however, has a more pronounced action on absorption

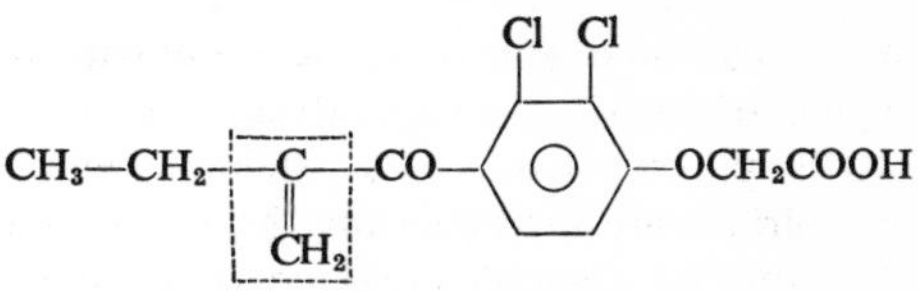

Ethacrynic acid

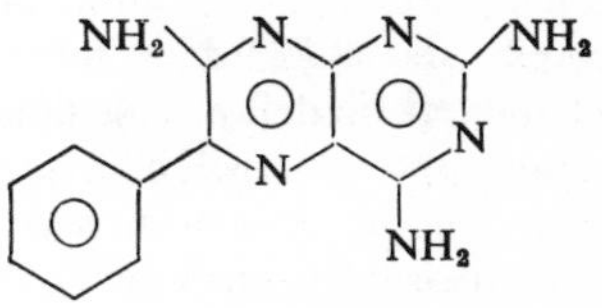

Triamterene

Fig. 16.4

in the loop of Henle than mercurials and is generally more potent as well as being orally active.

The clinical experience with ethacrynic acid is still slender but it appears highly effective and of slow toxicity. Like the thiazides it may precipitate gout.

One of the interesting things about ethacrynic acid is its marked species selectivity. It is highly active in man and the dog, but it is without effect in rats and only weakly active in the guinea-pig.

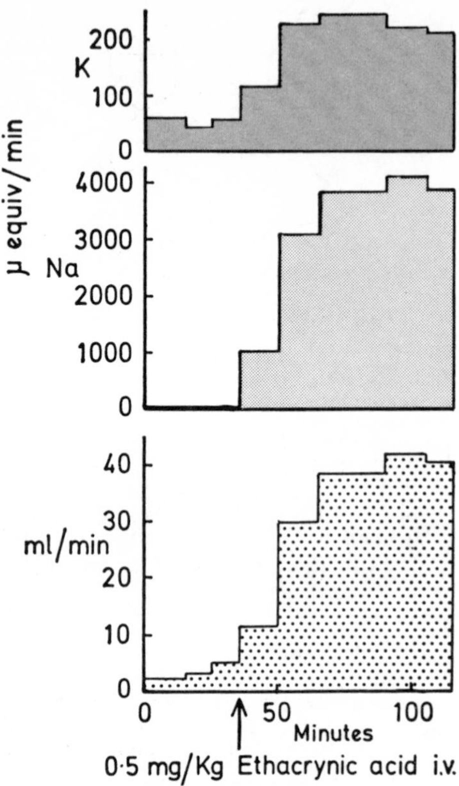

Fig. 16.5. The effects of an intravenous injection of ethacrynic acid on urine production, and sodium and potassium excretion in a patient with oedema due to cardiac failure.

Triamterene (Fig. 16.4)

Triamterene, in normal animals and subjects, produces a diuresis, increased excretion of sodium and bicarbonate, but a decreased excretion of potassium. At first it was thought that this was due to antagonism of the effects of aldosterone but the effects persist in adrenalectomized animals and in the presence of aldosterone antagonists.

Amiloride has very similar actions. Both drugs are rarely used alone, but in combination with diuretics causing potassium loss, they potentiate the diuresis while reducing the potassium loss.

Aldosterone and spironolactone

Aldosterone plays a physiological role in regulating sodium and water balance by its action on the renal tubule. Present evidence suggests this is mainly exerted in the distal tubule and stimulates sodium reabsorption and potassium secretion. The mechanism of action of aldosterone has been explored further in the toad bladder where it also increases sodium transfer. It appears that the main limiting factor to sodium transfer in this organ is the rate of passive entry of sodium into the cells and aldosterone increases this after a characteristic delay. This delay is due probably to a process involving the synthesis of a greater amount of a protein constituent of the cell which takes an hour or two to be effected. The amount of aldosterone secreted physiologically is controlled by a complicated process involving renin release by the juxtaglomerular cells of the kidney and the formation of angiotensin which stimulates the cells in the adrenal cortex which form aldosterone. Administration of aldosterone leads to a decrease in sodium excretion and an increase in potassium excretion but this effect rapidly decreases with repeated administration presumably due to a compensatory change in the proximal tubule. However, in adrenal insufficiency in Addison's disease aldosterone corrects the defect in renal handling of electrolytes. Aldosterone is not used clinically because it is inactive by the oral route and **fludrocortisone** (9α-fluorohydrocortisone) which is orally active is used instead. Most other corticoids with the exception of cortexolone have little mineralocorticoid action.

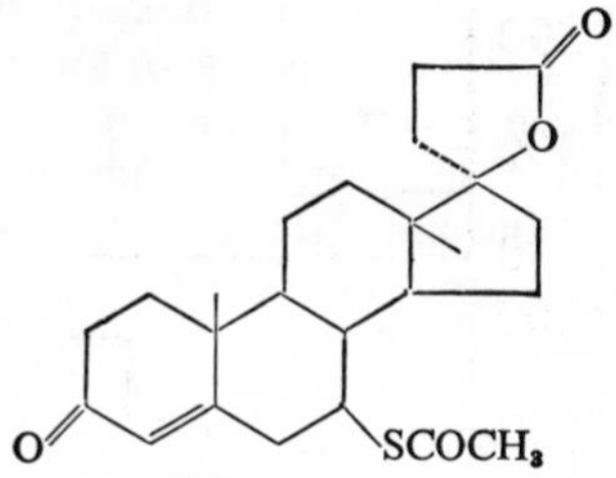

Spironolactone

Fig. 16.6. The structure of spironolactone.

Spironolactone

Spironolactone (Fig. 16.6) is one of a series of steroid derivatives having a lactone ring in the spiro arrangement at position 17. It appears to be devoid of direct effects as illustrated by its lack of effect on renal electrolyte excretion in adrenalectomized animals. However, it will antagonize endogenous and exogenous mineralocorticoids apparently by a simple competitive mechanism. Spironolactone is rather disappointing as a diuretic perhaps due to the compensatory process referred to above. When proximal tubule activity is reduced by other diuretics the effect of spironolactone is enhanced. Its use is restricted to refractory oedema which has not responded to other diuretics.

Osmotic diuresis

Diuresis can be produced by administration of large amounts of a substance readily filtered in the glomerulus but which is reabsorbed with difficulty in the proximal tubule. A simple example is the hexitol, **mannitol.** Normally, as sodium is reabsorbed in the tubule its concentration remains constant because sodium and its accompanying anions are the major osmolytes of the glomerular filtrate, and hence the passive reabsorption of water by osmotic equilibration maintains the sodium concentrations. When mannitol is present, as sodium is reabsorbed an increasing fraction of the remaining osmolyte in the tubule is mannitol and the sodium concentration falls. As the rate of sodium reabsorption is directly dependent on its concentration and ceases when the concentration falls to ~60 mEq/l a reduced reabsorption of both sodium and water occurs and hence a diuresis rather similar to that produced by mercurials results. A similar diuresis can be caused by excess filtered glucose in uncontrolled diabetes mellitus. Sodium sulphate produces a similar effect in a slightly different way. The sulphate ion is virtually non-absorbed and as it is passively concentrated in the tubules generates a concentration potential retarding sodium reabsorption.

Osmotic diuretics have a limited clinical use in poisoning (salicylates, barbiturates) where they may reduce passive reabsorption by reducing the concentration gradient and may also be used in acute renal insufficiency.

Drugs affecting uric acid excretion and metabolism

Uric acid is the main end-product of purine metabolism in man and the normal plasma level is precariously near the solubility limit at which crystals precipitate in the tissues. It appears that in the course of evolution man has lost the gene determining the enzyme uricase present in other mammals which metabolizes uric acid further to allantoin but he has retained a mechanism in the kidney for conserving uric acid. This is a complicated process in which both tubular secretion and reabsorption occur but the latter predominates so that urate clearance is normally less than 10 per cent of the filtration rate.

Gout results when the plasma urate rises and deposition occurs (mainly as monosodium urate) at selected sites in joints, subcutaneous areas (tophi), and the kidney. The increased plasma urate level in gout may be due to excessive urate production from an inborn error of metabolism, may be stimulated by drugs, such as acetazolamide, may be a consequence of increased nucleic acid breakdown in neoplasms, or it may be due to defective excretion by the kidney.

Uric acid excretion can be influenced by a large number of drugs which with one exception are acidic in character and are apparently excreted by the same transport process in the proximal tubule as hippurate, pencillin, the acid dyes of the phenol red type, and the radiographic contrast agents, diodrast, iopanoic acid, and diatrizoate.

Since the tubules both reabsorb and secrete uric acid and both these processes are sensitive to drugs, urate excretion may either decrease or increase. Most uricosuric drugs decrease clearance in small doses and increase it at greater dosage. In looking for improved uricosuric drugs the main objectives have been to favour the latter action and to produce prolonged effects. **Salicylates** decrease urate clearance except at high concentrations and are, therefore unsatisfactory. The related carboxylic acid **probenecid** is very effective in increasing urate clearance which may increase by 3–10-fold and its effects are sufficiently long lasting that dosage twice a day suffices. **Sulphinpyrazone,** a relative of phenylbutazone, is even more active and selective but is more toxic than probenecid. Uricosuric drugs cause a rapid excretion of urate but the immediate fall in blood level may be disappointing because of the large tissue reservoir of deposited urates in gout. The normal urate pool is only 1–2 g, equivalent to about 48 hours' production, but in gout excess excretion of over 100 g urate has been found after prolonged use of probenecid.

Recently it has become possible to influence plasma urate level by depressing uric acid synthesis by **allopurinol,** an analogue of hypoxanthine which inhibits xanthine oxidase, the enzyme responsible for the last stages of conversion of purines into uric acid. The levels of hypoxanthine and xanthine in the blood and urine are increased but since these latter are more soluble deposition in the tissues does not occur. Allopurinol is now established as an important drug in the control of gout (Fig. 16.7).

Alteration of urine pH

It is frequently useful to be able to alter the pH of the urine. This may be required to potentiate the action of a drug such as mersalyl, to provide the best milieu for chemotherapeutic action, or to control drug excretion. The latter action is of growing importance. Drugs that are weak bases exist in equilibrium between the charged, protonated form and the uncharged forms. The charged form is hindered by its hydrophilic character from easy transfer across cell membranes whereas the uncharged form is more hydrophobic and can often diffuse across cell membranes relatively rapidly. When a basic drug is filtered in the glomerular filtrate and concentrated in the renal tubules by reabsorption of part of the water in which it is dissolved, the drug will tend to diffuse back into the blood. The rate at which it can do so depends on the fraction which is uncharged and hence on the urine pH. Therefore the blood level of a basic drug that is

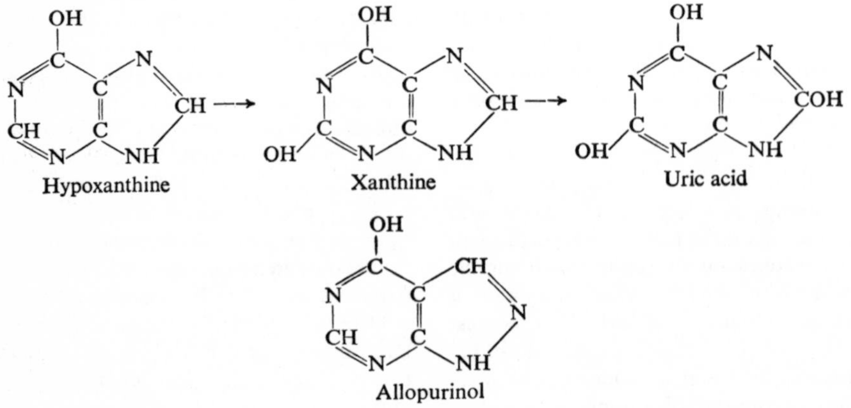

Hypoxanthine → Xanthine → Uric acid

Allopurinol

Fig. 16.7

Fig. 16.8. The structures of some uricosuric drugs.

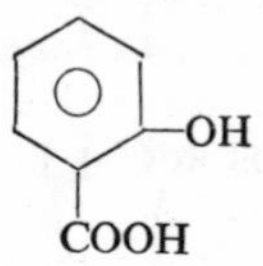

$SO_2N(C_3H_7)_2$

OH

COOH
Salicylic acid

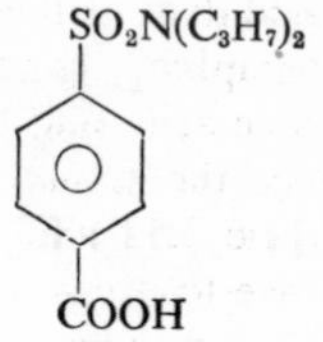

COOH
Probenecid

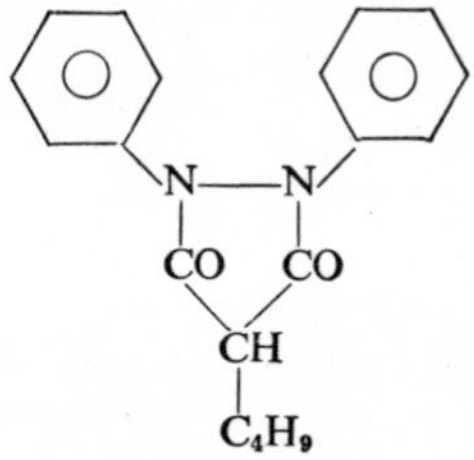

N—N
CO CO
CH
C_4H_9
Phenylbutazone

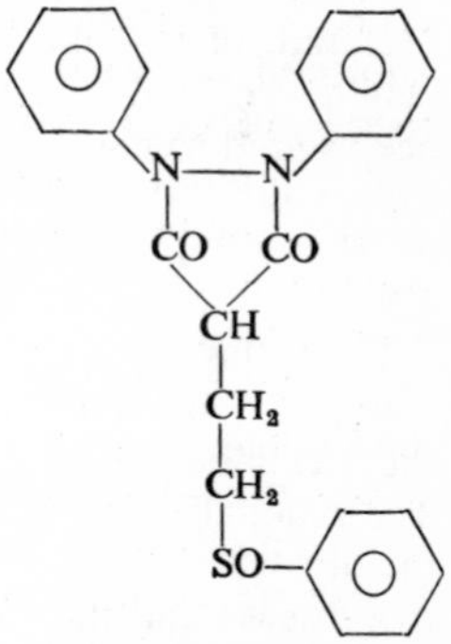

N—N
CO CO
CH
CH_2
CH_2
SO—
Sulphinpyrazone

mainly excreted unchanged will be significantly reduced by lowering urine pH (examples, amphetamine, mecamylamine). In the case of acidic drugs (such as salicylates or barbitone) excretion is increased by raising the urine pH.

The urine pH is most simply raised by giving **sodium bicarbonate,** or **sodium citrate,** the citrate ion being metabolized so that the final effect is equivalent to giving sodium bicarbonate but without the release of carbon dioxide in the stomach which may be undesirable. Acidification is usually achieved with **ammonium chloride.** In this case the ammonium ion enters into the ornithine cycle in the liver and is converted into urea and yields a hydrion; this reaction occurs rapidly and efficiently so that the administration of ammonium chloride has an effect equivalent to that of giving hydrochloric acid.

FURTHER READING

Baba, W. I., Tudhope, G. R., and Wilson, G. M. (1962). Triamterene, a new diuretic drug, *Brit. med. J.* ii, 756.

Bank, N. (1968). Physiological basis of diuretic action, *Ann. Rev. Med.* **19,** 103.

Berliner, R. W. and Orloff, J. (1956). Carbonic anhydrase inhibitors, *Pharmacol. Rev.* **8,** 137.

Beyer, K. H. and Baer, J. E. (1961). Physiological basis for the action of newer diuretic agents, *Pharmacol. Rev.* **13,** 517.

Beyer, K. H., Baer, J. E., Michaelson, J. K., and Russo, H. (1965). Renotropic characteristics of ethacrynic acid: a phenoxyacetic saluretic-diuretic agent, *J. Pharmacol. exp. Ther.* **147,** 1.

De Stevens, G. (1963). *Diuretics*, New York.

Gutman, A. B. (1966) Uricosuric drugs with special reference to probenecid and sulfinpyrazone, *Advanc. Pharmacol.* **4,** 91.

Kagawa, C. M., Sturtevant, F. M., and Van Arman, C. G. (1959) Pharmacology of a new steroid that blocks salt activity of aldosterone and deoxycorticosterone, *J. Pharmacol. exp. Ther.* **126,** 123.

Orloff, J. and Berliner, R. W. (1961). Renal pharmacology, *Ann. Rev. Pharmacol.* **1,** 287.

Pitts, R. F. (1959). *The physiological basis of diuretic therapy*, Springfield, Ill.

Pitts, R. F. (1958). *The physiological of the kidney and body fluids*, 2nd ed., Springfield, Ill.

Sharp, G. W. G. and Leaf, A. (1966). Mechanism of action of aldosterone, *Physiol. Rev.* **46,** 593.

17

CHEMOTHERAPY I: BACTERIA, FUNGI, VIRUSES

HISTORICAL

ALTHOUGH there are many remedies in the literature of folk medicine which purport to cure fevers and infected wounds, few have been found to contain active ingredients. An exception is the infusion of Peruvian bark which contains cinchona alkaloids highly effective in the treatment of malaria.

When this preparation was introduced into Europe, it became used indiscriminately in the treatment of all fevers (as opium was). The rationalization of its use came only after the discovery of the causative agents of infective disease and the subsequent classification of febrile illnesses according to their origin. The focus shifted accordingly from the alleviation of symptoms to the eradication of the cause. It was soon possible to grow bacteria in culture and it was then found that the organisms could be killed by carbolic, iodine, and heavy metal salts like silver nitrate and mercuric chloride. These agents provided the basis for the new antiseptic surgery introduced by Lister. They were used to sterilize instruments and suture material, to cleanse the skin, were sprayed in the air while operations were in progress, and were applied locally to wounds. It soon became apparent that severe limitations to their use were imposed by their toxicity for healthy animal and human cells which was comparable to their toxicity for the infecting organism. What was needed were agents which were selectively toxic against micro-organisms but with minimal toxicity for the host.

It was Ehrlich who first perceived one of the ways in which this might be achieved. In the course of experiments in which he was staining cells with the new synthetic dyestuffs, he noticed that some of these dyes were taken up selectively by particular cells or by organelles within the cells. He realized that if it were possible to find dyes that were selectively taken up by micro-organisms and were also toxic, then the selectivity of uptake might allow a toxic action on the micro-organism without significant toxicity to the host. While the initial idea applied to uptake of the antibacterial, the underlying general principle was one upon which all chemotherapy is based, viz. the discovery of biochemical difference between the infective agent and the host, and the search for toxic agents that can exploit this difference and are therefore selectively toxic.

Ehrlich's first success with his new approach was with the benzidine-azo dyes, Trypan Red and Trypan Blue. These were able to cure experimental infections with trypanosomes, but the margin between the therapeutic dose and the toxic dose was small. About this time (1905) Thomas found that an organic arsenic compound atoxyl (arsanilic acid) was highly effective in experimental trypanosomiasis and not very toxic. This finding was rapidly exploited by Ehrlich who made and tested many hundreds of organic arsenicals. Out of this programme came tryparsamide, soon shown to be effective in treating African trypanosomiasis in man, the arsphenamines and arsenoxides which revolutionized the treatment of syphilis and were the mainstay of the therapy of this disease until the advent of penicillin. The strategy of finding a lead in therapy, and then synthesizing large numbers of congeneric molecules for test in both culture and experimental infection, is now the general way in which new drugs are developed and it has been extremely successful in the development of chemotherapeutic agents for protozoal and parasitic diseases. It was curiously unsuccessful in bacterial chemotherapy until the discovery in 1932 by Domagk that the azo dye prontosil could cure streptococcal infections in mice, and in a sense this was a throwback to Ehrlich's starting-point, the azo dyes. Clinical trials soon showed its effectiveness in human streptococcal infections, but curiously enough its use was not widely exploited. This was because the medical thinking of the time favoured treatment with specific antisera. One anomalous feature of prontosil was that it was almost wholly ineffective in culture, but was effective in the whole animal. This anomaly was explained by Trefouel and his colleagues who showed that prontosil was metabolized *in vivo* to the simpler substance sulphanilamide which *was* active *in vitro* as well as *in vivo*. This made it clear that the activity of prontosil was nothing to do with its being a dye but depended on the sulphonamide group; the synthesis of congeners proceeded apace and out of the more than 4000 sulphonamides synthesized came agents of greater effectiveness, lower toxicity, and improved pharmacological properties. The first evidence of how the sulphonamides act came from the discovery by Woods and Fildes that the effectiveness of sulphonamides was much lower in some culture media compared to others. They were able to show that an antagonistic substance was present in these media which turned out to be 4-aminobenzoic acid (PABA), a bacterial growth factor. The structural analogies between PABA and the sulphonamides were evident and suggested that the basis of the chemotherapeutic was the inhibition of a reaction in the bacteria which utilized PABA.

The next great advance came from exploitation of the fact first noted by Pasteur that some bacteria could interfere with the growth of other bacteria. In 1939 the group led by Florey at Oxford started a systematic study of such 'antibiotics'. The second substance they studied had been originally discovered by Fleming in 1929. Fleming found that a green mould of the penicillin species which had contaminated a culture plate seeded with staphylococci caused lysis of the colonies in its neighbourhood. A filtrate of a culture of the mould was highly active in killing a considerable range of bacteria and could cure some infections in mice. The active material was, however, unstable and attempts to purify it failed. Florey's group soon confirmed these findings as well as the very low toxicity of the material to animals. They were able to partly purify the material and obtain enough to try in a patient. The result was spectacular and it soon became clear that penicillin, as the agent had been named by Fleming, was a chemotherapeutic agent of quite extraordinary effectiveness.

Within a short time the problems of large-scale production had been solved, and indeed use of penicillin confirmed that a new age in the treatment of infection had arrived. Widespread search for other antibacterial products produced by micro-organisms has revealed hundreds of new agents often with quite novel chemical structures. The phenomenon is a curious one that may be an evolutionary device that gives the organism that produces the antibiotic a competitive advantage. It is usually found that when organisms are growing in favourable conditions with abundant supplies of nutrients, only a trivial amount of antibiotic is produced, but when conditions are unfavourable to rapid growth the synthesis of antibiotic is increased, i.e. under the very conditions in which an improved survival might result if competitors were eliminated. We have seen that some antibacterial agents are natural products, others result from chemical synthesis, and some again from synthetic variants on natural products. The natural agents are often called antibiotics to distinguish them from the synthetic ones; this seems an absurd relic of a vitalistic past and we will not make this distinction but refer to all as chemotherapeutic agents.

PRINCIPLES OF CHEMOTHERAPEUTIC ACTION

As pointed out earlier the strategy of selective chemotherapy is to take advantage of biochemical differences between micro-organisms and the host to seek points of attack in the organism that are entirely absent in the higher organisms. Pathogenic micro-organisms represent an enormous range of species and it is, therefore, not surprising to find that antibiotics may attack a very wide or very narrow range of species. We shall discuss later the relative merits

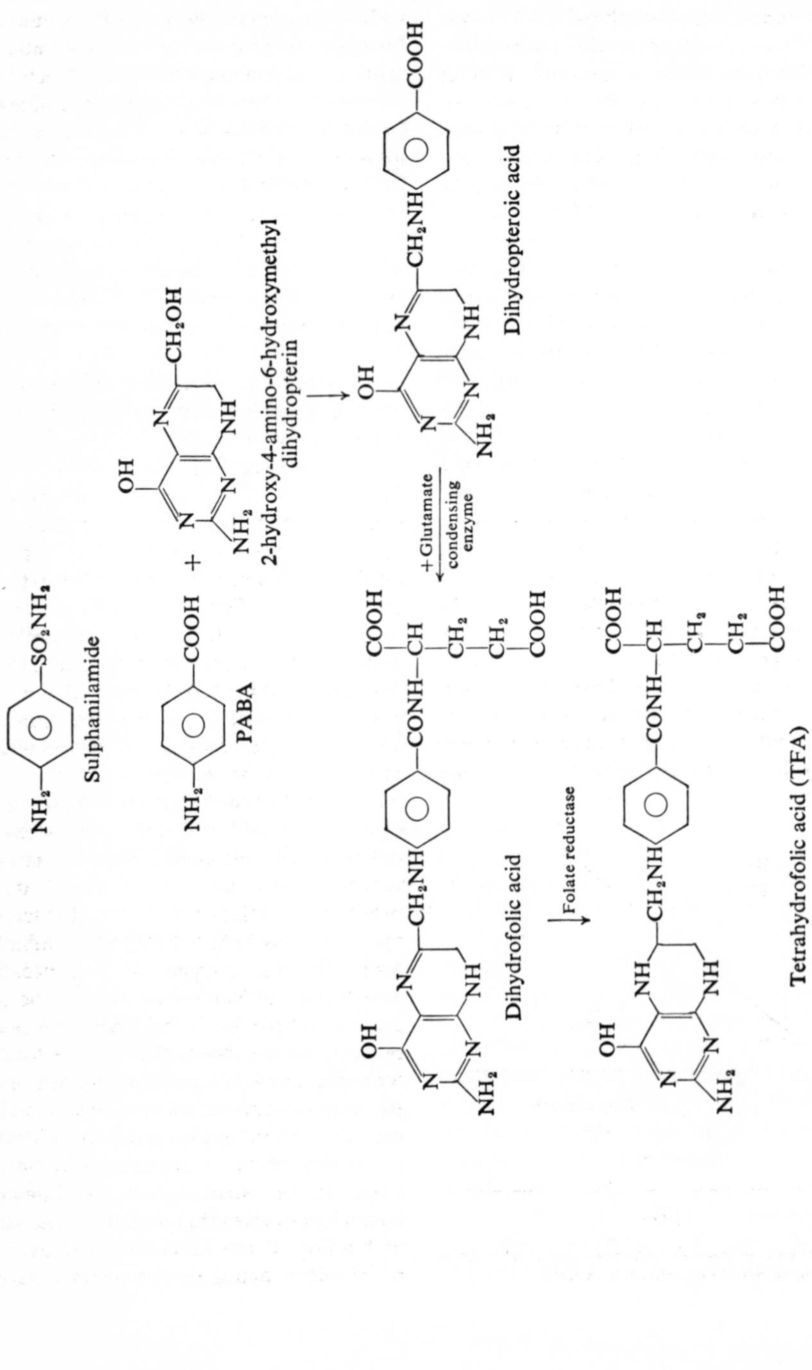

Sulphanilamide

PABA + 2-hydroxy-4-amino-6-hydroxymethyl dihydropterin → Dihydropteroic acid

+ Glutamate condensing enzyme

Dihydrofolic acid

Folate reductase

Tetrahydrofolic acid (TFA)

Fig. 17.1

of broad- and narrow-spectrum chemotherapeutics. We shall now consider in detail what these biochemical differences amount to.

We saw earlier that sulphanilamide interferes with the utilization of the growth substance PABA by micro-organisms. Further investigation showed that the bacteria condense PABA with a pteridine to form dihydropteroic acid and then add a terminal glutamic acid residue to form dihydrofolic acid. This is then reduced by folate reductase to tetrahydrofolic acid (TFA) which is an important coenzyme essential for the synthesis of nucleotides. In its absence the organism cannot make nucleic acid and is therefore unable to reproduce. Sulphonamides competitively inhibit the first of these steps, and thus reduce or completely block the synthesis of TFA.

The organisms are able to reproduce for a while on the pre-formed stores of TFA but these do not last long due to metabolic losses and dilution and then reproduction ceases, but the bacteria are *not* killed—the action is thus referred to as *bacteriostatic.* Now folic acid is a vitamin essential for the survival of man. Why does the sulphonamide not produce similar effects on the host? The reason is that mammals are unable to synthesize folic acid and are wholly dependent on preformed folic acid in the diet. On the other hand, the organisms that are sensitive to sulphonamides are unable to utilize the preformed folic acid in the tissue fluids because it is unable to penetrate the bacterial cell wall. Some organisms are able to utilize preformed folic acid and are consequently resistant to sulphonamides. The structural resemblance between sulphanilamide and PABA is obvious and it was one of the first inhibitory metabolic analogues to be discovered. For antibacterial action it is vital that an unsubstituted amino group is present in the 4 position but the amide group can be substituted by a variety of aliphatic, aromatic, and heterocyclic groups, thus allowing a considerable variation in potency, solubility, etc. (p. 208).

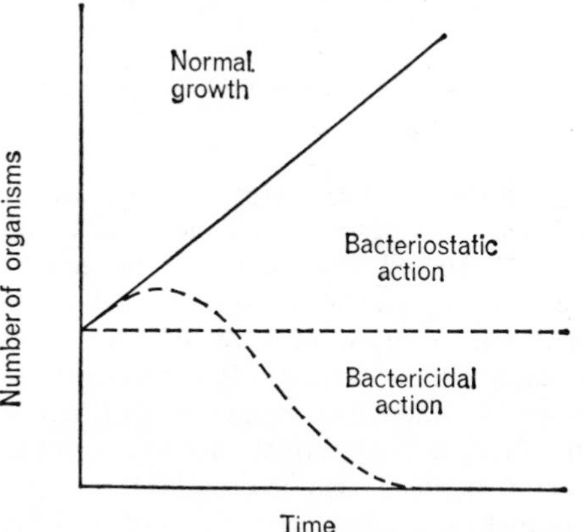

Fig. 17.2. Effects of bacteriostatic and bactericidal agents on bacterial multiplication in culture.

The metabolic pathway leading to TFA can also be interfered with by inhibition of folate reductase so arresting synthesis at the dihydrofolic stage: neither dihydrofolic acid nor folic acid can be utilized in thymidylate synthesis. The highly potent inhibitor of folate reductase, methotrexate, is a powerful antibacterial when tested *in vitro* and inhibits the growth of *Staph. aureus* at a concentration of 10^{-9} M. It is another very elegant example of a metabolic analogue. However, mammals, while relying on preformed folic acid from the diet, still need to reduce folic acid to TFA and so possess a folate reductase. Alas, methotrexate is equally good at inhibiting human folate reductase and because of this lack of selectivity is useless as an antibacterial. However, after a prolonged search agents have been found that are preferential inhibitors of the bacterial enzyme. For instance, trimethoprim inhibits the *Staph. aureus* enzyme at a concentration 100 000 times lower than acts on the human enzyme (Table 17.2). It is therefore perfectly possible to use doses that almost totally inhibit the bacterial enzyme, without affecting the human enzyme; trimethoprim is in consequence a useful antibacterial. In this case the selectivity of the action depends on differences in the structure of the human and bacterial enzymes that determine the strength of binding of the inhibitors. The availability of inhibitors acting on two distinct stages in a

Table 17.1. Spectrum of activity of commonly used antibacterial substances

	Bactericidal				Bacteriostatic	
	Benzyl-penicillin	Cloxacillin	Ampicillin carbenicillin	Streptomycin	Sulphonamides	Tetracyclines
Gram −ve cocci	+	+	+	−	−	+
Gram +ve cocci	+	+	+	+	+	+
Benzylpenicillin resistant staph.	−	+	+	+	−	+
Gram −ve bacilli	−	−	+	+	+	+
H. influenzae	−	−	+	−	+	−
Pseudomonas	−	−	+	−	−	−
Proteus vulg.	−	−	+	+	+	+
Gram +ve bacteria	+	+	+	−	+	+
Myco. tuberc.	−	−	−	+	−	+
Spirochaetes	+	+	+	−	−	+
Rickettsia	−	−	−	−	−	+
Yeasts and fungi	−	−	−	−	−	−

Table 17.2 Inhibition of folate reductase

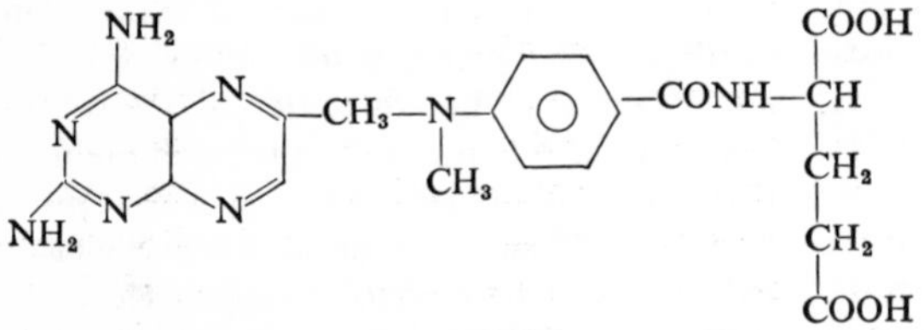

	Half inhibition of folate reductase (M)		
	Human	*E. coli*	*Staph. aureus*
Methotrexate	9×10^{-8}	6×10^{-9}	1×10^{-9}
Trimethoprim	3×10^{-4}	5×10^{-9}	5×10^{-9}

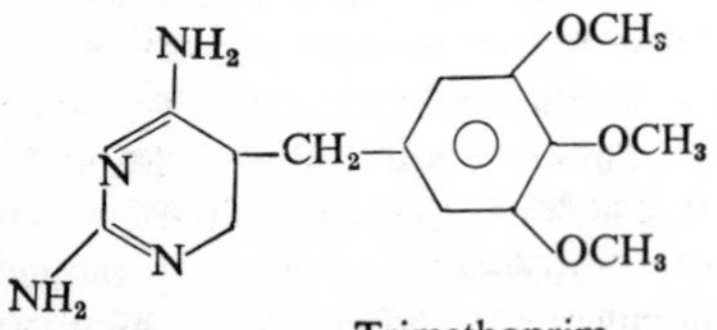

metabolic pathway raises the important question of how effective the two are in combination. This problem has been extensively studied. The combination is synergistic, i.e. the effects are greater than expected from the sum of the individual effects, so that in combination much smaller amounts of the two drugs are needed than either alone (Fig. 17.3).

Bacteria differ from mammalian cells in having a cell wall in addition to a lipoprotein cell membrane; the latter is probably basically similar to that of mammalian cells. The cell wall provides a strong mechanical support for the cell which not only protects the organism from mechanical damage but also enables it to survive in media of low osmotic strength without bursting. When bacteria are grown in sublethal concentrations of penicillin, they are abnormal in shape, being bloated and distorted. This led to the suggestion that the antibacterial effects of penicillin might be due to interference with the synthesis of cell wall structures. It was then found

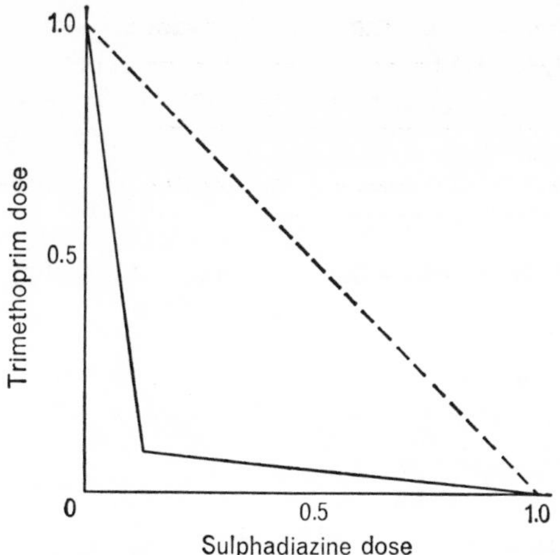

Fig. 17.3. Curative effect of combination of trimethoprim and sulphadiazine on mice infected with *Proteus vulgaris*. The solid line shows the concentration of both drugs needed to cure compared with the doses of either alone. The most effective combination is 8 per cent of the dose of trimethoprim with 12 per cent of the dose of sulphadiazine. The dashed line is the result expected if the drugs are just additive. (Hitchings and Burchall (1965) *Advanc. Enzymol.* **27,** 417.)

by Park and his colleagues that in these abnormal cells there was an accumulation of large amounts of a peculiar compound containing amino acids (called a 'Park peptide'). The reasonable suggestion was made that this peptide represented a building block for cell wall synthesis which accumulated because the inhibition of a later stage in cell wall production prevented its use.

Gradually the complex story of how the cell wall is made has become unravelled and the way in which penicillin works has become clearer. The Park peptide consists of UDP coupled to *N*-acetylmuramic acid (NAM) and then to a pentapeptide which in *Staph. aureus* consists of L-Ala–D-Glu–L-Lys–D-Ala–D-Ala. The terminus of the chain consists of the unusual D-isomer of alanine which is not found in animals. The first stage in construction of the cell wall polymer is the coupling of the NAM groups of the peptides by alternating *N*-acetylglucosamine (NAG) groups, and the second is by coupling of the peptide chains by a transpeptidation reaction in which the terminal D-Ala is lost (Fig. 17.4). The evidence suggests that it is mainly this latter stage that is inhibited by penicillin although the details still remain uncertain. Other antibacterials also interfere with the cell wall reactions. For instance, D-cycloserine (*Oxamycin*) also causes formation of abnormal cell forms and the accumulation of a different peptide, the product of reaction 3. D-cycloserine is an inhibitor of reactions 4 (*a*) and 4 (*b*) so that D-Ala and D-Ala–D-Ala are not found. Cycloserine (Fig. 17.5) can be regarded as a structural analogue of D-alanine.

Vancomycin and ristocetin have yet another way of interfering with cell wall synthesis; they have specific binding properties for peptides with a D-Ala–D-Ala terminus. The complex of peptide and antibacterial inhibits the cross linking process. Bacitracin also inhibits cell wall formation but the details of the process are obscure.

The inhibition of cell wall synthesis leads to the formation of unstable forms during reproduction which lyse and hence the antibacterials acting in this way are bactericidal. Since cell wall synthesis has no counterpart in mammalian cells the cytotoxic effect is specific. Although all bacterial cell walls appear to contain mucopeptide, those of Gram-negative organisms contain much less and depend mainly on an alternative structure (teichoic acid) which is therefore not susceptible to penicillin-type action. It is also possible that the resistance of Gram-negative organisms is partly due to the failure of the antibiotic to penetrate.

Some chemotherapeutic agents act upon the cell membrane. For instance, the macrolide polymers such as nystatin, amphotericin, and filipin have a specific lytic action on cells whose membranes contain cholesterol. Bacterial cell membranes do not contain appreciable amounts of cholesterol and are not affected but the cell membranes of fungi are rich in cholesterol, so that these substances are fungicides. Unfortunately, mammalian cell membranes also contain cholesterol, so that toxicity confines the use of these agents mainly to topical application. Gramicidin and tyrothricin have a more general action on cell membranes and are also only used topically.

1 UDP—NAM+L-Ala → UDP—NAM—L-Ala

2 UDP—NAM—L-Ala+D-Glu → UDP—NAM—L-Ala—D-Glu

3 UDP—NAM—L-Ala—D-Glu+L-Lys → UDP—NAM—L-Ala—D-Glu—L-Lys

4(*a*) L-Ala → D-Ala

4(*b*) D-Ala+D-Ala → D-Ala—D-Ala

5 UDP—NAM—Ala—Glu—Lys+D-Ala—D-Ala

→ UDP—NAM—Ala—Glu—Lys—D-Ala—D-Ala (PP)

6 PP+UDP—N-Acetylglucosamine →

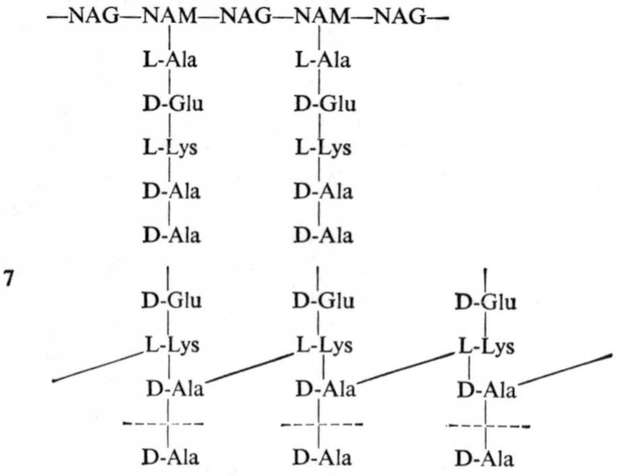

Fig. 17.4. Synthesis of bacterial cell wall.

The second major group of chemotherapeutic actions is on protein synthesis. So far actions on amino acid activation have not been seen and the site of action has been localized to the ribosome. A particularly clear action is that of puromycin which is a structural analogue of the terminal adenylic acid of a t-RNA. It appears that puromycin binds to the ribosome in place of the aminoacyl end of t-RNA, and then peptidyl transferase attaches it to the growing end of the peptide by its amino group. Since its structure is inappropriate for further growth of the peptide it acts as a terminator and the short peptide chain then detaches from the ribosome. The cell accumulates peptide fragments each terminated by puromycin. Since puromycin acts equally well on protein synthesis in mammalian cells, it is not a practical antibacterial.

A related mechanism is that of chloramphenicol and tetracycline which bind directly to the ribosome preventing the peptide bond-forming reaction. These agents are selective for bacterial ribosomes and do not bind to the larger ribosomes of animal cells.

Both chloramphenicol and tetracycline are bacteriostatic and their effects are quite rapidly reversible. Streptomycin and the related neomycin, kanamycin, and gentamicin also inhibit protein synthesis as a result of binding to the ribosome and in this case the binding has been shown to depend on a single structural protein (P10) on the 30S subunit. The binding of streptomycin distorts the ribosome so that t-RNA binding is defective, and not only is the rate of amino acid incorporation slowed but a mis-reading of the

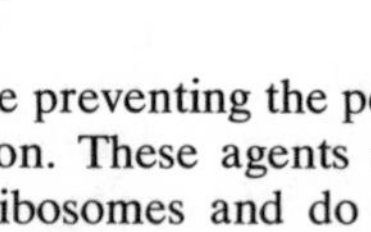

Fig. 17.5. Cycloserine.

genetic code occurs. This means that errors are made and the wrong amino acids incorporated; the proteins produced are useless and it is probable that these abnormal proteins account in some way for the fact that streptomycin is bactericidal unlike the other inhibitors of protein synthesis.

Combinations of antibacterials

We have already referred to one case, sulphonamides and trimethoprim, where combined use is synergistic. This is a common feature when antibacterials act on the same process, e.g. penicillin and ristocetin, or chloramphenicol and tetracycline, but when the drugs act on entirely different systems the results are often more difficult to predict. For instance, sulphonamide and penicillin are often less effective in combination than either alone and chloramphenicol also reduces the effectiveness of penicillin. In general it is not wise to combine bacteriostatic and bactericidal drugs.

RESISTANCE

The development of resistance to chemotherapy is a major problem not only as a source of failure in a particular case but because it will lead to the state where the majority of organisms that are isolated in disease are resistant to one or more antibacterials, as is now the case with staphylococci isolated in hospitals. Resistance develops as a result of the presence of natural mutants which are selected out as a result of the killing of the susceptible population. Resistance is *not* caused by the drug. Resistant strains are readily obtained by culturing in the presence of the antibacterial drug. Commonly, if a high concentration of drug is used no resistant colonies are found and it is necessary to culture in the presence of successively rising concentrations, so that resistance is then the result of a number of mutations. In the case of streptomycin, completely resistant strains can be isolated from mixed populations.

Resistance can be due to several causes. It may be that in the resistant strain the target enzyme is produced in greatly increased amounts so that, even though strongly inhibited, enough residual total activity remains. This is the major cause of resistance to folate reductase inhibitors; the enzyme concentration may be several thousand times as great in resistant as in sensitive strains. A more radical change is where as a result of a change in its structure the target molecule is no longer able to bind the antibacterial. This is clearly the case with streptomycin, where ribosomes from resistant organisms no longer bind streptomycin and this is due to a mutation affecting the P10 binding protein. Reconstitution of ribosomes from resistant organisms with P10 from sensitive organisms restores sensitivity. Binding of chloramphenicol to ribosomes of resistant strains is similarly lost. In the case of sulphonamide resistance the pteroic synthetase seems to become less sensitive to inhibition, although this may not be the only cause of resistance. In some instance, it appears that resistant organisms are less permeable to the antibacterial. This has been reported with tetracyclines, sulphonamides, methotrexate, and some antitrypanosome drugs. In other cases the organism develops the ability to detoxify the antibacterial, a classic example being in the case of penicillin where resistant strains of staphylococci contain the enzyme penicillinase which opens the β-lactam ring of penicillin to form the inactive product penicilloic acid. The enzyme can be so active that resistance is very great. Inactivation of chloramphenicol can occur as a result of *O*-acetylation, and streptomycin can be converted to an adenylate.

A recent discovery has been the development of transferable resistance. This was first noted in Japan where dysentery organisms became resistant simultaneously to three or four antibacterials (sulphonamides, streptomycin, tetracycline, chloramphenicol). This was shown to be due to exchange of genetic material between bacteria in a manner similar to the transfer in bacterial sexual conjugation. The transfer of DNA probably occurs through conjugation tubes (pili) and can rapidly infect a sensitive population. These R-factors can also cross species so that for instance R-factors in coliforms may infect other enterobacteria such as *Shigella* or *Salmonella*. The resistance from R-factors is due either to increased metabolism, i.e. the R-factors carry the genes for the metabolic enzymes, or to reduced permeability. There are few organisms that will not develop resistance under appropriate conditions and it is very important that therapy should be designed to minimize the evolution of resistance. The most important factor is adequate dosage over a relatively short period (normally less than 7–14 days). Frequently two or more chemotherapeutics together may reduce the risk of resistance. If resistance depends on mutants, the chances of a mutant resistant to two or more antibacterials appearing is extremely small (this is not true with infective R-factor resistance). A case where multiple therapy has especial significance is in the chemotherapy of tuberculosis. These sluggish organisms multiply very slowly and prolonged therapy for periods up to 2 years is needed. This provides very favourable conditions for development of resistance when either streptomycin or isoniazid is used alone but is rare when they are used in combination and especially so when the weak antimycobacterial *p*-aminosalicylic acid is added to the combination.

CHEMOTHERAPEUTIC SPECTRA

Some chemotherapeutic agents act only on a single species or a limited group of organisms. These are referred to as narrow-spectrum. Examples are isoniazid active only against mycobacteria, nystatin active only against yeasts, or griseofulvin active against fungi. At the other extreme are drugs which affect a very wide range of species and are referred to as broad-spectrum. Examples are tetracycline and ampicillin. Other agents may have an intermediate range, such as penicillin, which kills cocci and Gram-positive bacilli, but is ineffective against most Gram-negative bacilli. The purported advantage of the wide-spectrum agents is that they reduce the need for identifying the causal organism and testing it for sensitivity. On the other hand, they violently alter the normal saprophytic bacterial flora as well as attacking the pathogens and are liable to lead to serious problems from superinfection by organism such as *Candida* which are normally kept in check by the competitive pressure of surface saprophytes.

The present view is that except where treatment is very urgent it is better to isolate the organism to test its sensitivity to a range of antibacterials and select the most appropriate one even if of narrow spectrum.

DOSAGE SCHEDULES

In Chapter 2 the value of measuring blood levels of drugs and determining the biological half-life in determining dosage schedules was emphasized. In the case of chemotherapeutics these guide lines need careful consideration. For instance, the biological half-life of penicillin is less than one hour. Does this mean that penicillin must be given at very frequent intervals to exert its effects? In the early days of penicillin, this was thought to be the case and dosage every 3–4 hours was used, but gradually it came to be realized that dosage once or twice a day was adequate. Why is this? In the first place, if a drug is bactericidal as long as the dose is great enough to kill most of the organisms this action does not need a maintenance dose (they stay dead!); repeated does are needed only to deal with the small fraction of organisms which were not killed (possibly because they were not in the division cycle) and it may be advantageous to allow these organisms to enter the division cycle. Secondly, the reaction between some chemotherapeutics such as penicillin and the organisms is pseudo-irreversible so that even after removal of the agent by washing, it takes many hours for the organisms to be able to recommence growth—it is this process rather than the fall in blood level that dictates the appropriate interval between doses.

In general, then, the dose schedule must be

worked out on rational grounds related to considerations of this kind.

ANTIBACTERIAL AGENTS

Penicillins

Penicillins are acyl derivatives of 6-amino penicillanic acid. The original penicillin introduced by the Oxford workers was a mixture in which the most effective component was the phenacetyl derivative of 6-APA referred to as **benzylpenicillin** (or penicillin G). It was then found that by adding phenylacetic acid to the culture medium a greatly increased yield of virtually pure benzylpenicillin was obtained. This is a very active antibacterial which kills a wide range of Gram-negative and positive cocci; streptococci remain highly sensitive, but the majority of staphylococci isolated nowadays are resistant penicillinase-producing strains. Most strains of gonococci and pneumococci are sensitive. *Clostridia, B. anthracis, Fusobacteria,* and *Actinomycetes* are also sensitive. The spirochaete of syphilis (*Treponema pallidum*) is extremely sensitive, and the introduction of benzylpenicillin revolutionized the treatment of syphilis.

The absorption of penicillins from the oral route is dependent mainly on their stability in acid. Benzylpenicillin is acid labile and not suitable for oral administration. Subcutaneous dose is usually in the range 0·1–2 g/day (1 μg = 1·6 units) and is rapidly absorbed so that the peak concentration is reached within 30 minutes, but the half-life is brief, due to the rapid excretion of penicillin in the urine by tubular secretion. The excretion rate can be reduced by probenecid (Chapter 16), but this is rarely worth employing since penicillin is cheap and of very low toxicity so that large doses can be employed and also, on the other hand, most organisms are sensitive to 0·1 μg/ml or less. If prolonged action is needed a depot preparation such as **procaine penicillin** can be used which produces blood levels for 18–36 hours. This may be used where there is little prospect of giving repeated doses, as in the treatment of venereal diseases. Another depot preparation **ben-**

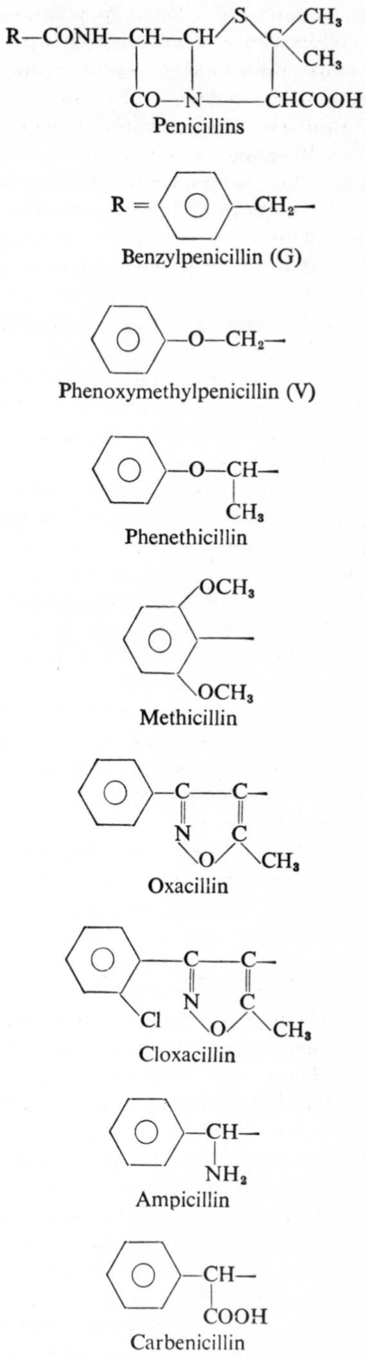

R—CONH—CH—CH—S—C(CH_3)(CH_3); CO—N——CHCOOH

Penicillins

R = C_6H_5—CH_2—

Benzylpenicillin (G)

C_6H_5—O—CH_2—

Phenoxymethylpenicillin (V)

C_6H_5—O—CH(CH_3)—

Phenethicillin

2,6-(OCH_3)$_2$$C_6H_3$—

Methicillin

C_6H_5—C=N—O—C(CH_3)=C—

Oxacillin

2-Cl-C_6H_4—C=N—O—C(CH_3)=C—

Cloxacillin

C_6H_5—CH(NH_2)—

Ampicillin

C_6H_5—CH(COOH)—

Carbenicillin

Fig. 17.6. Structure of penicillins.

zathine penicillin is much more insoluble and produces appreciable blood levels for a week or more and is used mainly as a prophylactic against infections by *Streptococcus haemolyticus* (an extremely sensitive organism) in rheumatic fever.

Penicillin penetrates the cerebrospinal fluid and serous cavities poorly—to some extent this penetration is increased in inflammation, but it is unwise to rely on this in treating meningitis. Penicillin is poorly tolerated in the subarachnoid space and readily produces convulsions.

Penicillin is an extraordinarily non-toxic drug and almost all the untoward reactions to the drug are due to hypersensitivity. These may appear as skin rashes of many kinds, angioedema, serum sickness, and anaphylaxis. The high antigenicity of penicillin seems to be due to the readiness with which penicillin can acylate plasmaproteins to form penicilloyl or penicillenyl derivates which are excellent antigens. In such a situation it is to be expected that allergic reactions will be more common on the second or later course of treatment. Since the hypersensitivity reactions may be serious and indeed fatal, their presence is normally an indication to stop therapy and warn the patient against subsequent treatment.

The main disadvantages of benzylpenicillin are its susceptibility to hydrolysis by acid and penicillinase and a good deal of effort has been put into finding penicillins lacking these disadvantages. The addition of phenoxyacetic acid to the culture medium in place of phenylacetic acid leads to the formation of **phenoxymethyl-penicillin** (Penicillin V) which is much more resistant to acid hydrolysis and can therefore be relied upon to give good blood levels when administered by mouth. Phenoxyethyl-penicillin (**phenethicillin**) is very similar. Both have a range of activity and potency very similar to benzylpenicillin, but also share its susceptibility to penicillinase. Further advance came from the development of the semisynthetic penicillins. These are made by direct acylation of 6-APA. These became possible after the discovery of a strain of penicillium which formed an amidase which splits the side chain of penicillin thus allowing the large-scale production of 6-APA. The first important semisynthetic penicillin was **methicillin** which is very resistant to penicillinase and so attacks strains resistant to benzylpenicillin, but it is not acid resistant and must be given by injection. Resistant staphylococci are highly susceptible to methicillin but it is less effective against other cocci, it is thus a narrow-spectrum antibacterial reserved for treating resistant staphylococcal infections. **Oxacillin**, **cloxacillin** and **fluoxacillin** are both acid and penicillinase resistant, they can thus be used as orally active drugs for sensitive and resistant strains; they have a broader spectrum than methicillin but are less active on sensitive strains than benzylpenicillin. **Ampicillin** is surprisingly a broad-spectrum agent and is effective against many Gram-negative bacilli such as *E. coli*, *Shigella*, and *Salmonella*, notably *Salmonella typhi.* It is also very active against *Haemophilus influenzae* and is much used in respiratory infections. It is well absorbed by mouth but is hydrolysed by penicillinase. **Carbenicillin** has an even broader spectrum and is notably effective against *Pseudomonas* and *Aerobacter.* It is resistant to both penicillinase and acid but is poorly absorbed and must be given by injection. Unfortunately these semisynthetic penicillins are just as likely to cause hypersensitivity as benzylpenicillin.

A new and interesting penicillin derivative is **mecillinam** which has a novel side chain (hexahydroazepinylmethyleneamino-P) and appears to have a different mechanism of action. It does not inhibit the mucopeptide cross-linking reaction although it does depress wall synthesis. Mecillinam is effective against a wide range of Gram-negative bacteria; it is especially useful against *Salmonella* (*typhi* and *paratyphi*) and *Shigella.* Since it is excreted in high concentration in the bile it should be useful in carriers. Mecillinam is sensitive to penicillinase and therefore not useful for strains producing this enzyme; however, there is little cross resistance with ampicillin. Mecinillam is not absorbed by mouth but the pivaloyloxymethyl ester (pivmecillinam) is well absorbed and is rapidly hydrolysed *in vivo* to free mecillinam.

Cephalosporins

Cephalosporins are closely related to penicillins, having a nucleus 7-aminocephalosporanic acid that differs only in the replacement of the thiazole ring by a dihydrothiazine ring. Substituents in the 3 position allow for a greater range of chemical manipulation. In general, they are broad spectrum agents, and although they are susceptible to penicillinase, this is less than most penicillins. Their mechanism of action appears to be the same as for penicillin, and there is some cross over of hypersensitivity reactions between the two groups. In general cephalosporins are alternatives to penicillin and the two most commonly used are cephalothin which must be given by injection and cephaloridine which is active by mouth (Fig. 17.7).

Sulphonamides and cotrimazole

The sulphonamides were the first of the modern anti-bacterials, and as newer agents have come into use their importance has declined, but with the introduction of the combination with **trimethoprim** (Table 17.2) as **cotrimazole** they have regained an importance that is second only to the penicillins. Sulphonamides can be modified by substitution on the amide group by various heterocycles; these change the potency (but not significantly the range of organisms affected), the binding to plasma proteins, the rate of excretion, and the solubility in body fluids. When a partner sulphonamide for trimethoprim was sought one was chosen that was highly active and soluble and that had a similar biological half-life to that of trimethoprim (16 hours) so that when the two drugs were administered together the ratio of their concentration in the body would stay nearly constant. The choice fell on sulfamethoxazole (biological half-life 10 hours). The combination is given in the ratio 400 mg sulfamethoxazole to 80 mg trimethoprim. Cotrimazole is a very wide range antibacterial, and not only does the combination reduce the probability of the development of resistance but organisms that are not sensitive to either agent alone have proved sensitive.

While cotrimazole can be used very generally it has proved of special value in urinary infections due to *E. coli* and *Proteus mirabilis* and in respiratory tract infections such as acute and chronic bronchitis and bronchiectasis.

Toxic effects with sulphonamides are more common than with penicillins and include skin rashes, leukopenia or thrombocytopenia and the gastrointestinal symptoms, nausea and vomiting.

Sulphasalazine (salicylazosulphapyridine), a sulphonamide related to the original prontosil, is used in the treatment of ulcerative colitis; its mechanism of action is unknown.

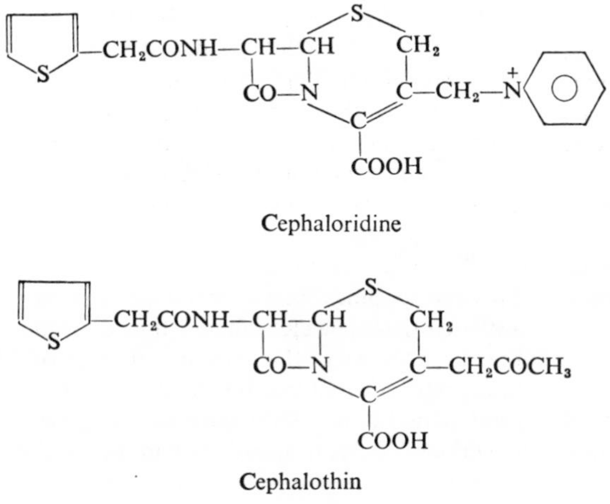

Cephaloridine

Cephalothin

Fig. 17.7. Cephalosporins.

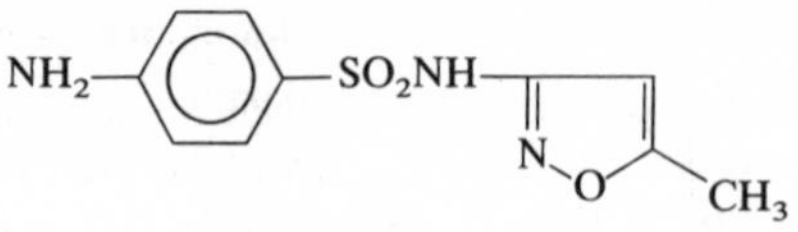

Sulfamethoxazole

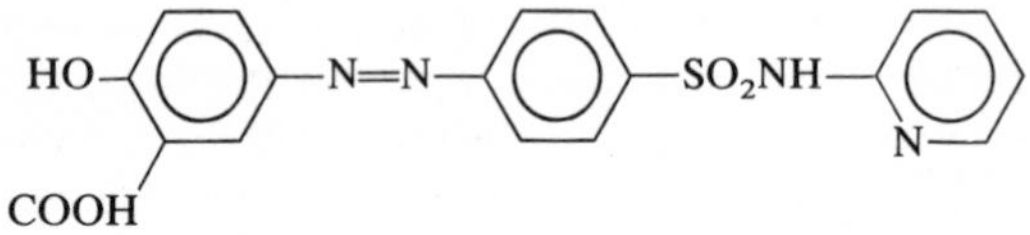

Sulphasalazine

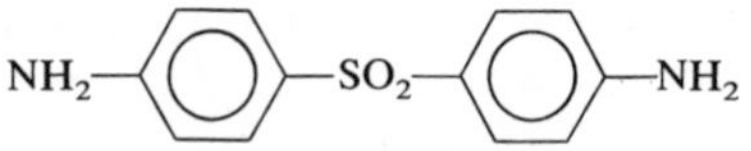

Diaminodiphenylsulphone (dapsone)

Fig. 17.8

ERYTHROMYCIN

Erythromycin is classed as a macrolide, so named because its structure contains a very large cyclic lactone. Like penicillin it is of fungal origin (*Streptomyces erythreus*). It is most effective against Gram-positive cocci but many Gram-negative organisms are also sensitive. It has activity against mycoplasma, brucella, and rickettsia.

Erythromycin acts by interfering with protein synthesis by interaction with the large 50S subunit of the bacterial ribosome (overlapping the site of interaction of chloramphenicol). The free drug is poorly absorbed but esters such as the stearate, estolate, or ethylsuccinate are well absorbed. The drug has few toxic effects and is widely used for treating infections due to penicillin-resistant staphylococci. It is very useful in dealing with carriers of diphtheria and highly effective against *Clostridium tetani.* It is also one of the most useful drugs in pneumonia due to mycoplasma. **Lincomycin** and **clindamycin,** while not macrolides, have a similar range of action.

Gentamicin

Gentamicin is the most important member of the aminoglycoside group of antibacterials which includes **streptomycin, neomycin, kanamycin,** and **paronomycin.** All of this group act on ribosomes depressing protein synthesis and resistance may develop due to a mutation in the P10 protein. All are toxic and liable to produce degeneration of the auditory nerve, but gentamicin is safe provided precautions are taken to prevent excessive blood levels. This means that if renal function is depressed, the dose must be suitably reduced and the blood level must not be allowed to exceed 10 μg/ml. Gentamicin is a broad-spectrum agent which finds its main use in serious infections where its action against *Staph. aureus, proteus,* and *pseudomonas* is important. The use of streptomycin is now almost exclusively in tuberculosis (see below), both because of its toxicity and the readiness with which resistance develops. None of this group are absorbed from the gut.

Tetracyclines

The tetracyclines are very broad-spectrum antibacterials that after their initial introduction found a very wide use in general infections, and still do in some countries but in most parts of the world their use in general infections has been replaced by more specific

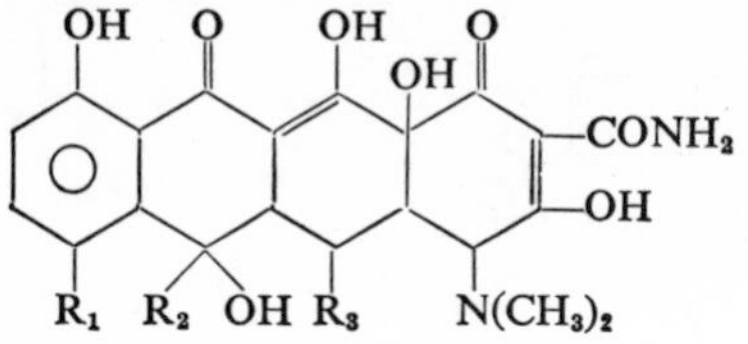

Tetracyclines

R_1	R_2	R_3	
H	CH_3	H	Tetracycline
Cl	CH_3	H	Chlortetracycline
H	CH_3	OH	Oxytetracycline
Cl	H	H	Demethylchlortetracycline

Fig. 17.9. Structures of tetracyclines.

and less toxic agents, and they are used mainly in some of the infections in which they have a special value. After penicillin (and hence in penicillin-resistant cases) tetracyclines are useful in venereal diseases since they are effective in gonorrhoea, less so in syphilis, and also in granuloma inguinale chancroid and in non-gonoccoccal urethritis (aetiology uncertain). Tetracycline is very effective against cholera, in brucellosis due to both *Br. abortus* and *Br. melitensis*, and in rickettsial infections such as typhus and Rocky Mountain spotted fever. Tetracyclines either alone or in combination with chloroquine are effective agents against amoebiasis. They are active by mouth although the absorption is somewhat irregular. Toxic effects are not uncommon, usually due to allergic type of reactions in the skin; gastrointestinal upsets are common, including diarrhoea. Tetracycline should not normally be used in patients with kidney disease or in pregnancy.

Chloramphenicol

Chloramphenicol is a fairly broad-spectrum antibacterial which originally found wide usage; unfortunately it produces a fatal aplastic anaemia in about 1 case in 10 000. With the abundance of other safer agents this risk is unacceptable except in severe illness, where this risk is small compared with other risks. In practice, chloramphenicol is now used only in typhoid, typhus, and in meningitis due to *H. influenzae.*

The choice of antibacterial agent

Such a wide range of antibacterial agents is available that it is not always easy to see how a particular agent is chosen. In many cases the choice is not difficult because the clinical diagnosis provides a strong indication of the likely causative organism and recent experience with the organism will give indications of its sensitivity to different drugs. It will be sensible, if feasible, to isolate the organism and test its sensitivity but it will often be necessary to start treatment before the results of such tests are known. In textbooks of clinical pharmacology elaborate lists are to be found of the best choice of antibacterial for various diseases. In some hospitals it is possible to call up the computer for such advice!

Chemotherapy of tuberculosis

The introduction of streptomycin for treatment of tuberculosis radically changed the handling and prognosis of patients with this disease. From a condition in which the mortality was high, with treatment by prolonged bed rest combined with drastic surgery, it has become amenable to simple treatment, much of it in the home or while ambulant, with a very high recovery rate. Chemotherapy in tuberculosis raises special problems because of the avascular nature of the lesions and the sluggish reproduction of the organism; in consequence therapy needs to be continued for a prolonged period in most cases. Such prolonged treatment highlights problems of drug toxicity and of the development of resistance.

When streptomycin was administered alone it was found that a considerable fraction of the tubercle bacilli isolated acquired resistance. It was found that if the patient also received ***p*-aminosalicylic acid (PAS),** a feeble bacteriostatic, the emergence of resistance was reduced to negligible proportions. This combination was effective but very unpopular, largely due to the PAS which needed to be taken in large amounts, was expensive, and frequently caused gastrointestinal upsets, nausea, vomiting, abdominal pain, and diarrhoea. In 1952 the simple

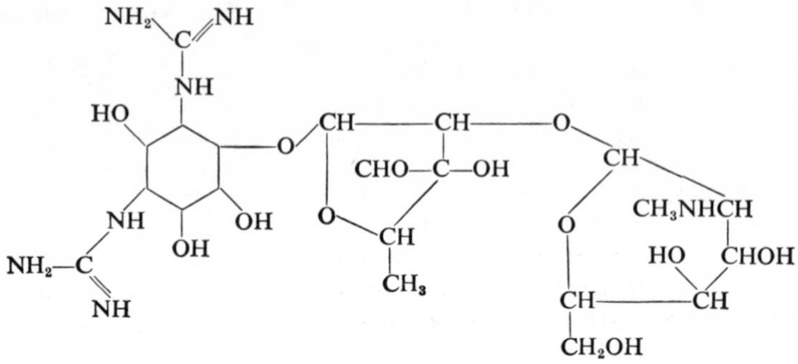

Streptomycin

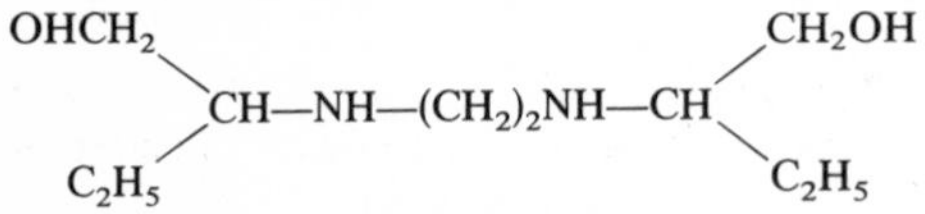

Ethambutol

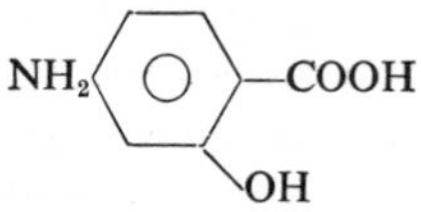

p-Aminosalicylic acid (PAS)

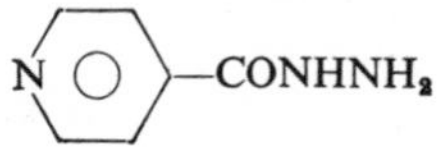

Isoniazid

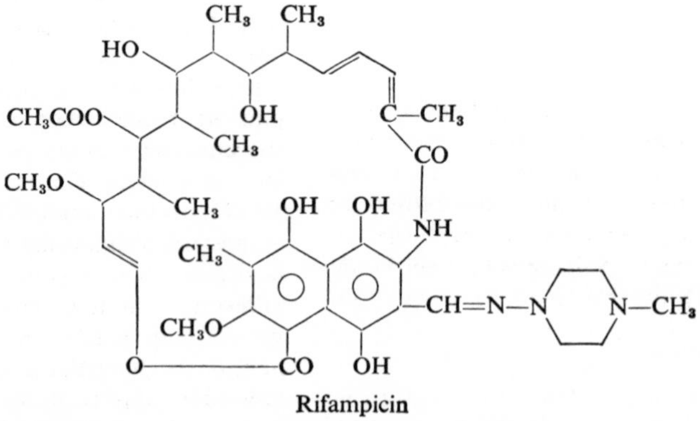

Rifampicin

Fig. 17.10. Drugs used in the treatment of tuberculosis.

compound **isoniazid** was found to be an extremely effective antimycobacterial at low dosage. It is active by mouth (streptomycin must be injected) and of relatively low toxicity. The most common toxic effect is peripheral neuritis although optic neuritis, ataxia, convulsions, a toxic psychosis, and hypersensitivity reactions may also occur.

Rifampicin (rifampin) is a macrocyclic antibiotic with a novel action in inhibiting DNA-directed RNA synthesis, and is highly active as a mycobactericidal agent (all the other substances are mycobacteriostatic). It is relatively non-toxic although jaundice and a variety of hypersensitivity reactions occur. It is the most rapidly acting drug and the quickest at stopping live bacteria being excreted in the sputum.

Ethambutol is an active mycobacteriostatic of very low toxicity that has effectively displaced PAS. **Pyrazinamide** is increasingly used as a secondary agent, less frequently **ethionamide, cycloserine,** or **viomycin,** all of which have troublesome toxic effects.

As indicated earlier, regimens for treating pulmonary tuberculosis used to consist of streptomycin, isoniazid, and PAS and these were usually given for a period of 1–2 years. Recently two major changes have occurred; first, it has been found that a course of 9 months is adequate, and that patients are treated as well or better when ambulant as when in bed, and secondly the combination of drugs has altered. A recent trial showed the superiority of rifampicin 600 mg and isoniazid 300 mg orally supplemented in the first two months by ethambutol 25 mg/kg orally each day. In other regimens streptomycin 1 g was given once a week and pyrazinamide was found useful.

Leprosy

This disease is caused by another mycobacterium, *M. leprae*. The standard chemotherapeutic agent is **dapsone,** which is bacteriostatic. Treatment must be carried on for many years and resistant organisms are becoming common. **Rifampicin** is bactericidal and probably the treatment of choice, but unfortunately is expensive.

ANTIFUNGAL AGENTS

Griseofulvin is a systemic fungicide active against mycotic diseases of the skin, hair, and nails (ringworm, athletes' foot) due to *Epidermophyton*, *Trichophyton*, and *Microsporum*. The drug is very poorly absorbed by mouth but is, nevertheless, effective by this route. The main side-effects are headache and nausea and vomiting. Equally good effects can often be obtained by local application of a cream containing a synthetic compound **tolnaftate,** a compound that appears quite non-toxic.

Serious systemic infections with *Histoplasma*, *Coccidioides*, *Blastomyces*, and *Candida* can be treated with **amphotericin B** which acts on organisms whose cell membranes contain cholesterol. It is poorly absorbed from the gut and is therefore given by slow intravenous infusion. It is a very toxic drug and a large range of serious side-effects have been recorded but it is life-saving in these infections.

Nystatin is a related polyene that is used topically particularly for *Candida* infection of the vagina and gut (it is not absorbed).

ANTIVIRUS AGENTS

It can be seen from the foregoing account that so many good antibacterial agents are available that we can afford to be eclectic; in contrast is the poverty of effective antiviral agents. This is mainly because the available points of attack on viruses are so few—a virus is little more than a package of genes with a protective coat and penetrative apparatus that relies for its metabolic functions on the host cell. In order to be an effective parasite its metabolic needs must match what the host can provide. Nevertheless, there are several ways in which antiviral agents might act. Firstly they directly attack the free virus or prevent it adhering to or penetrating the host cell. There is some evidence that **amantadine** acts at this stage on some influenza viruses and an effect has been demonstrated in man in A_2 influenza. **Phenoxymethylisoquinolines** appear to act as inhibitors of viral neuramidinase and interfere with attachment. Trials in human influenza are promising. They may also act on myxoviruses and enteroviruses but full trials have not yet been reported.

Actions on replication have been shown in the case of **idoxuridine**, which is incorporated into the virus DNA and may lead to coding errors. Idoxuridine has been successfully used in the treatment of corneal herpes by local application but is not practical for systemic use. Two other nucleotide derivatives have shown promising antiviral activity. One, **ribavirin** (1-ribityl-triazole-3 carboxamide), has shown activity against the viruses of herpes, hepatitis, and influenza. Topically applied to the vesicular lesions of herpes zoster, ribavirin reduced pain and shortened the course of the disease. Systematically it accelerated recovery in hepatitis A. Side effects are few but general use is unlikely because ribavirin is teratogenic. The other nucleotide is **vidarabine** (9-β arabinosyladenosine; ara A), which is also active against herpes. A very simple compound **phosphonoacetic acid** has also been shown to be active against herpes viruses and appears to have very low toxicity. **Methisazone** is a thiosemicarbazone of *N*-methylisatin and appears to inhibit the synthesis of the viral structural proteins necessary for assembly of completed pox viruses. Trials in India have established that methisazone is highly successful in reducing the incidence of smallpox among contacts but it is of no value in treating the established disease **Interferons** are small proteins formed by many cells after infection with DNA or RNA viruses and which inhibit virus growth relatively unselectively. Great difficulties have been encountered in preparing interferon and effort has been concentrated more on methods of stimulating endogenous production. It has been found that a non-pathogenic virus DNA extracted from penicillium (statolon) and some synthetic polynucleotides are capable of stimulating interferon formation but they are unfortunately rather toxic. In Chapter 9 it was mentioned that levamisole potentiated many antibody responses and this includes antiviral antibodies.

ANTISEPTICS

A very large number of substances have been used for killing bacteria outside the body, unhampered as this process is by requirements of being harmless to the host. In fact, nearly all antiseptics are protein denaturants and act on enzymes, etc. in the bacteria and for the same reason the effectiveness of most antiseptics is considerably reduced in serum, blood, or pus. Antiseptics are used for the following purposes:

1. *Instrument and material sterilization*

Some instruments are too delicate to be boiled or autoclaved; suture material and implantable materials, e.g. plastic vascular grafts, middle-ear inserts, may also need other methods. The most effective sterilizing system used is **ethylene oxide** in gaseous form. A simple related method uses an aqueous solution of **glutaraldehyde.** Cationic agents (benzalkonium, cetyltrimethylammonium, cetrimide) and chlorinated phenols are also used for cold sterilization of instruments, thermometers, oxygen masks, etc.

2. *Cleaning of the skin before operations*

Cleaning of the skin is no easy matter because of the bacteria resident in sweat and sebaceous glands and in hair follicles. **Ethanol** and **isopropanol** are both used at 70 per cent concentration and are effective but not persistent; they are improved by the addition of 0·5 per cent **chlorhexidine**, a chlorinated phenyl-biguanide or of benzalkonium. The organic mercurial **thiomersal** (*Merthiolate*) is also very effective. Two per cent iodine in isopropanol is a very efficient skin disinfectant but caution is needed since some individuals are sensitized to iodine.

3. *Coarse disinfection*

Disinfection of contaminated glassware, bed pans, benches, floors, etc. is most usually carried out with phenolics such as Lysol which is a mixture of cresols and soap, or Dettol, a chlorinated xylenol. Bath water is often made antiseptic by the addition of hexachlorophane.

4. *Water*

Drinking-water and swimming-baths are usually sterilized with gaseous chlorine or sodium hypochlorite.

FURTHER READING

Barber, M. and Garrod, L. P. (1963). *Antibiotics and Chemotherapy*, Edinburgh.

Busch, H. and Leme, M. (1967). *Chemotherapy*, Chicago.

Doyle, F. P. and Nayler, J. H. C. (1964). Penicillins and related structures, *Advanc. Drug Res.* **1,** 1.

Gale, E. F. (1963). Mechanism of antibiotic action, *Pharmacol. Rev.* **15,** 481.

18

CHEMOTHERAPY II: PROTOZOA AND METAZOA

MALARIA

MALARIA is a disease affecting many millions of people and despite the availability of very effective drugs, it has not yet proved possible to devise a strategy for its eradication. The intermediate host and vector are mosquitoes of the *anopheles* species which on biting the victim inject sporozoites into the blood stream. These are taken up by the parenchymal cells of the liver where they mature into merozoites which are released into the blood stream; most of them penetrate into red blood cells, there to start a further development cycle through trophozoites and schizonts to merozoites which are released by rupture of the erythrocyte, together with modified proteins that are responsible for the febrile reaction. Since the development cycle is synchronized from the time of infection, the release of showers of merozoites occurs at regular intervals. In malaria due to *Plasmodium vivax* this occurs every three days, hence the name tertian (usually called benign tertian because the mortality is low); with the less common *Pl. malariae* the periodicity is over four days, hence quartan. Infections due to *Pl. falciparum* are very severe and fulminating and periodicity is less apparent. A proportion of the trophozoites in the erythrocytes undergo differentiation into sexual forms called gametocytes—these forms are infective for the mosquito and in the mosquito's gut sexual fertilization occurs, giving rise to sporozoites and hence completing the cycle.

In tertian and quartan malaria a proportion of the merozoites released from the erythrocytes reinfect the tissue cells so that a persistent exoerythrocytic infection occurs. This does not occur in falciparum malaria, which is a purely erythrocytic infection after its initial stage. The characteristic of tertian and quartan malaria is their very chronic, nature with recurrences occurring sometimes after long intervals but a low fatality rate. On the other hand, falciparum malaria is very acute and severe—the large amount of modified blood pigments appearing in the urine giving it the name of blackwater fever. The fatality rate in untreated susceptible individuals is very high, but in endemic areas a low level of immunity develops which does not prevent attacks occurring but greatly reduces the mortality.

Action of chemotherapeutic drugs

The most satisfactory way of preventing the development of malaria would be by killing the pre-erythrocytic forms of the parasite either as injected by the mosquito or in the tissues. No agents are known which kill the sporozoites, but the later pre-erythrocytic forms of falciparum malaria are killed by **pyrimethamine, chlorguanide,** and **primaquine**; none of these drugs is very effective against this stage of quartan or tertian. Drugs acting in this way are said to be *causal prophylactics.*

Drugs which prevent the erythrocytic stage of development are called *suppressants.* This treatment is started before entering a malaria region and continued for some weeks afterwards and prevents the development of a clinical attack. When the treatment ceases a proportion of those infected with tertain or quartan parasites may develop an attack due to the persistence of the exoerythrocytic forms; this does not occur with falciparum. The drugs used are **chloroquine, chloroguanide,** and **pyrimethamine.**

Clinical cure of an *attack* of malaria is produced by schizonticides, of which **chloroquine** and **amodiaquine** are most useful and produce a rapid response. Chloroguanide and pyrimethamine, although highly active in killing schizonts, are less useful in treating

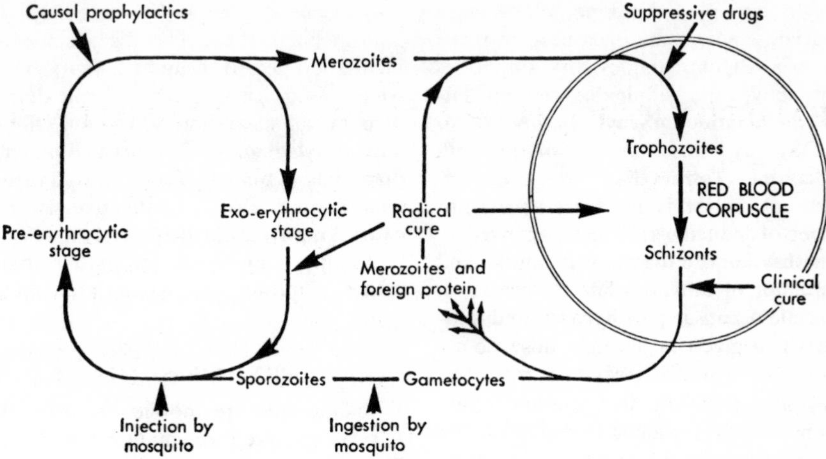

Fig. 18.1. The malarial parasite life cycle.

attacks because their action develops rather slowly.

A radical cure of tertian or quartan fevers depends on destroying the exo-erythrocytic forms as well as the erythrocytic forms; this can be accomplished with **primaquine,** a drug of the 8-aminoquinoline series.

Unfortunately, resistance to these drugs, particularly in falciparum malaria, is on the increase and so secondary drugs may need to

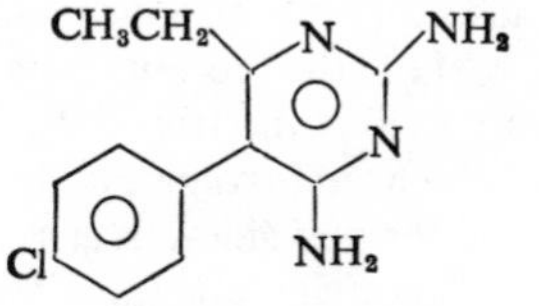

Pyrimethamine

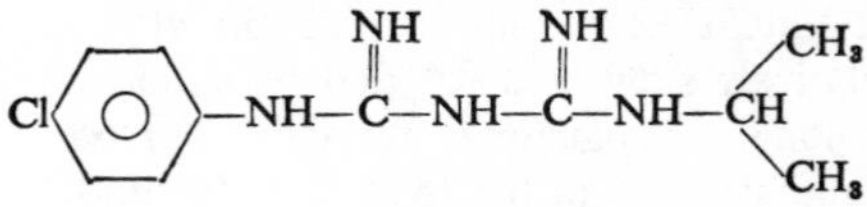

Proguanil

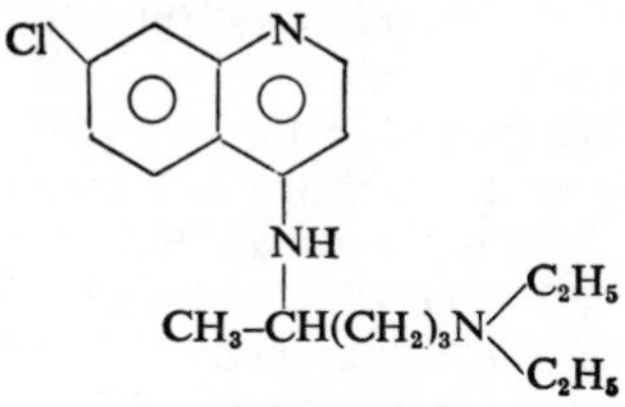

Chloroquine

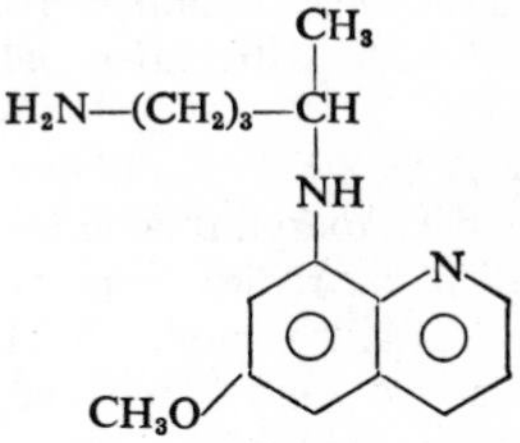

Primaquine

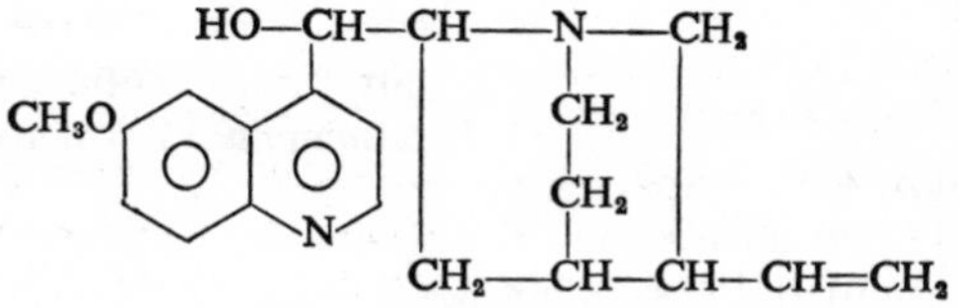

Quinine

Fig. 18.2. The structures of drugs used in the treatment of malaria.

be brought into play. **Quinine,** the earliest antimalarial, is now sometimes used in resistant malaria. Sulphonamides and sulphones are also active and **sulphadoxine** and **sulphalene** or **diaminodiphenylsulphone** (dapsone, DDS) may be used in combination with **pyrimethamine. Tetracyclines** are occasionally used, but caution is necessary because of the danger of inducing resistant bacteria.

Pyrimethamine is a diaminopyrimidine and is an inhibitor of dihydrofolate reductase. It is an excellent causal prophylactic and suppressant when given in a single dose 25 mg by mouth once a week. Toxicity is rare.

Chloroquine is a 4-aminoquinoline effective against the erythrocytic forms of all the malarial parasites. It is very rapid in action and quickly controls acute clinical attacks. It is also active against the gametocytes of *P. vivax.* Chloroquine is well tolerated and toxicity is rare unless the dose is very high and prolonged, when retinal damage may occur. **Aminodiaquine** is a closely related drug especially active in falciparum infections.

Proguanil (chloroguanide) is a biguanide which is an effective causal prophylactic and suppressant. Like pyrimethamine, its effects are relatively slow in onset and its action is not prolonged. Proguanil is not active *in vitro,* but is metabolized in the liver to a diaminotriazine analogous to pyrimethamine and which is also a reductase inhibitor. Toxicity is uncommon although gastro-intestinal upsets may occur.

Primaquine is an 8-aminoquinoline and is active against the exoerythrocytic forms and hence is used in the radical cure of tertian and quartan malaria. It is more toxic than the other antimalarials. Gastrointestinal symptoms are not uncommon, so is some degree of methaemoglobinaemia and cyanosis.

LEISHMANIASIS

Leishmaniasis is caused by various species, *L. donovani* (*Kala-azar*), *L. brasiliensis*, and *L. tropica* which are transmitted by sandflies. The primary lesion is usually in the skin and from thence spreads to the lymph nodes and may become general through the reticulo-endothelial system. The disease has a long incubation period of up to 2 years. The most widely used drugs are the organic derivatives of pentavalent antimony, **sodium stibogluconate, ethylstibamine,** and **urea stibamine.** The diamidines **pentamidine** and **hydroxystilbamidine** are also very effective. In resistant cases **Amphotericin B** (p. 211) may be used. Antimony compounds are rather toxic and rashes, vomiting, and pyrexia are common.

TRYPANOSOMIASIS

Trypanosomes are mobile protozoa, and in Africa there are three main species, *T. brucei, T. gambiense*, and *T. rhodesiense*; the disease is transmitted by tsetse flies (*Glossina* sp.). The disease is characterized by a febrile phase followed by an encephalomyelitis (sleeping sickness). The drugs most commonly used in treatment are **pentamidine** and **suramin.** Pentamidine is the treatment of choice for early cases, and it has low toxicity but it is less effective in the cerebral phase. Suramin is also mainly used in the pre-cerebral stage. For the cerebral stage the most commonly used is the trivalent arsenical **melarsoprol,** which unfortunately is rather toxic. The most serious side-effect is an encephalopathy, although colic and vomiting are common. An alternative is the pentavalent arsenical **tryparsamide** which, while less active, penetrates reliably into the central nervous system.

The American form of trypanosomiasis is due to *T. cruzi* and is transmitted by bugs, the disease it causes being called Chagas' disease. The clinical disease manifests as a local swelling around the site of the bite, followed at a later stage by a severe cardiomyopathy and occasionally by a meningo-encephalitis. The best drugs available are a nitrofurazone **nifurtimox** and the antimalarial **primaquine,** but neither is very satisfactory.

TRICHOMONAS

Infections of the vagina and the urethra by *Trichomonas homines* are very common and

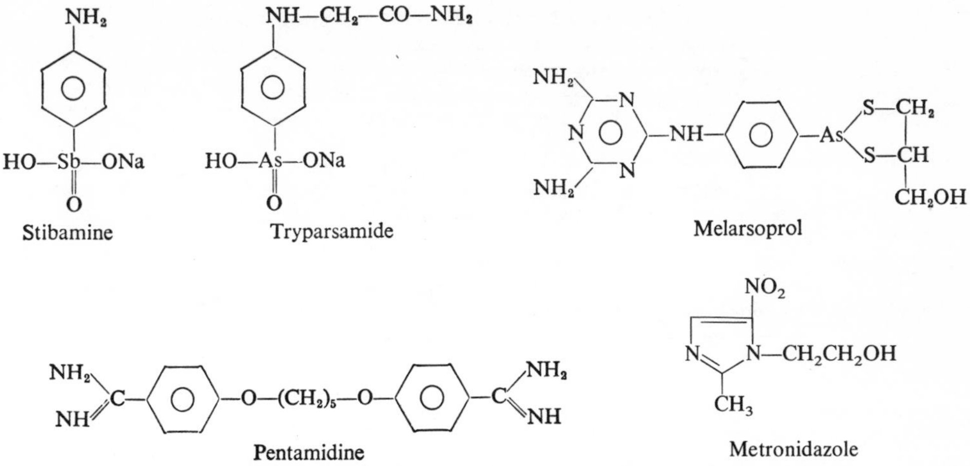

Stibamine Tryparsamide Melarsoprol

Pentamidine Metronidazole

Fig. 18.3. The structures of drugs used to treat protozoal infections.

troublesome. They are effectively treated by **metronidazole** by mouth. The drug, which is of low toxicity, can also be used in intestinal infections due to *Giardia lamblia.*

AMOEBIASIS

Infections with *Entamoeba histolytica* occur primarily in the large intestine, where ulcers are produced, causing a dysentery syndrome with frequent motions and abdominal pain. In chronic cases ulceration around the anus and tissue abscesses, notably in the liver, occur. **Metronidazole** is very effective in both the intestinal and metastatic forms of the disease. It is free of toxic effects and simply administered (2·4 g per day for three days) and has almost completely displaced **emetine. Paromomycin** is also effective in the intestinal form. **Diloxanide furoate** is used mainly for asymptomatic intestinal amoebiasis and as a prophylactic.

HELMINTHIASIS

The treatment of intestinal worms depends primarily on finding agents that cause the worms to release their attachment in the intestine so that they are swept out in the faeces. This is achieved usually by paralysing the worm, but sometimes by making it convulse, taking advantage of the different neurotransmitters found in invertebrates. For instance piperazine blocks inhibitory transmission to the body musculature of ascaris and the anticholinesterase dichlorvos has a selective action on the acetyl cholinesterase of the worm. One of the remarkable things about anthelminthics is that so often cure is produced by a single dose.

Piperazine is a very simple and safe drug which has a selective effect on *Ascaris* (roundworms) but also has an effect on pinworms (*oxyuris*). It is given as the citrate or phosphate salt by mouth. **Trichlorethylene,** another very simple compound, is used against the hookworms (*necator* and *ankylostoma*). It is given as the liquid in gelatine capsules. Side-effects are mainly intestinal but include headache and temporary unsteadiness and confusion. **Mebendazole** is a very effective agent against roundworms, whipworms, and hookworms and is virtually non-toxic. **Bephenium** is also highly effective against roundworms and hookworms and is the agent of choice for the latter. **Pyrantel-pamoate** and **levamisole** are very effective in roundworms. **Thiabendazole** is used mainly for threadworms and guinea-worm (*dracunculus*) but has a very wide range and hence is particularly useful in mixed infections.

Table 18.1. Drugs used in the treatment of intestinal worms

Type of worm	Drugs of choice
Roundworm	Piperazine, pyrantel pamoate, levamisole, mebendazole
Hookworm	Bephenium, pyrantel pamoate, thiabendazole trichlorethylene
Tapeworm	Niclosamide, dichlorophen
Pinworm	Pyrantel pamoate, piperazine pyrviniumpamoate
Threadworm	Thiabendazole, pyrvinium pamoate
Whipworm	Mebendazole, thiabendazole

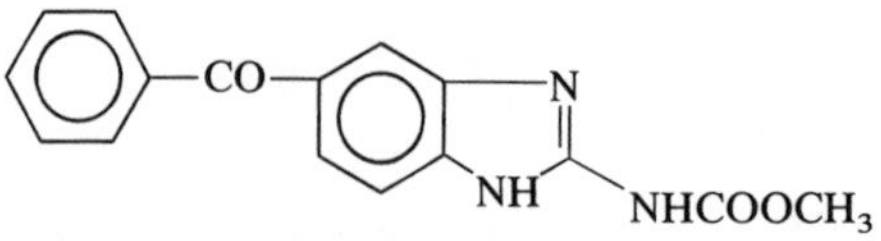

CO N NH $NHCOOCH_3$

Mebendazole

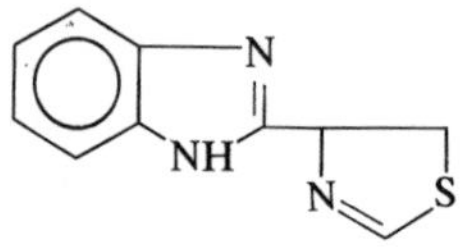

N NH N S

Thiabendazole

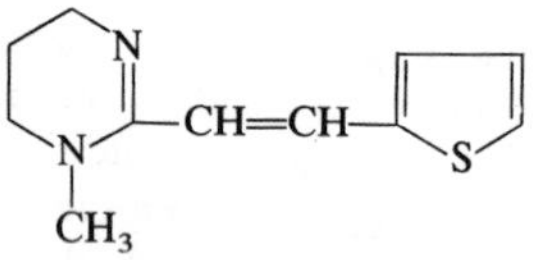

N N CH_3 —CH=CH— S

Pyrantel

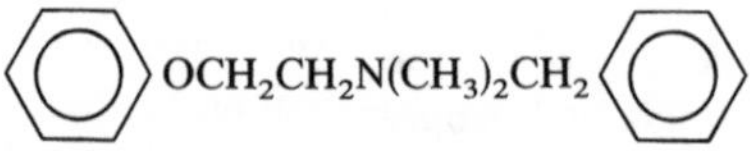

$OCH_2CH_2N(CH_3)_2CH_2$

Bephenium

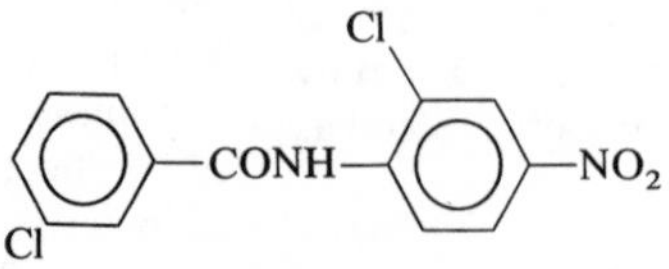

Cl CONH NO_2 Cl

Niclosamide

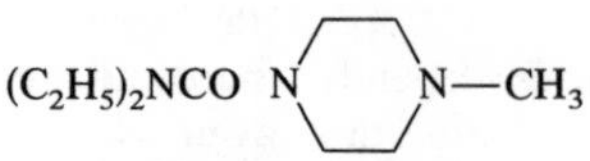

$(C_2H_5)_2NCO$ N N—CH_3

Diethylcarbamazine

Fig. 18.4. Anthelminthics.

Tapeworm infestations are best dealt with by **niclosamide** or **dichlorophen.**

FILARIA

Filaria are blood worms. The *Wuchereria* sp. migrate into the lymphatics and cause severe lymphoedema and hence elephantiasis of the limbs and scrotum. By the time the disease has reached this stage most of the worms are dead and the pathology is due to a reaction to the dead filaria and hence anthelminthics may worsen the disease temporarily. The circulating microfilaria are killed by **diethylcarbamazine** (hetrazan), and this drug is used for mass chemotherapy in control campaigns. The chronic disease can be treated with **melarsonyl** (trimelarsan) or **suramin.** The filarial worm *Onchocerca volvulus* which is widespread in Africa also causes lesions due to microfilaria in the eye (both in the choroid and retina) and in the skin. Although the microfilaria are very sensitive to diethylcarbamazine, treatment is hazardous owing to the very severe allergic reactions that develop to the dying or dead worms.

SCHISTOSOMIASIS

Schistosomiasis is acquired by working or bathing in water in which snails infested with schistosomes are discharging cercariae, a free-swimming form which rapidly penetrates the skin and changes into a schistosomula which in the case of *S. mansoni* make their way to the portal veins and there undergo sexual differentiation and maturation. The mature female fluke then discharges enormous numbers of eggs which are discharged with the faeces and by contaminating water supplies complete the parasitic circle. In the case of *S. haematobium* the adult worms settle in the veins around the bladder and the eggs are discharged in the urine. *S. mansoni* infections are very effectively treated with either intramuscular **hycanthone** or oral **oxamniquine;** both these agents selectively kill the male fluke.

S. haematobium is not sensitive to either of these agents, the most useful drug being **niridazole.** Where this is ineffective the older (but toxic) drugs such as **stibophen** and **sodium antimony dimercaptosuccinate** may be needed.

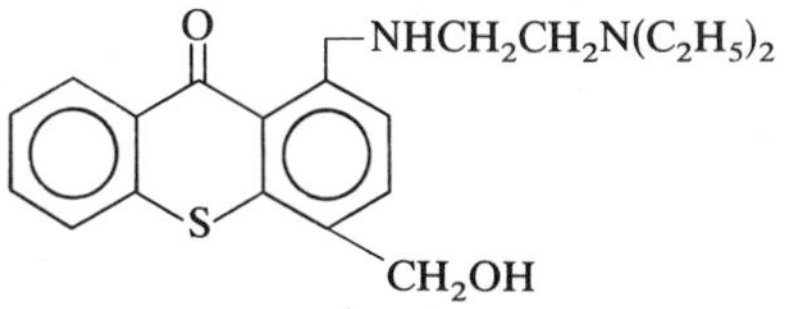

$NHCH_2CH_2N(C_2H_5)_2$; CH_2OH ; O ; S

Hycanthone

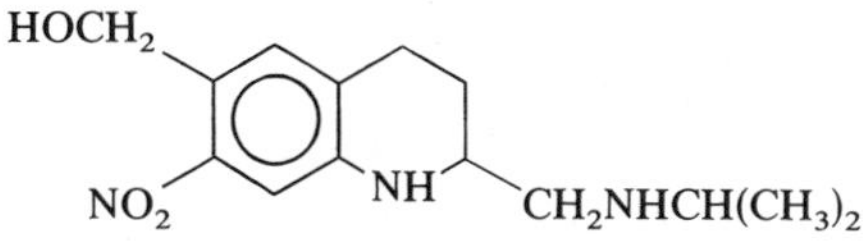

$HOCH_2$; NO_2 ; NH ; $CH_2NHCH(CH_3)_2$

Oxamniquine

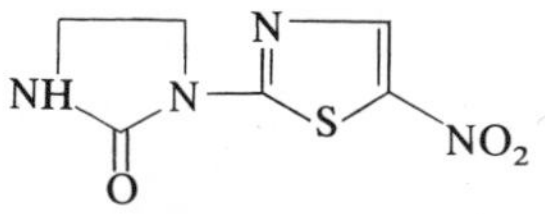

NH ; N ; N ; S ; O ; NO_2

Niridazole

Fig. 18.5. Drugs used in schistosomiasis.

FURTHER READING

Brown, H. W. (1969). Anthelmintics, new and old. *Clin. Pharmacol.* **10.**

Katz, N. and Pellegrino, J. (1974). Experimental chemotherapy of schistosomiasis mansoni. *Adv. Parasitology*, **12.**

Peters, W. (1970). *Chemotherapy and drug resistance in malaria*, London.

Powell, S. J. *et al.* (1966). Metronidazole in amoebic dysentry and amoebic liver abscess. *Lancet*, ii.

Rollo, I. M. (1964). Chemotherapy of malaria, in *Biochemistry and physiology of Protozoa*, New York.

Wilcocks, C. and Manson-Baker, P. E. C. (1972). *Tropical diseases*, London.

19

CHEMOTHERAPY III: CANCER

GENERAL PRINCIPLES OF CANCER CHEMOTHERAPY

THE rational design of cancer chemotherapy really requires a full understanding of the way in which tumours differ from the host tissues. We have already pointed out in connexion with bacterial chemotherapy that the aim is, if possible, to find some unique metabolic difference between the invader and the host—this was well exemplified by the action of penicillin on bacterial cell walls built up from muramyl peptides which do not occur in animal tissues. Uniqueness in tumour cells is more elusive. Normal tissue cells divide and differentiate according to a predetermined genetic plan probably controlled by local growth-controlling substances. In tumour cells this control system has been abrogated either by mutation, by foreign nucleic acid of viral origin, or by interference by chemical carcinogens. The resulting tissue shows varying degrees of regression to a more undifferentiated state with defective organization and balance of growth. The extent of these changes varies with the type of tumour, and is rarely homogeneous, i.e. a tumour frequently contains areas of quite different orders of maturity. In many respects the regression of these cells is to a state comparable to that found in the embryo in which many enzyme systems are absent since the relevant operons are not activated till a later stage of development. Tumours also differ in the response induced in the surrounding tissues which may range from indifference to an active fibrotic, phagocytic response not dissimilar to that in inflammation. From this description it may be judged that metabolic differences in tumours may be largely deletive, i.e. restrictive of substrate utilization so that tumours are frequently at a natural disadvantage compared with normal cells and growth rate is limited by the turnover of particular metabolic pathways. In addition the cells are actively dividing whereas the majority of adult tissue cells show only the occasional mitoses. Obvious exceptions are the haemopoietic cells, skin, gut mucosa, and gonadal tissue all of which are involved in rather rapid turnover and have a partially differentiated stem cell population whose general characteristics are not very dissimilar to those of the tumour cells. It will be recalled that in bacterial chemotherapy there are two main classes of effective agents, those that kill, and those that control growth, the latter being effective mainly because the phagocytes are able to deal with restricted numbers of organisms. Since phagocytic destruction of tumour cells is less effective, growth control is less effective in tumours unless it can be kept up indefinitely. In a few cases this is so, for instance some mammary cancers retain the sensitivity to oestrogens of the parent cells and their growth can be depressed by lowering oestrogen levels by ovary or pituitary ablation, or by feedback control with androgens. Some prostatic cancers are correspondingly dependent on androgens and can be controlled by androgen suppression with oestrogens. In general the aim in tumour chemotherapy is therefore to kill the tumour cells, and to produce as complete a destruction as possible.

With most antitumour agents there is a logarithmic relationship between the survival of cells and the dose of drug (Fig. 19.1); this means that if a certain dose kills 99 per cent of cells, twice this dose will be needed to kill 99·99 per cent. This very steep dose-response curve is favourable to killing tumour cells but also to the destruction of the host cells. Most antitumour agents have a

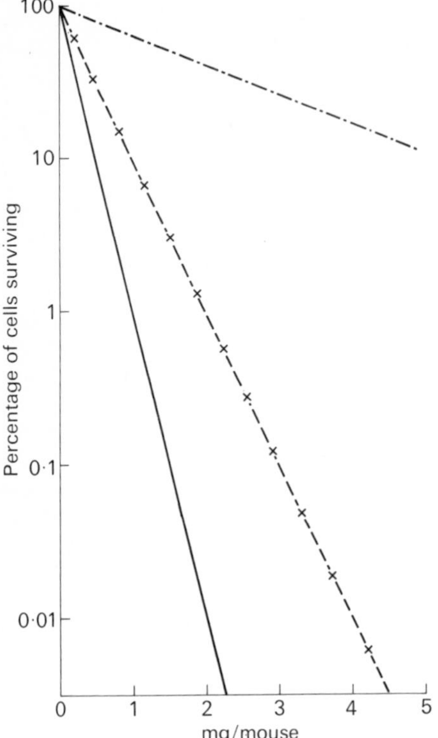

Fig. 19.1. Cells surviving after administration of 5-fluorouracil to mice.

— - — normal marrow cells
—— lymphoma
×--× proliferating

greater effect on cells in an active state of cell division than on those in a resting phase. This is illustrated in Fig. 19.1 where it can be seen that the normal bone marrow population is relatively insensitive to 5-fluorouracil and much less sensitive than the cells in the lymphoma, but if the bone marrow cells are shifted into rapid proliferation by preliminary depopulation their sensitivity to 5-fluorouracil is greatly increased and is comparable to that of the tumour. Therefore, in planning cancer chemotherapy we need to consider the cell cycle and where in this cycle drugs act. In any cell population some cells are not in a dividing state and are said to be resting (G_0; Fig. 19.2); others are in a division cycle which begins with a phase G_1 in which DNA is not synthesized and goes through a DNA synthesis phase (S) and then into another non-synthetic phase (G_2) before the morphological changes identified with mitosis occur. After cell division the daughter cells may go into a resting phase or re-enter the division cycle. G_0 is insensitive to antitumour agents which mostly act on the S phase (i.e. on DNA synthesis) or on mitosis either by interfering with the structure of DNA by intercalation or cross linking, or by blocking metaphase (the separation of the chromosome pairs) by interfering with spindle development or contraction (Fig. 19.3). The factors switching cells from G_0 into G_1 are not understood but in normal tissues must be concerned in regulating the normal cell mass. This means that when the dividing cell population has been largely eliminated by an antitumour drug, many of the cells in G_0 are switched into the division cycle; similar behaviour seems to operate in many tumours. This can be taken advantage of in planning chemotherapy. Thus the initial treatment may attack a majority of the cells in a rapidly growing tumour; following this, the resting cells start to divide and become susceptible to follow up treatment. On the other hand, in a slowly growing tumour few cells will be in the division phase and the strategy may be to use a relatively small dose

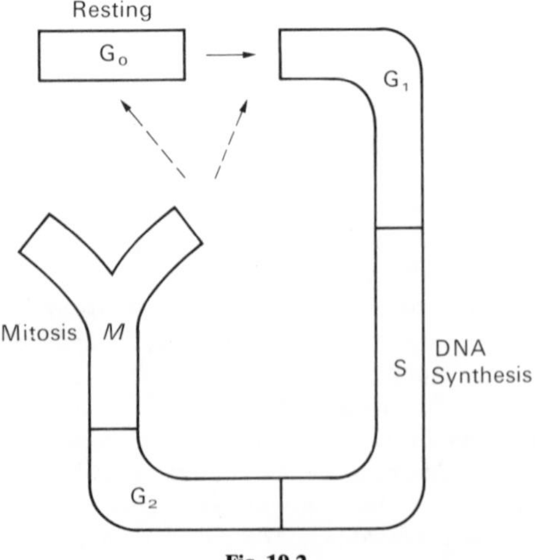

Fig. 19.2.

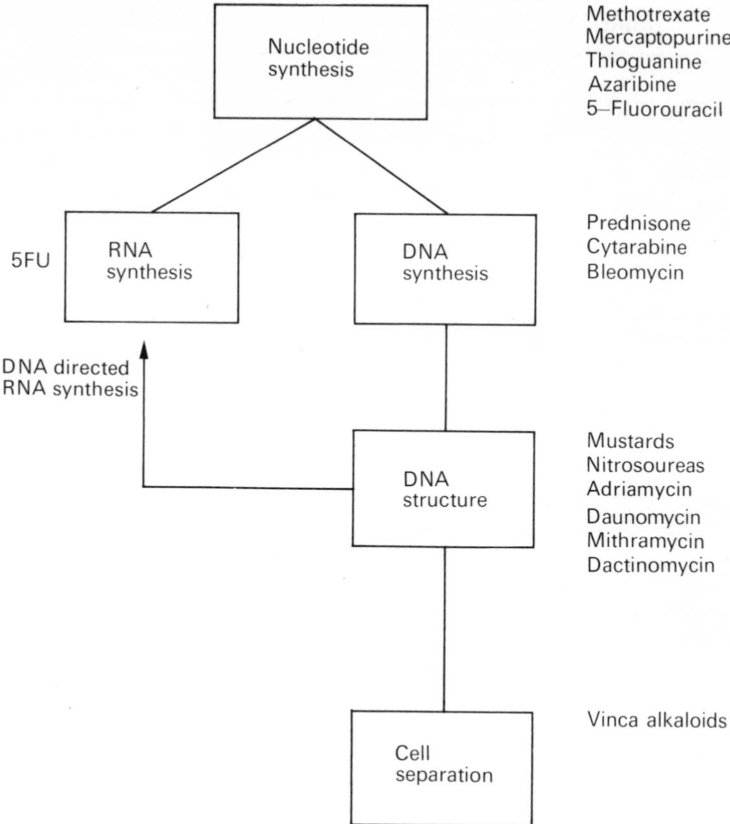

Fig. 19.3. Sites of action of antitumour drugs.

of drug to kill most of the dividing cells but to induce a large population of the resting cells to go into division with a follow up of a larger dose of drug. Fig. 19.1 makes it clear that similar problems apply to the host cells, so that matters of timing of the courses of chemotherapy is of great importance and of very considerable difficulty.

The availability of antitumour drugs acting on different aspects of cell function suggested that in analogy with the value of combining agents already discussed in the case of co-trimazole, this might be beneficial in the case of cancer. Table 19.1 shows some results obtained in the treatment of acute lymphoblastic leukaemia with five antitumour drugs alone and in combination—it can be seen that some combinations are very effective, not only in the percentage of patients going into remission, but also in increasing the duration of the remission. What is a remission? It may be a complete cure, but more often the tumour cell mass has been reduced to a very small amount that slowly regrows and when a clinically apparent mass reappears the disease is said to be in relapse. Let us look at a few figures. Suppose the tumour mass is initially 1 kg; this corresponds to about 10^{12} cells. Suppose that the chemotherapy has killed 99·9999 per cent of cells; the residual cell mass will be 10^6 cells or 1 mg of cells, but nevertheless if these cells can double only once a week the cell mass will have returned to 1 kg after 5 months. This indicates that after the initial therapy, a maintenance regime should be established and this has been

Table 19.1. Treatment of acute lymphoblastic leukaemia

	Remissions (per cent)	Duration (months)
MTX	22	—
MP	27	—
ADR	33	—
VCR	57	2
Pred	63	1·5
MTX+MP	45	—
Pred+MP	82	—
Pred+VCR	85	2
Pred+VCR+ADR	97	10·5
Pred+VCR+MTX+MP	94	5

MTX, Methotrexate; MP, mercaptopurine; ADR, adriamycin; VCR, vincristine; Pred, prednisone.

very successful—for instance, whereas the duration of remission after the prednisone and vincablastine combination was only 2 months, with the simple addition of intermittent methotrexate it was extended to 18 months and with increasing sophistication in the procedures it has recently been extended to 5 years. Rather similar results have been achieved in Hodgkin's disease. In other solid tumours the results have been less encouraging but this appears to be due, at least in part to the philosophy of treating early tumours by surgery and/or radiotherapy and reserving chemotherapy for those cases that cannot be treated in that way, or for cases that have recurred. This certainly produces a rather biassed view of the results of chemotherapy. The present approach takes into account a fact very well established with experimental tumours, namely that the probability of cure depends on the initial size of the lesion. The logical implication of this to remove as much of the tumour as possible by surgery or radiotherapy and combine this with multi-agent chemotherapy to deal with local residues and with early metastases. This approach is proving successful in many kinds of cancer, even in ones such as mammary carcinoma previously regarded as very resistant to chemotherapy; the best combination of chemotherapy at this date seems to be 5-fluorouracil, methotrexate, vincristine, cyclophosphamide, and prednisone.

ANTIMETABOLITES

The antimetabolites act either directly or indirectly on the synthesis or introduction of purines and pyrimidines into nucleic acid.

METHOTREXATE

This an analogue of folic acid (see Chapter 17) which is an inhibitor of the enzyme dihydrofolate reductase which is responsible for reducing dietary folic acid to its two reduced forms, dihydrofolate (DHF) and tetrahydrofolate (THF). THF is the form of the coenzyme that can act as a carrier of methyl, methylene, or formyl groups which can be transferred as one carbon fragments in purine biosynthesis. If the synthesis of THF ceases, then as the cellular store of THF falls so purine synthesis declines and eventually ceases. Even more important is the fact that when methylated THF is used in the biosynthesis of the pyrimidine nucleotide thymidylic acid from its precursor deoxyuridylic acid, the THF is oxidized back to DHF so that to keep this reaction going requires continuous reduction of DHF to THF. It appears that this latter action is the key to the powerful action of methotrexate on dividing cells. Methotrexate binds to dihydrofolate reductase very strongly so that it can produce virtually complete inhibition of the enzyme. In sensitive tumours the dose of methotrexate needed may not be sufficient to inhibit cell multiplication in the gastro-intestinal tract or the bone marrow, but in the case of the more resistant tumours very high doses are needed and severe toxic effects may result. The acute toxic effects can be reversed rapidly by a suitable form of THF—a stable form is 5-formyltetrahydrofolate (leucovorin, folinic acid). **Leucovorin** acts partly by providing a fresh supply of THF but also by competitively displacing methotrexate from the enzyme so that its excretion is accelerated.

Methotrexate is a major drug in almost all treatment schedules, and by itself it is curative in chorionepithelioma.

Aminopterin and **dichlormethotrexate** are related compounds.

FLUOROURACIL

5-Fluorouracil (Fu) is not itself an active antimetabolite but in the tissues it is converted enzymatically into 5-fluorouridylate which is incorporated into RNA and which thereby affects RNA synthesis and its functional capacity as well as ribosomal stability. However, it also undergoes a further metabolic change through ribonucleotide reductase to the deoxynucleotide 5-fluorodeoxyuridylate which is a very powerful inhibitor of thymidylate synthetase. In general, these metabolic reactions are more extensive in tumour cells than in normal cells, so giving some selectivity. Fu has a wide usefulness.

CYTARABINE

Cytarabine (cytosine arabinoside, ara-C) is an interesting substance in which the ribose of cytidine is replaced by the stereoisomer arabinose. This substance must also be activated *in vivo* to form Ara C phosphates which inhibit DNA polymerase (especially the RNA-dependent enzyme) and can also be incorporated into RNA and DNA. A related substance is **5-azacytidine**.

MERCAPTOPURINE

Mercaptopurine (MP) can be regarded as an analogue of adenine in which the amino group is replaced by sulphur. MP undergoes a complicated series of metabolic changes in which the most important products are probably thioinosinate and its methylderivative, 6-methylmercaptopurineribonucleoside. Major effects of these compounds are on the synthesis of adenylate and guanylate. Rather little MP is incorporated into DNA. MP is a major first-line drug in the treatment of acute leukaemia. **Thioguanine** is a closely related drug in which the only difference is the NH_2 in the 2-position which makes it an analogue of guanine.

ALKYLATORS

The alkylating antitumour drugs all derive from the observation that nitrogen mustards (nitrogen analogues of mustard gas) caused agranulocytosis. A great variety of compounds of this series have been made with the objective of either directing the alkylator to a specific site, or controlling its action through effects on the metabolic pathway of the drug. The active drugs are all bifunctionals, i.e. have two active groups, and it is now generally accepted that they act by alkylating the 7-position of guanine (Fig. 19.4) and then, by alkylating a guanine on an adjacent position in the other strand of double-stranded DNA, forming a cross link that prevents the strands separating. Single alkylations in guanine (e.g. produced by methylnitrosamine) are relatively easily excised and replaced by DNA repair enzymes; this is less possible with cross links.

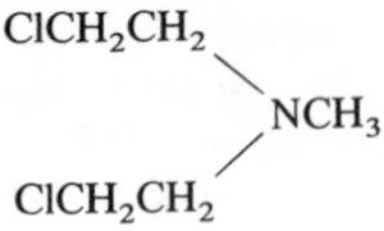

$ClCH_2CH_2$ / $ClCH_2CH_2$ \ NCH_3

Mustine

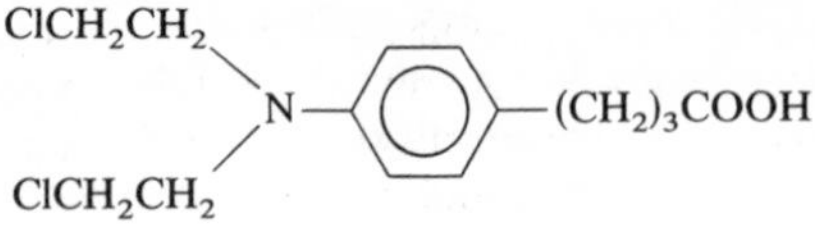

$ClCH_2CH_2$ / $ClCH_2CH_2$ \ N—C_6H_4—$(CH_2)_3COOH$

Chlorambucil

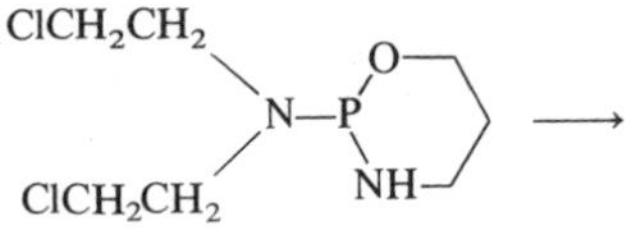

$ClCH_2CH_2$ / $ClCH_2CH_2$ \ N—P (O, NH ring)

Cyclophosphamide

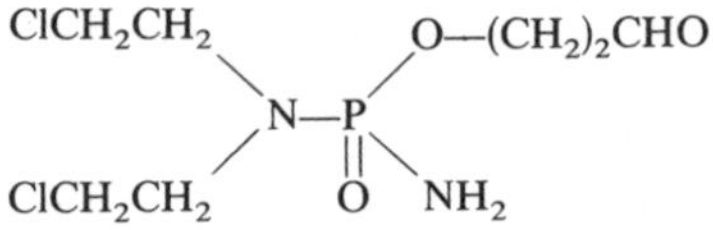

⟶

$ClCH_2CH_2$ / $ClCH_2CH_2$ \ N—P(=O)(O—$(CH_2)_2CHO$)(NH_2)

Aldophosphamide

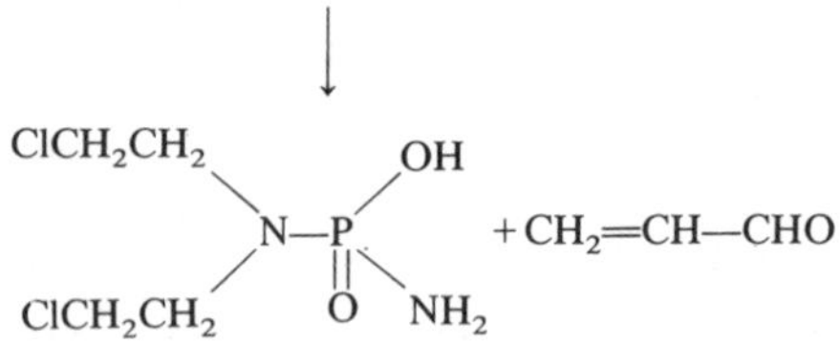

↓

$ClCH_2CH_2$ / $ClCH_2CH_2$ \ N—P(=O)(OH)(NH_2) + CH_2=CH—CHO

Phosphoramide mustard + Acrolein

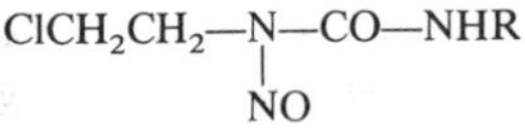

$ClCH_2CH_2$—N(NO)—CO—NHR

Nitrosoureas

BCNU	R = CH_2CH_2Cl
CCNU	R = Cyclohexane
McCCNU	R = *p*-methylcyclohexane

Fig. 19.4. Alkylating agents.

Mustine (mechlorethamine, mustargen)

Mustine is unstable in solution and must be made up fresh and given intravenously. It is of great value in early Hodgkin's disease and lymphomas and is used as a part of combined therapy for late Hodgkin's disease. It is not often used in other cancers. **Chlorambucil** is a more stable substance that can be taken orally. It is slower in action and the least toxic of the nitrogen mustards; it is the main drug used in treating chronic lymphocytic leukaemia. **Melphalan** is similar but is also used in multiple myeloma and some solid tumours.

CYCLOPHOSPHAMIDE

Cyclophosphamide, while it has the characteristic *bis*(chlorethylamine) structure, is not directly active. After administration it is oxidized in the liver by the mixed function oxidase to the 4-hydroxy derivative. This is in equilibrium with the open-chain aldophosphamide which breaks down spontaneously to phosphoramide mustard and acrolein (Fig. 19.4), both of which have strong anti-tumour activity. In many tissues the aldophosphamide is further oxidized enzymatically to the non-toxic carboxyphosphamide, but the necessary enzyme is deficient in most tumour cells. Cyclophosphamide is relatively less toxic than mustine, particularly severe CNS side effects do not occur, and there is less damage to megakaryocytes. Cyclophosphamide is a valuable drug that is a component of many of the combination regimes.

BUSULPHAN

Busulphan belongs to a different series of alkylators, the sulphonic esters, and is the *bis*(methylsulphonate) of tetramethylene glycol. It has a highly selective action in chronic myeloid leukaemia for which it is the drug of first choice.

NITROSOUREAS

These compounds are hybrids between the nitrogen mustards and the alkylating nitresoureas. **BCNU** (carmustine) is unstable and must be administered like mustine but **CCNU** (lomustine) and **methyl CCNU** (semustine) can be given by mouth. They are highly active against a wide range of experimental and human tumours.

ALKALOIDS ACTING ON DNA

Adriamycin and **daunomycin** are fungal products that are chemically related to the tetracyclines. They intercalate, i.e. the ring becomes inserted between adjacent turns of the DNA helix. The unwinding of the helix leads to inhibition of DNA polymerase and DNA-directed RNA polymerase; activity is greatest in the *S*-phase. They are the most active agents currently available for soft tissue sarcomas and thyroid carcinoma and are useful components of treatment schedules for carcinoma of the lung and breast. The main toxic action is on the heart and heart failure due to myocardial degeneration may occur.

DACTINOMYCIN

Dactinomycin is another intercalating drug derived from a fungus, and its mode of action is similar to adriamycin. However, it is very toxic and its use is restricted to a few tumours.

BLEOMYCIN

Bleomycin is a mixture of polypeptides derived from a fungus. Through mechanisms that are still unknown bleomycin is able to cause breaks and fragmentation in DNA and is able to interfere with repair mechanisms. It has minimal activity on the bone marrow and activity against squamous cell carcinomas and malignant lymphomas. Unfortunately, its usefulness is limited by its liability to produce severe pulmonary fibrosis.

VINCA ALKALOIDS

The alkaloids **vinblastine** and **vincristine** are derived from the periwinkle, *Vinca rosea.* They arrest mitosis in metaphase (as does colchine) through interfering with the spindle protein, tubulin, and are exceedingly active substances. They produce beneficial results in a wide range of sarcomas, and carcinomas as well as in leukaemia and Hodgkin's disease. The most important toxic effect is on the leucocytes, although a wide range of other effects are seen. Nevertheless, they are a valuable component of most multiple drug schedules.

PLATINUM DIAMMINES

Amongst the most simple anti-cancer drugs are the planar *cis*-diammines of platinum II. The *trans* isomers are inactive. In many of their properties, they resemble the alkylators and it seems likely that they cross link the amino groups of adenine. The drug has a wide range of activity, but has toxic effects on the kidney and causes deafness.

GLUCOCORTICOIDS

It was noted earlier that glucocorticoids such as **prednisone** had important tumour-suppressant effects. These seem to be exerted through cytoplasmic receptors which migrate to the nucleus inhibiting DNA synthesis. Toxicity is low.

IMMUNOSUPPRESSION

Most of the antitumour drugs are also capable of suppressing the immune response. This can be shown most simply in the response of circulating immunoglobulins to the injection of an exogenous antigen.

Immunosuppression is used clinically in organ transplantation to suppress histocompatibility respones; without immunosuppression kidney transplants from all except identical twin donors are rapidly rejected. With effective immunosuppression transplants can survive for many years.

Immunosuppression is also used in autoimmune diseases such as haemolytic anaemia, thrombocytopenic purpura, systemic lupus erythematosus, and the nephrotic syndrome.

Glucocorticoids and a derivative of mercaptopurine, **azathioprine,** are most widely used. Cyclophosphamide is also widely used and occasionally vinblastine.

FURTHER READING

Chabner, B. A. *et al.* (1975). The clinical pharmacology of antineoplastic agents. *New Engl. J. Med.* **1107,** 1159.

Connor, T. A. (1975). Drugs used in the treatment of cancer. *FEBS Letters.* **57,** 223.

Heffter, A. (1974). *Handbook of experimental pharmacology. Antineoplastic and immunosuppressive agents, Berlin.*

Marsh, J. C. (1976). Effects of cancer chemotherapeutic agents. *Cancer Research* **36,** 1853.

20

QUANTITATIVE AND HUMAN PHARMACOLOGY

BIOLOGICAL ASSAY

BIOLOGICAL methods of assay are used to detect, and measure the concentration of, substances by observing their pharmacological effects on living animals or tissues. They are usually more troublesome, and less accurate, than physical or chemical methods and are only used when there is no other reliable way, or when the physical or chemical methods are too insensitive. Most bacteriological products, such as toxins, antitoxins, and sera, can only be detected biologically. Some of the biological tests for hormones, chemical transmitters, and vitamins have been largely replaced by chemical and physical methods, and this process will doubtless continue; but it is probable that biological methods will always be necessary for some of the hormones, and few of the new methods are so well established that it is possible to dispense with the biological method altogether. When biological methods and chemical methods for the assay of a pharmacologically active substance disagree so widely that the disagreement cannot be due to the error of the tests, the biological method is, by definition, right and the chemical method is wrong.

Biological assay is often very important, since drugs such as insulin could not be used unless it was possible to ensure a uniform product. If there was much variation between different supplies of the drug patients would die from overdosage or underdosage when they started to use a new supply. Accurate biological methods of testing insulin and other such substances have been developed in recent years, so that it is now theoretically possible by using sufficiently large numbers of animals, to attain any required degree of accuracy; but this has only been achieved through the acceptance of certain general principles governing the design of the experiments.

Bioassays are also used in diagnosis and in clinical research. The concentration of gonadotrophins in the blood or urine may be estimated quantitatively by injecting these fluids into animals. Other hormones can also be estimated in the same sort of way, but chemical methods are generally preferred when these are available.

The strength of a preparation can be stated in animal units. For example, a Unit of insulin was originally defined as the quantity of insulin which reduced the blood sugar of a normal rabbit by a certain arbitrary amount. This depends, of course, on a number of factors such as the weight of the rabbit, its state of nutrition, and the room temperature, but even when all known causes of variation have been standardized, rabbits still vary in their response to insulin, and an animal unit must always be subject to large errors of unknown size, since a London rabbit is not necessarily the same as an American rabbit or a Cambridge rabbit or even as another London rabbit. The use of rabbit units or rat units has been compared with the convention, once adopted, that a cubit was the length of the king's forearm and was liable to vary with the size of the king.

These large and unknown errors have been reduced to reasonable and known proportions by the use of standard preparations, consisting of actual samples of various biological products, adopted and preserved by the 'Expert Committee on Biological Standardization' of the World Health Organization and issued to suitable persons for biological assay. A Unit is defined as a definite weight of one of these standard preparations, and assays involve comparisons of the tested preparations with the standard preparation. The error of the test still depends largely on the variability of the animals, but it is reduced because the variability involved is that between animals coming from the same stock and brought up together, instead of the general variability of animals of the same species. Even more important advantages of the use of a standard preparation are the facts that the error of the result can usually be calculated, and that it can be indefinitely reduced by the use of more animals. The methods of calculation are discussed below.

Accurate biological assays are only possible when the active principle of the standard preparation is identical with the active principle of the preparation compared with it. Methods of assay which did not fulfil this requirement have often been proposed in the past, but have never proved satisfactory. For example, it was found that posterior pituitary extracts and potassium salts both caused a contraction of the isolated uterus of a guinea-pig, and it was proposed that pituitary extracts should be compared with the potassium chloride on this preparation and that their activity should be expressed in terms of their potassium equivalent. It was found, however, that when the assay was repeated it did not give constant results because the sensitivity of uteri to potassium did not always vary in proportion to their sensitivity to pituitary extracts. The only satisfactory standard for the assay of the active principle of the pituitary which produces this effect is a stable preparation of the active principle itself.

So long as the standard preparation is suitable, there is no reason why the effects observed in an assay should be the same as those desired when the drug is used in therapeutics. Insulin can be assayed by its power to cause convulsions in mice, and the value of the result is not impaired by the fact that the production of convulsions will not be the usual purpose for which the insulin will be used in practice.

CALCULATION OF THE ERROR

Generally speaking, the best method of estimating the error of any measurement is to repeat the measurement several times, and to see how closely the results agree among themselves. When precision is important, and the experimenter is not content to accept the nearest round number as the result, repeated measurements of any kind always show a certain amount of variation, and the error can be calculated from the size of this variation. These principles are generally recognized by everyone who takes the trouble to make duplicate determinations of a measurement. Duplicate determinations are sufficient to show that the error of many simple physical measurements is small enough to be neglected, but the error of biological measurements is often so large that more attention must be paid to it. Duplicate determinations give only a very crude estimate of the error, since the actual size of the discrepancy between any particular pair of measurments is largely due to luck. At least a dozen parallel measurements or pairs of duplicate measurements are required for anything like a reliable estimate of the error. In the case of biological measurements this may involve a prodigious amount of work, and it is sometimes preferable to calculate the error indirectly from the variability of the animals themselves. This variability is usually responsible for most of the error, which depends on which individual animals are chosen for any particular test. Such errors are called errors of sampling because they are due to the assumption that the animals chosen are a typical sample.

The mathematical methods used in calculating errors may appear arbitrary and unnecessarily complicated, but they fit the facts and can also be justified by theoretical arguments. The following argument is crude, but it illustrates the kind of principle involved.

A certain rich man had 64 friends and gave each of them 100 marbles. He then tossed a coin with each friend, and the loser of each toss paid one marble to the winner. Since the tossing was done fairly, half his friends lost and half of them won, so that after the first round of tossing 32 of his friends had 101 marbles and 32 of them had 99. They then tossed again and half of each group won again, so that there were 16 friends with 102 marbles, 32 with 100 marbles, and 16 with 98 marbles. The left

Fig. 20.1. Theoretical frequency distributions, in which the vertical scale denotes the frequency of the values shown on the horizontal scale. This figure can only be understood by reading the text. The curve on the right is a normal curve.

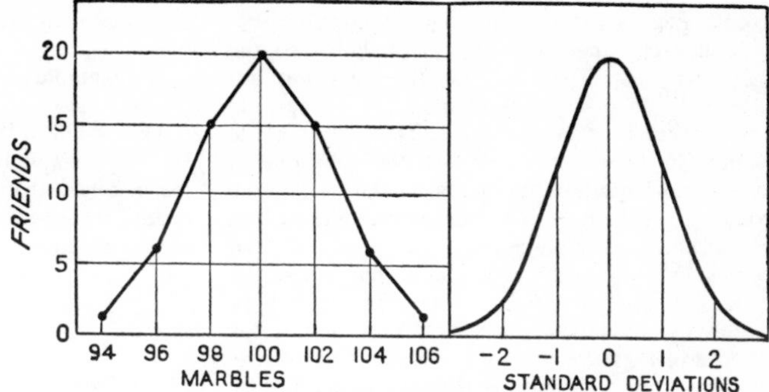

part of Fig. 20.1 shows the distribution of marbles that might be expected according to this argument after 6 rounds of tossing. The number of marbles is plotted on the horizontal scale against the number of friends that might be expected to have that number of marbles on the vertical scale. These calculations only give expectations, and in actual practice these expectations would not be exactly fulfilled, but that is another story.

This distribution is known as the binomial distribution, because the probability of each possible result (number of wins) is given by one of the terms of the binomial expansion of $(p+q)^n$, where p is the probability of a win and $q=1-p$, and n is the number in a sample (the number of rounds of tossing). In the case of the rich man it is assumed that $p=q=0{\cdot}5$.

If the process is continued, the curve approximates more and more closely to a smooth curve whose shape can be calculated and which is known as the normal curve and is shown in the right part of Fig. 20.1. The size of an animal (or any other measurement) may be considered to depend upon a large number of chances, each corresponding to a round of tossing, so that the distribution of sizes should, on this theory, be similar to the distribution of marbles among the friends of the rich man. The theory would, however, be worthless were it not for the fact that, if a large number of animals are measured and divided into groups so that all the animals in the same group are about the same size, and if the number in each group is plotted against the size, an approximately normal curve actually is obtained.

In biological measurements there is, however, a complication. The effect of each chance is likely to depend upon the size of the animal. A warm day which adds a hundredth of a ton to a 5-ton elephant will not add the same weight to a 5-milligram maggot; it is more likely to add a hundredth of a milligram. The effect of each chance on the weight of the animal is, in fact, likely to be proportional to the weight itself. Allowance can be made for this fact by calculating the weight of the animal in logarithms, since the difference between log 5 tons and log 5·01 tons is the same as the difference between log 5 mg and log 5·01 mg; and this holds true whatever units of weight are used.

One of the advantages of this method of calculation is illustrated in Fig. 20.2, which is based on measurements of the blood pressure of normal university freshmen. The curve on the left was obtained by dividing the scale of blood pressures into a number of small ranges at the points 80, 85,

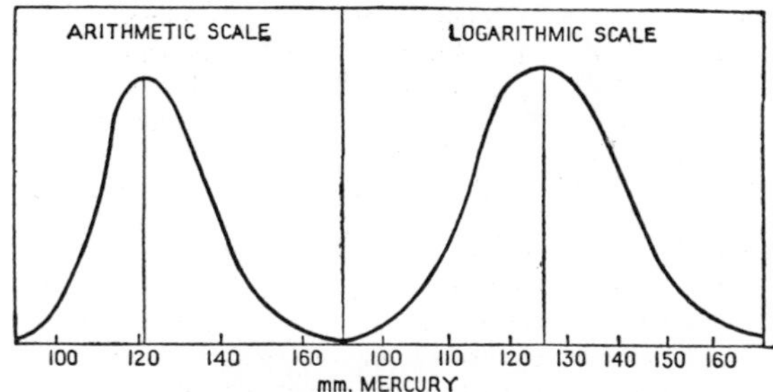

Fig. 20.2. Frequency distribution of systolic blood pressures. The vertical scale is proportional to the relative frequency with which different blood pressures occurred. The logarithmic scale of blood pressures gives a normal curve. The arithmetic scale does not. (From data by Alverez (1923) *Arch. intern. Med.* **32,** 17.)

90, 95, etc., mm of mercury. The number of readings in each range was then plotted against the blood pressure. The curve on the right was obtained by converting each reading into a logarithm and repeating the same process. This second curve is more like a normal curve than the other one is. When the variations in biological data are large compared with the mean, the logarithmic method of calculation usually gives more nearly normal curves than the simpler method, but when the variations are small compared with the mean, both methods give equivalent results, and in these cases the use of logarithms is an unnecessary complication and only desirable for the sake of uniformity with the curves where the variation is large. It was found in these experiments that blood pressures over 180 and below 90 mm of mercury were observed occasionally in healthy young men of 18 years of age. Such blood pressures are not necessarily an indication of disease, but may be merely due to the inevitable variability of all populations.

When an assay, or any other measurement, is repeated many times, the individual results vary in the same way as the weights of individual animals and are distributed in normal curves. It is therefore impossible to give the error in the form of a definite value which is never exceeded, but possible to estimate the the value which is exceeded once in 100 times or once in 1000 times.

The error is proportional to the breadth of the curve and is measured in terms of the standard deviation (σ). This can be estimated from a set of n observations by calculating first the mean of the observations ($\bar{x}$) and then the deviation (difference) of each observation from this mean (d). The expression

$$\sqrt{\left(\frac{\sum d^2}{n-1}\right)}$$

then gives an estimate of the standard deviation. The square of the standard deviation is called the variance; the use of this term is sometimes convenient because it eliminates square-root signs from the formulae.

The standard deviation of the logarithms of the result (λ) is calculated by writing down the logarithms of the results, finding the mean logarithm, calculating and summing the squares of the deviations from this mean, dividing this sum by $(n-1)$, and taking the square root.

When several sets of observations, distributed about different means, are available for calculating the standard deviation the appropriate formula is

$$\sigma \quad (\text{or } \lambda) = \sqrt{\left(\frac{\sum d^2}{\sum(n-1)}\right)},$$

and in applying this formula the summation is extended over all the values of d and n in all the different groups.

An example of the practical application of these formulae is given on p. 233.

The standard deviation (σ) is a measure of the error of a single observation: the standard error of the mean of n observations is $\sigma/\sqrt{n}$; its variance is σ^2/n. The standard error of the sum or difference of two means is

$$\sqrt{\left(\frac{\sigma_1^2}{n_1}+\frac{\sigma_2^2}{n_2}\right)},$$

where σ_1 and n_1 refer to one set of observations and σ_2 and n_2 refer to the other; the variance of the sum or difference is

$$\frac{\sigma_1^2}{n_1}+\frac{\sigma_2^2}{n_2},$$

that is, the sum of the variances of the two means separately.

The main use of the standard deviation depends on the fact that the shape of the normal curve is known. The range of results between $\bar{x}-\sigma$ and $\bar{x}+\sigma$ includes about $\frac{2}{3}$ of all the results; the range $\bar{x}\pm 2\sigma$ includes about 95 per cent and the range $\bar{x}\pm 2{\cdot}576\sigma$ includes 99 per cent of the results. This fact was used in the *British Pharmacopoeia* 1948, from which the following clear statement is taken by permission.

> In expressing the limits of error of biological assays the term 'limits of error ($P=0{\cdot}99$)' is used. The statements of the errors of these assays are based on the convention that, for practical purposes, a probability of 0·99 is equivalent to certainty. In other words, it has been estimated that the result of the assay will be within the stated limits 99 times out of every 100 times that the assay is made. These limits are given as percentages of the true result. Thus, the statement 'limits of error ($P=0{\cdot}99$) 95 and 105 per cent' means that it has been estimated that in 99 assays out of 100 the result will be greater than 95 per cent, and less than 105 per cent, of the true result.
>
> If the error of the test, or its logarithm, is normally distributed, the stated limits of error correspond to the range covered by ±2·576 times the standard deviation.

METHODS OF ASSAY

There are three methods of interpreting the result of a biological assay.

Method 1. Threshold dose measured on each animal

These assays are those in which a drug is administered slowly to an animal until some observable effect is produced. The assay of digitalis by means of cats is an example of such a test. The cat is anaesthetized with chloralose, its blood pressure is recorded, and a suitable extract of digitalis is allowed to run into a vein at a rate of 1 ml per minute. At the moment when the heart stops beating and the blood pressure falls to zero the volume of fluid which has run in is recorded. This volume contains the dose necessary to kill that particular cat under the conditions of the experiment. Two series of such experiments, using the standard separation of digitalis and the unknown preparation respectively, are carried out and the potency calculated from the average results.

The results shown in Table 20.1 illustrate the best general method of calculating the result and its error.

The ratio of the potencies of the tinctures was estimated as antilog (1·27 − 1) or 1·86. Since the standard tincture contained 1 unit per ml, the unknown tincture was estimated to contain 1·86 units per ml. Direct calculation without logarithms gives an estimate of 1·88 units per ml.

Since it is unlikely that the variability depends on which tincture is used, the standard deviation of the logarithm of the estimate for one cat (λ) is estimated from both sets of figures together from the expression

$$\sqrt{\left(\frac{\Sigma d^2}{\sqrt{(n-1)}}\right)}$$

which is

$$\sqrt{\left(\frac{0{\cdot}0059+0{\cdot}0109}{5+5}\right)} \text{ or } 0{\cdot}041.$$

This is equal to log 1·10, and is thus equivalent to a standard deviation of 10 per cent.

The standard error of the logarithm of the estimate of the ratio of the potencies is

$$\sqrt{\left(\frac{\lambda_1^2}{6}+\frac{\lambda_2^2}{6}\right)}$$

or 0·0237. This is equal to log 1·056 and is thus equivalent to a standard error of 5·6 per cent. Direct calculation without logarithms gives an estimate of 5·9 per cent. In cases like this, where the standard deviation is not greater than 10 per cent, the two methods of calculation give practically identical results. When the error is large the method using logarithms is the only one which gives accurate results.

Method 2. Responses recorded or measured

Sometimes the effect of the drug can be observed repeatedly on the same tissue. The two samples of the drug are given alternately and the doses adjusted until they give equal effects. Fig. 20.3 shows the result of an assay of this kind. This is a record of the contractions of a piece of guinea-pig's intestine

Table 20.1. The individual lethal dose (ml per kg of cat) of tinctures of digitalis diluted 1/20 with saline

Standard tincture				Unknown tincture			
Lethal dose	log dose	d	d^2	Lethal dose	Log dose	d	d^2
18·2	1·26	0·01	0·0001	12	1·08	0·08	0·0064
19·6	1·29	0·02	0·0004	10	1·00	0·0	0·0
17·0	1·23	0·04	0·0016	9·5	0·98	0·02	0·0004
17·4	1·24	0·03	0·0009	8·7	0·94	0·06	0·0036
19·7	1·29	0·02	0·0004	10·2	1·01	0·01	0·0001
21·1	1·32	0·05	0·0025	9·6	0·98	0·02	0·0004
	6 | 7·63		0·0059		6 | 5·99		0·0109
Mean	1·27				1		

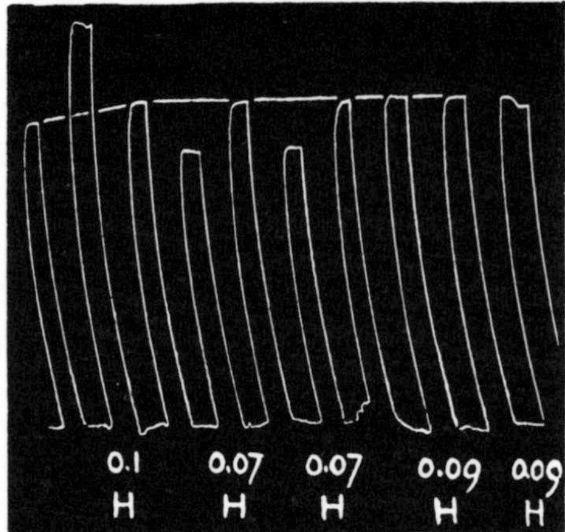

Fig. 20.3. Assay of histamine by its action on guinea-pig's intestine in a 2 ml bath, showing ten independent contractions. The drum was stopped after each contraction and the solution changed. H = histamine. The figures denote ml of a 0·2 μg per ml solution added to the bath. The alternate doses are 0·1 ml of an extract, which was equivalent to 0·09 ml of the histamine solution. (From Gaddum (1936) *Proc. roy. Soc. Med.* **29,** 1373.)

which was suspended in a bath of salt solution similar to that shown in Figure 1.1. When doses of a standard solution of histamine or of an extract of blood were added to the bath in small volumes of fluid they caused a contraction of the muscle which was recorded on the drum. When each contraction was complete the drum was stopped and the salt solution changed so that the muscle relaxed again. The effects labelled *H* were due to the histamine solution, and the volumes of this solution are given in millilitres (ml). The other effects whose summits are joined by a white line are all due to 0·1 ml of the extract. It will be seen that the effect of this volume of the extract was less than that of 0·1 ml *H*, and greater than that of 0·07 ml *H*, and about equal to that of 0·09 ml *H*. The concentration of histamine in the extract was therefore about 0·18 mg per litre.

Since 2·5 ml of extract had been made from 10 ml of blood, the original concentration of histamine in the blood was 0·045 mg or 45 μg per litre. Such small quantities of histamine can only be detected by methods such as this.

Similar methods are used for the assay of the principle in the posterior lobe of the pituitary which causes a contraction of the uterus and for adrenaline, acetylcholine, and other substances.

Accurate estimates of the potency and the limits of error can be made by using methods of calculation originally designed for assays in which the standard and unknown preparations are tested on different animals. A simplified method of calculating the error in this case was described by Bliss.

Many of the vitamins and hormones can be assayed by methods of this class. One group of animals receives the standard preparation and a similar group receives the unknown preparation which is being tested. After a suitable interval of time the animals, or parts of the animals, are weighed and the result is calculated from the average weights in the two groups.

The calculation of the results of such assays and their errors generally depends on a consideration of the relation between dose and effect. Fig. 20.4 shows the results of a comparison between two steroid hormones found in extracts of adrenal cortex. These two substances both have the effect of increasing the amount of glycogen in the liver. Groups of fasting adrenalectomized mice received various doses of each of them by subcutaneous injection and were killed after a suitable interval. The vertical scale shows the average amount of glycogen in the liver (mg per 100 g body weight) and the horizontal scale shows the total dose (mg) given to each mouse (in a series of seven injections). On the left side of the figure the doses are plotted on an ordinary arithmetic scale, and on the right side they are plotted on a logarithmic scale. This means that the logarithm of each dose is plotted instead of the dose itself.

The use of logarithms has the following effects:

1. When each dose is double the preceding dose, they are plotted at equal intervals on the logarithmic scale. If the largest dose is many times as large as the smallest, the smaller doses are apt to be huddled too closely

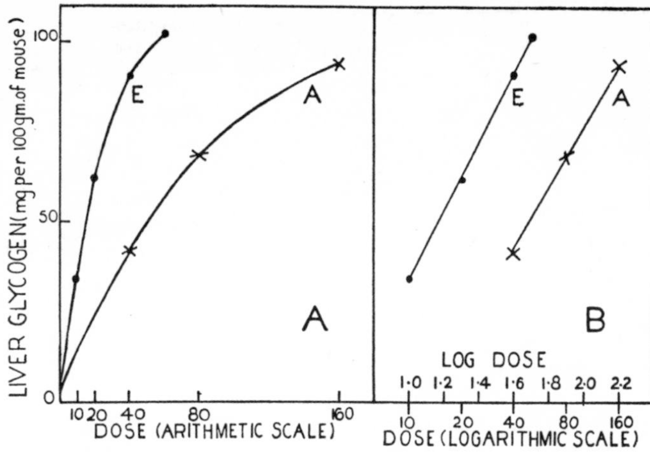

Fig. 20.4. The effects of 11-dehydrocorticosterone (A) and cortisone (E) on liver glycogen in mice. The dose–effect lines (*A*) are not parallel. The log-dose–effect lines (*B*) are nearly straight and parallel. (Venning *et al.* (1946) *Endocrinology*, **38,** 79.)

together on an arithmetic scale. The logarithmic scale avoids this trouble.

2. The two lines on the right side of the figure are parallel and the two curves on the left are not. In this case the result of the test is that E is about 3·5 times as active as A. This means that, for any given effect, the dose of A is about 3·5 times as large as the dose of E. On the arithmetic scale the distance from the vertical axis at any given height is 3·5 times as large for A as for E. On the logarithmic scale the horizontal distance between the two lines is about constant and equal to log 3·5.

3. The points can be fitted by straight lines when plotted on a logarithmic scale, but not when plotted on an arithmetic scale. These straight lines, of course, cannot be extended indefinitely in either direction, but it is commonly found that straight lines can be used to represent the middle part of the curve and that this device works best when logarithms are used. When necessary, the lines can sometimes be straightened by measuring the effect in some other way, or by using some function of the effect (such as its square or logarithm) instead of the effect itself.

4. When arithmetic scales are used, the error of the test is generally not normally distributed, and increases as the dose increases. If logarithms are used the error is generally normally distributed and independent of the dose.

In all these ways the calculations are simplified by the use of logarithms, and this has been enough to induce those concerned with biological assays to overcome any initial distaste they may have felt, and to regard logarithms as a very useful tool.

Simpler designs. The experiment whose results are shown in Fig. 20.4A may be called a (4 and 3) dose assay. In routine testing it is generally more convenient to use fewer doses. The simplest satisfactory design is known as a (2 and 1) dose assay and is illustrated in Fig. 20.5a which shows some of the same data as Fig. 20.4. In this figure the effects of 40 and 80 mg of A are plotted against log 40 and log 80 and the straight line through these points is taken as the dose–effect curve for A. A dose of 20 mg of E caused an effect of 62 and the graph shows that this corresponds to 1·82 on the line. The antilog of 1·82 is 66·1 so that the ratio of the potencies is 66·1/20 or 3·3. Calculation from simple geometry gives the result as 3.336.

Fig. 20.5b which is taken from the same data, illustrates a (2 and 2) dose assay. In this case the two lines are very nearly parallel and the result can be obtained simply, and with reasonable accuracy, by actually drawing a horizontal line at some convenient place and measuring its length. This method gave the result as 3·34, but the actual figure depends on the place where the line is drawn, and on the skill of the draughtsman. It is really more

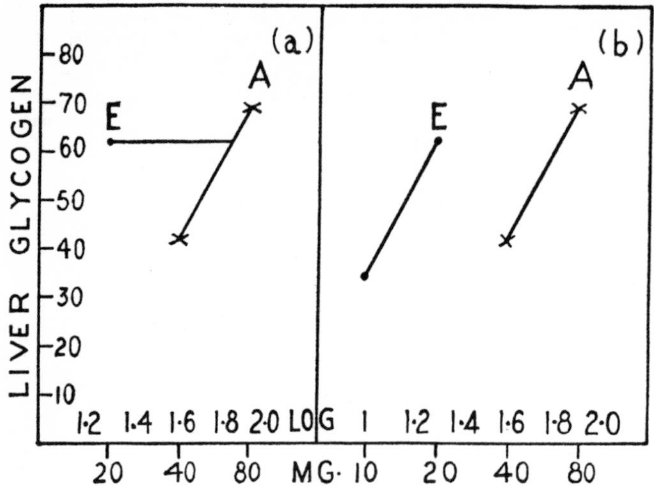

Fig. 20.5. Same data as Fig. 20.4 to show (*a*) a (2 and 1) dose assay, and (*b*) a (2 and 2) dose assay.

satisfactory to calculate the result, and this raises difficulties because the lines are not exactly parallel even in Figs 20.4B and 20.5b, and are often much less nearly parallel than this. In such cases it is necessary to find lines which fit the results as well as possible. This can be done roughly on graph paper by drawing parallel curves which appear by eye to give the most satisfactory fit. This simple procedure is not ideal, since no two persons would fit exactly the same curves to a given set of results. In order to avoid this error, mathematical formulae are used for calculating the result. These formulae give not only the best possible estimate of the result of the assay and its error, but also the equations of the straight lines which provide the best fit for the observatons as judged by the 'method of least squares'. When the number of doses is large the formulae are complicated, but they can be reduced to a simple form when (2 and 2) doses are used.

Consider an imaginary experiment to compare an unknown solution (U) with a standard solution (S). The design of the experiment depends on some assumption or other about the potency of U, based either on preliminary tests or previous experience. The solution U is adjusted so that it would be equal to S if these preliminary assumptions were exactly correct. Two groups of animals receive two different volumes of S and two other groups receive the same two volumes of U. The results are plotted in Fig. 20.6 in which S_1 and S_2 are the effects of S, U_1 and U_2 are the effects of U, and D is the logarithm of the ratio of the two volumes used. The sloping lines show the log-dose–effects curves which fit the observed points as well as possible, while still remaining parallel to one another. The vertical distances of the observed results from these lines are all equal.

If the slope of a line is estimated as the tangent of the angle it makes with the base line, the slopes of the lines through the observed points are $(S_2-S_1)/D$ and $(U_2-U_1)/D$. The true slope (b) is taken as equal to the average of these figures, so that $b=(S_2-S_1+U_2-U_1)/2D$. The difference between the effects of the two preparations is estimated as either (U_1-S_1) or (U_2-S_2) and the average of these is taken as an estimate of this difference, which is equal to the distance h on the graph. The result of the test (M) is the logarithm of the ratio of the activities (U/S).

Now $b=h/M$.

$$\therefore M=h/b=\frac{U_1-S_1+U_2-S_2}{S_2-S_1+U_2-U_1}D.$$

This formula is the same as that given by the method of least squares.

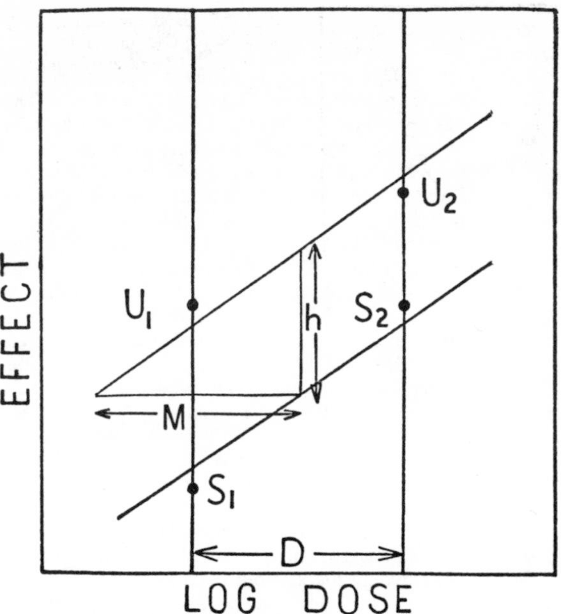

Fig. 20.6. Theoretical log-dose–effect lines to illustrate the calculation of the result of a (2 and 2) dose assay (see text).

The error of this estimate consists of two parts since both the numerator and denominator are subject to error. It may be approximately estimated from the formula:

$$s_M^2 = \text{variance of } M = \frac{V}{b^2}\left(1 + \frac{M^2}{d^2}\right)$$

where $V =$ the mean of the variances of the four estimates of the mean effect. The number 1 in the bracket represents that part of the error due to the estimate of the difference of the mean effects of U and S, and the M^2/d^2 represents that part due to the error of the estimate of the slope.

When the animals are few, or very variable, this formula becomes unreliable and it is then necessary to calculate the 'fiducial limits' by means of a more elaborate formula.

The term is not easy to explain, but if the fiducial limits ($P = 0{\cdot}95$) are calculated for each assay, the true result should be within these limits in 95 per cent of assays. If, for example, the fiducial limits are 80 and 125 per cent, it is reasonable to assume that the true result lies in this range. Such an assumption should be correct 95 times out of 100.

In microbiological assays the dose–effect curve is sometimes straight without the use of logarithms and in this case different methods of calculation are used.

Cross-over test. When the effect of a drug can be observed and measured more than once in the same animal, the accuracy may be very greatly increased by arranging the experiment as a cross-over test, which is carried out in two stages. On the first day one group of animals receives the standard drug and another similar group receives the unknown preparation and the effects are measured; on another day the drugs are crossed over, so that the first group receives the unknown preparation and the second group receives the standard. The average effect of each preparation, for both stages of the experiment together, is then calculated and the result interpreted by the methods discussed above using a dose–effect curve. The advantage of this arrangement is that it eliminates errors due to the difference between one animal and another, since both drugs are tested on the same animals. The effect of the difference between one day and another disappears in the calculation of the mean response of each dose-group. Cross-over tests were introduced by Marks, who used them for the assay of insulin on rabbits.

Method 3. Percentage of positive effects measured

The most familiar example of a test of this class is a toxicity test, in which a poison is injected into a group of animals and the percentage mortality determined. Fig. 20.7 shows the type of curve obtained when the percentage mortality is plotted against the dose given; the same methods of calculation can be used when the observed effect is not death, but some other effect such as oestrus, or hypoglycaemic symptoms.

The curve shown in Fig. 20.7 is sigmoid (**S**-shaped). The doses are given as percentages of the dose causing a mortality of 50 per cent. This dose is usually called the LD 50, in which the letters stand for 'lethal dose'.

The term ED 50 for effective dose is used in all cases except when the observed effect is death.

In the interpretation of an assay of this type each percentage is converted into a probit by means of special tables. If these probits are plotted against the logarithm of the dose the results can be fitted with straight lines and the results can then be interpreted as described above for method 2. In this case the error is calculated from theoretical considerations. The logical basis of the probit is outlined below.

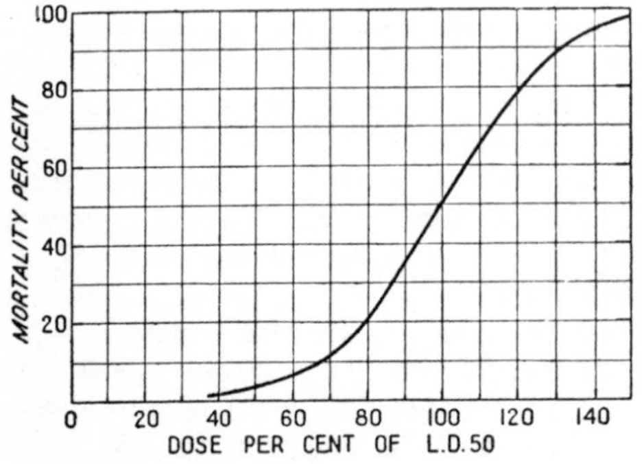

Fig. 20.7. The relation between the dose of digitalis and the percentage mortality among frogs. The curve is based on data given in the *British Pharmacopoeia* 1932.

If all the facts were known about each animal, the distribution of individual effective doses (I.E.D.) could be plotted as a frequency curve similar to those shown in Figs. 20.1 and 20.2. This has been done on the left of Fig. 20.8, in which the horizontal scale is a scale of doses and the vertical scale is a scale of frequencies. If any given dose is injected into a group of animals it will be effective in all those animals whose I.E.D. is equal to, or less than, the given dose. The percentage of responses (*AB*) will therefore be proportional to the area of the frequency curve to the left of a vertical line through the point corresponding to the given dose (the area *FGH*). In mathematical language the dose–percentage curve is the integral of the frequency distribution. This means that the exact theoretical shape of the sigmoid dose–percentage curve can be calculated, on the assumption that the distribution is normal. It is found that theory agrees with practice so long as the doses are plotted on a logarithmic scale.

This conclusion has been reached by plotting the results in a special way which has the effect of straightening the sigmoid curve. For this purpose, not only are the doses plotted on a logarithmic scale, but the percentages are plotted on a probability scale. The simplest way of doing this is to use logarithmic probability paper such as is shown in Fig. 20.9. The results of a test can be plotted on this paper and then interpreted as in method 2.

If logarithmic probability paper is not available it is necessary to convert the doses into logarithms and the percentages into probits, and then to plot the logarithms against the probits.

The probit is best defined in terms of the normal equivalent deviation (N.E.D.). The N.E.D. corresponding to any given percentage is calculated from the shape of a normal curve whose standard deviation is one. The N.E.D. is the deviation (from the mean) equivalent to the given percentage of the area of the curve. The probit is equal to the N.E.D. plus 5.

The relationship between percentages and probits is shown in Fig. 20.10. This curve is an integrated normal frequency curve. An interval of one unit on the scale of probits corresponds to one standard deviation, and the midpoint of the curve, corresponding to a mortality of 50 per cent is arbitrarily taken as 5. If the distribution of individual lethal doses is normal, the relation of the dose to the observed mortality (as shown in Fig. 20.7) will be the same as the relation of the probit to the mortality (Fig. 20.10). Both these quantities (dose and probit) are thus related to the mortality in the same complex way, and that is why their relation to one another is so simple that it can be expressed as a straight line (Fig. 20.9), about which the actual observations are distributed with deviations due to the sampling error.

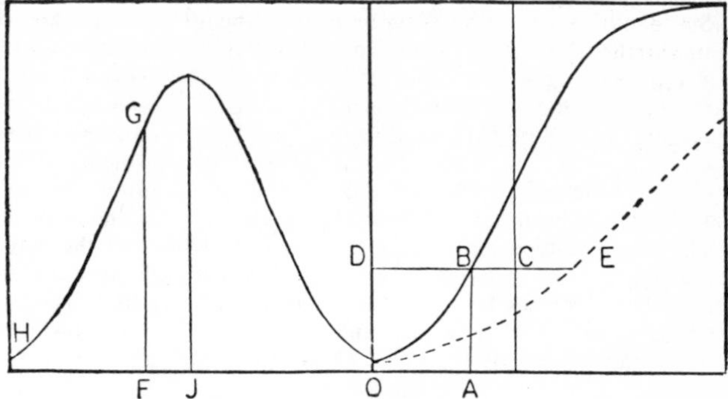

Fig. 20.8. The curve on the left is a normal frequency distribution like those shown in Figs. 20.1 and 20.2. The curve on the right is a dose–mortality curve like that shown in Fig. 20.7. The diagram illustrates the theoretical discussion of the relation of these two curves to one another. (From Gaddum (1933) *Spec. Rep. Ser. med. Res. Coun.* (*Lond.*) No. 183.)

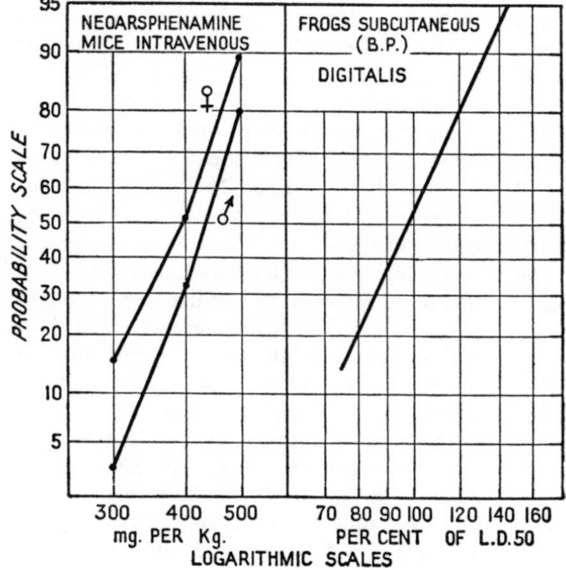

Fig. 20.9. Logarithmic probability paper. The horizontal scale is a logarithmic scale of doses. The vertical scale denotes percentage mortality and the lines are spaced in a way that depends on the shape of a normal curve. The distances are proportional to the corresponding probits. The right-hand figure portrays the same data as Fig. 20.7. The effect of using this paper is that the results lie approximately on straight lines.

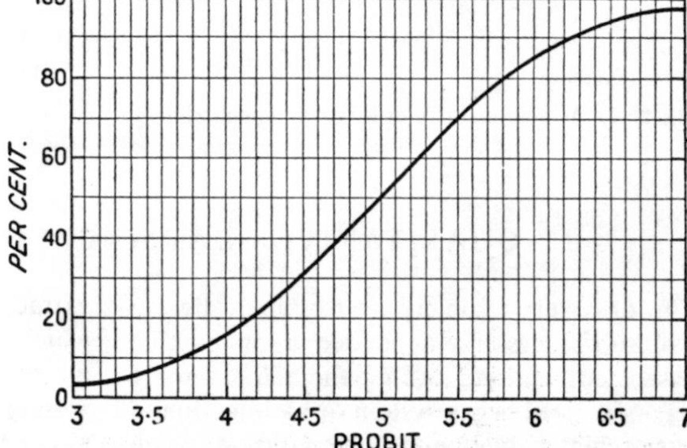

Fig. 20.10. Curve showing the relation between probits and mortality. The main object of this diagram is to clarify the explanation of probits given in the text. It can be used to determine roughly the probit corresponding to any given mortality. If mortalities are converted to probits and doses to logarithms the results can be plotted on ordinary graph paper, and the result is the same as if they had been plotted on the special paper shown in **Fig. 20.9.**

Straight lines are only obtained by the above method when the I.E.D. is normally distributed, but a similar argument applies to the more usual case where the log of the I.E.D. is normally distributed instead of the I.E.D. itself so that log I.E.D. gives a straight line when plotted against the probit. In practice the value of the probit is obtained from tables instead of from Fig. 20.10.

The whole relationship of dose to percentage is completely defined in terms of two quantities that can easily be estimated. One of these quantities is the ED 50, and the other is the standard deviation of the logarithms of the individual effective doses, which is known as λ and is approximately equal to the difference between the logarithms of the ED 69 and the ED 31. Its reciprocal is known as b and is equal to the slope of the curve. Those who determine the shapes of these curves should always estimate and state the values of these two quantities.

The error of a test of this kind can be calculated from theoretical considerations which will not be discussed here. It depends on the fact that the percentages observed with small groups vary widely owing to the chances associated with choosing animals for the experiment.

SEQUENTIAL ANALYSIS

In trials of drug action the basic principles of analysis are very similar to those we have already described. However, in evaluation of a new drug in the first place all that we may want to know is whether the drug has significant activity. It is important to find this out with the minimum number of subjects. If the drug is not active, it is not justified to continue to expose subjects to possible toxicity with no expectation of benefit. The method used in this case is called a sequential trial. In this method the effects of the test drug and of a placebo are compared. A preference for the drug or the placebo is developed either by the patient's subjective assessment or through some biochemical or physiological variable. The preferences for successive cases are plotted in the form shown in Fig. 20.11. When the preference is in favour of the alternative above the line, this is indicated by a short line of unit length plotted at 45° above the abscissa and conversely below the abscissa for preferences in the other direction. The data shown are from a study by Snell and Armitage of the effects of drugs on suppressing coughs. When pholcodine was compared with a placebo, results reached the level of 5 per cent significance after the study had been undertaken on only 18 subjects. A comparison of heroin with placebo was equally effective in demonstrating the efficiency of heroin. The method was used to compare pholcodine and heroin. In this the plot emerges at the angled end which is the zone of non-significance, i.e. the test was unable to show a superiority of pholcodine over heroin.

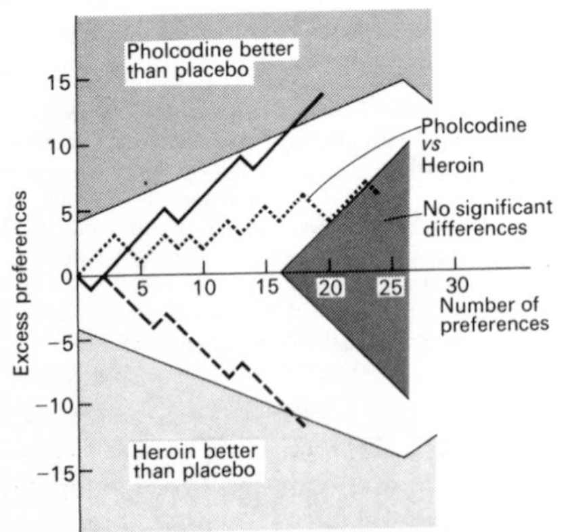

Fig. 20.11 A sequential trial of heroin and pholcodine in suppressing cough.

QUALITATIVE PHARMACOLOGICAL ANALYSIS

The discovery of many new biologically active substances has depended upon making tissue extracts and testing them for activity on an isolated organ system or by injection in a suitable whole animal preparation. Such extracts contain a number of constituents which may be contributing to the pharmacological activity. The classical method for sorting these out was by use of chemical and biological properties. For instance, if a tissue extract which causes a fall of blood pressure on injection is briefly boiled with decinormal caustic soda and the activity is markedly diminished, this may be due to loss of the alkali-labile ester acetylcholine, but it may also be due to other alkali-labile substances. This can be settled by seeing if a similar reduction of activity can be produced by pretreating the animal with atropine, which is of course a highly selective antagonist of acetylcholine and other muscarinic agonists. By a series of such tests it can be established in a preliminary way whether the activity is due to known or unknown agents.

A further biological test of identity is to compare the activity of the extract in a number of different test objects (e.g. blood pressure, contraction of intestine, vas deferens, uterus) with the supposed substance—if the quantitative assessment of the amount of substance present in the extract is always identical this is strong presumptive evidence that the substance in the extract is the same as the substance it is being compared with. However, biological methods do not have the same power of discrimination as physical methods. The simplest of these is liquid chromatography on paper, thin-layer, or column, the latest variant of which is called high-pressure liquid chromatography. The material separated by these methods can be tested further biologically. The material, if volatile enough, may also be separated in the gas phase by gas–liquid chromatography (G.L.C.) and finally identified by mass spectrometry or nuclear magnetic resonance.

An excellent example of this approach is seen in the recent work that led to the isolation and identification of enkephalins. It was first found that an acid-acetone extract of brain had an action on the guinea pig vas deferens that resembled that of morphine. The activity could not be extracted out of an aqueous phase by ethylacetate or ether. The activity could be purified by column chromatography on the ion-exchange resins CG-120 and CG-400 and then purified further by thin-layer chromatography on silica gel sheets. At this stage it was found that the activity was rapidly destroyed by exposure to the enzymes carboxypeptidase A or leucine aminopeptidase. It evidently had a peptide structure necessary for activity. Gel chromatography on Sephadex established that its molecular weight was in the region of 600. After derivatization it could then be separated by GLC and identified as a mixture of two pentapeptides by mass spectrometry. The sequence was confirmed by examining the partial hydrolysis products and the final structure confirmed by synthesis of the two enkephalins.

THE DISCOVERY OF NEW DRUGS

The original drugs in our pharmacopoeia were mostly of vegetable origin. They were discovered when it was found that certain plants had actions that were disagreeable or dangerous or had actions that were pleasant and helpful. By this means the purgative action of cascara sagrada, the ebrifuge action of cinchona, the analgesic action of opium, and the paralytic action of curare were found. The pharmacological activities of many minerals were found mainly in the Middle Ages by a similar process of trial and error. The evaluation of the plant remedies was very uncertain and active and inactive materials had actions ascribed to them which rarely could be substantiated by more careful studies.

Advances came rapidly in the nineteenth century when, with the development of chemistry, active principles, the alkaloids, were isolated in a pure state and their structure determined. It was then possible to relate actions to well-defined substances and gradually the idea developed that the kind of activity found was related to particular chemical structures. In parallel with these discoveries, the new process of synthetic organic chemistry was producing entirely new groups of compounds that had never been found in nature and as the biological activity of these compounds was tested, so new pharmacological actions were discovered. Gradually the principles discussed in Chapter 1 began to be applied, i.e. if an activity was found in a particular compound, related derivatives were prepared in a systematic way and tested for activity and the rules for structure activity worked out. The modified structure might lead to a less toxic drug, or a more active one, one that is active by mouth, with an altered duration of action, or a different selectivity. These principles can also be applied to natural compounds and have, for example, led to orally active steroids auch as ethinyloestradiol or the synthetic analogues of atropine or morphine. There is no schism between compounds of natural or synthetic origin—they are equally susceptible to molecular modification. It is interesting to find that when a series of analogues of a substance that has been found active is made, the most useful activity is frequently found amidst the first few synthesized. It is rare that a very long series of compounds needs to be made before the best is found, so that Ehrlich's famous studies on organic arsenicals in which the 606th member was arsphenamine and 912th neoarsphenamine is not at all typical; indeed even in this case the ultimately most useful member of the series, arsenoxide, was discovered early on.

When a new drug is put into clinical use, new findings may provide clues for drug improvement. The sulphonamides provide a very interesting case history in this respect. Soon after the azo dyes had been discovered it was found that sulphonic and sulphonamide groups increased the fixation of the dyes to fabrics. In the 1930s, following the idea originated by Ehrlich that dyes had chemotherapeutic effects, a number of azo dyes were tested for antibacterial action; one of them, prontosil, turned out to have considerable activity *in vivo* against strepococci. It was soon found that the azo linkage was unnecessary and that the active moiety was 4-aminobenzene-sulphonamide (sulphanilamide)—chemical modification of this molecule produced highly active antibacterial substances (see Fig. 20.12). It was noticed that when sulphanilamide itself was given to patients it had a mild diuretic activity and the urine became more alkaline. It was also found that sulphanilamide was a powerful inhibitor of a newly discovered enzyme, carbonic anhydrase. This became the starting point of a new effort in chemical synthesis and soon much more powerful substances exhibiting both these activities were found, an example of which was acetazolamide. However, as active exploration of the series continued, it was noticed that the two activities did not always proceed hand in hand and that it was possible to produce very active diuretics which were practically devoid of any activity in inhibiting carbonic anhydrase. Furthermore, they had little activity on acid–base balance but produced a dramatic loss of sodium and chloride in the urine; an important member of this new group is chlorothiazide.

Yet another new group of drugs arose from the continued development of antibacterial sulphonamides. During the clinical trial of sulphanilamido isopropylthiadiazole, an unpleasant side-effect appeared—the patients became weak, trembling, and sweaty. The physician concerned recognized these as the signs of hypoglycaemia and this supposition was readily confirmed by measurement of the blood sugar. Subsequent studies showed that an alkyl group was necessary but that the ring structure was not and eventually the structures that emerged were the sulphonyl-ureas which are very effective oral antidiabetic agents.

By an even more complex route the observation that sulphadiazine was an active substance in curing malaria in birds led through other substituted pyrimidines to the very active antimalarial, chloroguanide. On the other hand, some of the 2,4-diaminopyrimidines that had been found to be very active antifolates on bacteria were seen to be possible structural analogues of chloroguanide and when tested were found to be highly active, thus leading to pyrimethamine.

Even this semi-logical tale is an unusual one in drug development, although the discovery of new actions of drugs being used for

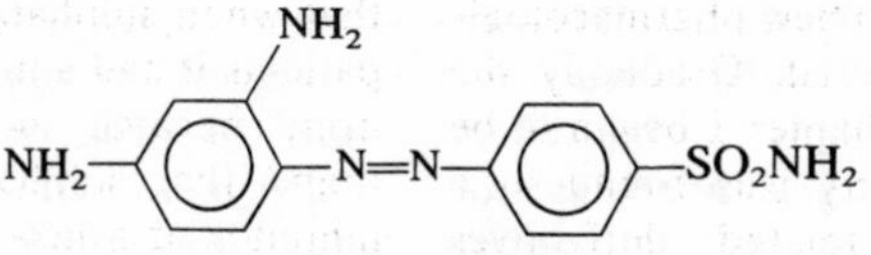

Prontosil

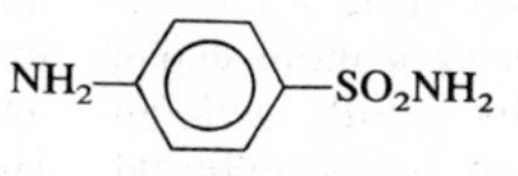

Sulphanilamide

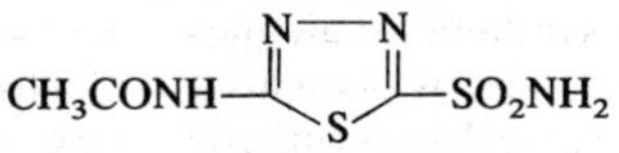

Acetazoleamide

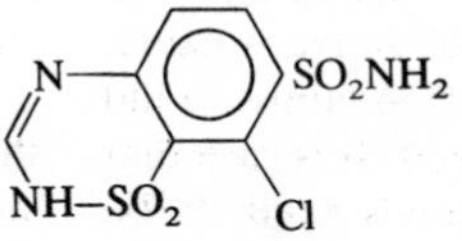

Chlorothiazide

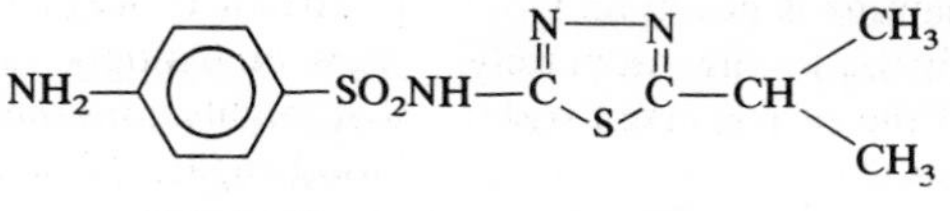

Sulphanilamidoisopropylthiadiazole

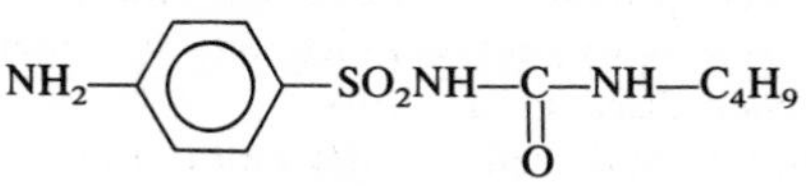

Carbutamide

Fig. 20.12

some established purpose is not that uncommon. For instance, the very important group of phenothiazine antipsychotics resulted from their use as anti-emetics when it was noted clinically that there was a striking improvement in the mental state of a psychotic patient receiving the drug. Similarly, the discovery that chloroquine was effective in improving systemic lupus erythematosus was an incidental finding in a patient being treated for malaria. However, in most instances, new drugs are identified through the use of *screening procedures.* What this means is that in the pharmaceutical industry each new compound is tested on a series of biological tests ranging from simple isolated organ preparations designed to identify particular kinds of action, such as contraction of the uterus or vas deferens, dilation of the coronary arteries, or inhibition of the release of histamine, or biochemical tests such as effects on protein synthesis, or cyclic adenylate formation, or on much more elaborate animal preparations, including tests of behaviour and a careful examination of a conscious animal injected with the substance.

The breadth of this battery of screening tests will depend partly on the resources available and also on the interests of the company who may have specialized interests in, say, bacterial chemotherapy, psychotropic drugs, or oral contraceptives. The synthesis of new compounds may be directed towards finding better variants of existing drugs or drugs of a particular type, usually dictated by an estimate of the available market, or towards the synthesis of entirely novel chemical structures in the hope that they may also show entirely new kinds of biological activity. Two interesting examples of the latter are the adamantane derivatives that have shown activity both as antiviral agents and in the treatment of parkinsonism, and the benzodiazepines, such as chlordiazepoxide, which have become important tranquillizers and hypnotics. The method of exploration of homologous series for improving the basic drug has been put on a more systematic basis in recent years by the development of the method called *quantitative structure activity relationships* (*QSAR*).

In this method, as well as studying the biological activity in the drugs series, some physical properties of the compound are either measured or calculated. The most generally useful properties studied are the partition of the substance between a lipophilic phase (usually octyl alcohol or chloroform) and water, the electronegativity of any aromatic or heterocyclic ring in the substance, and the strength of ionization of any charged group. When these properties have been evaluated in a few members of the series a correlation equation is set up to measure the relationship of these parameters to the drug potency. This equation will often make it possible to predict the biological activity of compounds not yet synthesized—the result may be that it is not necessary to synthesize the missing compounds or to direct attention to particular compounds. This procedure can lead to great economies in the drug development programme. It is also very interesting that the application of such procedures has emphasized the importance of hydrophobic groups in determining drug potency. It can be seen that the discovery of new drugs remains largely an empirical process in which the three Princes of Serendip have a dominant role. It is hoped that the development of *molecular pharmacology* will eventually lead to drug discovery purely from molecular arguments but the successes in this field are at present very few indeed.

THE DEVELOPMENT OF NEW DRUGS

When a promising new drug action has been found, there follows an intensive study of its pharmacology in animals designed to explore both the characteristic action and any additional pharmacological actions in a variety of species. It is usual at the same time to examine the alterations produced by different routes of administration both on actions and on the acute toxicity; in most cases chemical methods will need to be developed for detecting the drug and its major metabolites so that duration of action and comparison of metabolism in several species can be carried out.

A preliminary study of chronic toxicity is usually carried out at this stage. The drug is given at just sublethal dose for several weeks, usually in rats and dogs, and the effects on behaviour, growth, and on some simple biochemical parameters such as haemoglobin, blood sugar, and urine composition, examined together with histological examination of the major tissues. If the drug passes these hurdles consideration must now be given to what potential uses the drug may have in man and whether these merit a preliminary trial. This should be a joint evaluation of all the evidence by the developers of the drug and the clinical pharmacologists. If it is agreed to proceed there follows a careful study in single individuals starting with very cautious dosage to assess how well the drug is tolerated after single doses and, if the drug is of the kind that produces direct physiological effects, whether the effects are similar in character and magnitude to those already revealed in animals. If this is all right, it is then usual to proceed to a limited therapeutic evaluation in man, at the same time extending the examination of chronic toxicity over a longer time and a wider range of situations; in particular, since the thalidomide disaster, to administer the drug both to young animals and to mating pairs continuing through pregnancy.

It is as well to be clear about what is attempted in designing and carrying out animal toxicity tests. Ideally animal tests should predict toxic effects occurring in man; this pre-supposes that the same type of toxic effects do occur, but in fact there are several rather curious human toxic effects for which no animal tests are known. These are blood dyscrasias, skin effects, allergy, and most central nervous effects. Excluding these one can make a comparison and in Table 20.2 is shown a retrospective evaluation of six drugs that went to a full-scale clinical trial. It can be seen that toxicity in the rat was a poor indicator of toxicity in man and that the dog was a good deal better but still only detected a little over half the toxic effects found in man. What is more disturbing is that in both species toxic effects were found that did not arise in man. These results indicate first that study of animal toxicity is only a rough indicator of toxicity in man and further that some potentially valuable drugs may be damned

Table 20.2

Detectable toxic signs (6 drugs)		234
Found in man		53
Rat	toxic effects also found in man	18
	toxic effects not found in man	19
Dog	toxic effects also found in man	29
	toxic effects not found in man	24
Toxic effects in man detected in neither dog nor rat		23

for toxicity that would never appear in man. The classic case here is penicillin which has a low toxicity in man and most other species but produces a lethal haemorrhagic enteritis in guinea-pigs. Fortunately this was not known when penicillin was introduced into therapeutics. The present position is therefore that animal testing will normally reveal gross toxicity precluding use of a drug in man, and experienced toxicologists develop a feeling for the animal data which can be a valuable guide in deciding whether to proceed. The clinical pharmacologist is now ready to proceed with a carefully planned trial to establish therapeutic usefulness under conditions in which the patients can be kept under close surveillance so that unexpected toxic effect or unexpected therapeutic effect can be picked up quickly. The kind of action exerted by the drug will determine the character and duration of the assessment at this time. It is usual to use some sort of sequential trial in which the effects of the drug can be compared with a placebo or with some established treatment so that a decision on effectiveness can be reached as early as possible. This initial trial may be broadened out into a multicentre trial so that sufficient experience is obtained and the probability of encountering the less common drug hazards is increased.

Common toxic effects should have been picked up by the procedure described and thereafter it is the uncommon toxic effects that need to be looked for. For instance, chloramphenicol produces serious blood dyscrasias in about 1 patient in 10 000. Such a toxicity is unlikely to be detected even in large-scale clinical trials, and the best machinery for alerting attention to such a hazard is by adverse-reaction reporting. Doctors report any unusual reaction that has occurred when a patient is on a drug to a central agency which collates the reports and can rapidly spot an unusual clustering of toxic results. It was through this kind of reporting that it was noted that women taking oral contraceptives which were a combination of progestagen and oestrogen had a higher frequency of intravascular thrombosis than the general public and that the incidence of thrombosis was related to the amount of oestrogen in the pill.

In Britain the responsibility for regulating the introduction of new drugs and for monitoring drug safety falls on the Committee for Safety of Medicines (similar organizations, such as the Food and Drug Administration in the USA, operate in other countries). The CSM is responsible for the three phases of drug introduction which can be summarized as:

Phase I Initial studies in a few normal human volunteers.
Phase II Limited clinical trials in patients
Phase III A full-scale clinical trial

If Phase III yields acceptable results the drug may be given a Product Licence and the pharmaceutical firm may decide to put it on the market for general use. The new drug, like others, will be kept under surveillance through the adverse reactions reporting procedure.

In recent years the possibility that drugs (particularly those used for long periods of time) might induce cancer has given particular concern. The testing of drugs in animals for carcinogenic activity is not easy. If the potential for producing tumours is relatively low tests on enormous numbers of animals would be needed, so that practical animal tests are only likely to pick out substances of high carcinogenic potential. This problem has led to intense effort to discover *in vitro* tests that are both more effective and less costly. A considerable number of such tests are now available, the best known and validated of which is the Ames test. The principle of the test is the use of a mutant of a bacterium (*Salmonella typhimurium*) that has a metabolic defect that makes it unable to synthesize an essential nutrient, which must be provided in the culture medium if the organism is to multiply. For instance, the mutant may not be able to make the amino acid histidine and it will not multiply if histidine is not present in the growth medium. If a large number of the bacteria (say 10^9) are plated on an agar plate in a medium lacking any histidine, the vast majority will be unable to grow. However, there will usually be ten or twenty colonies and these can be shown to be due to organisms in which spontaneous reversion to the wild type (which does not need histidine) has occurred. The reversion is due to random mutation. If a mutagenic substance is included in the medium the reversion rate is increased. For instance, in a test of 2-aminoanthracene (2-AA), the control number of revertant colonies was about thirty but in the presence of 1 ng of 2-AA these increased to sixty and in the presence of 500 ng of 2-AA increased to more than 10 000. There is in general a linear relationship between the concentration of mutagen and the reversion rate.

Many substances that are known to be carcinogenic in animals fail to give a positive response in the Ames test. This is because these substances need to be activated by metabolism to produce mutagenic metabolites. It has proved possible to include a metabolic system from the liver in the Ames test to take care of this and when this is done the correlation between potency *in vitro* and *in vivo* becomes very good. The present position is thus that any candidate drug is now subject to one of these *in vitro* tests and if it shows up positive, it is unlikely to be taken further. This in fact proves to be a useful further test for evaluating the effects of molecular modification, since some members of a series may be positive and others negative. The application of this test to drugs that have been in long-standing use has revealed some valuable drugs that are positive. It is not easy to recommend the withdrawal of a valuable drug that has been in long use.

FURTHER READING

Ariens, E. J. (ed.) (1971). *Drug design*, New York.

Armitage, P. (1960). *Sequential medical trials*, Oxford.

Armitage, P. (1971). *Statistical methods in medical research*, Oxford.

Burn, J. H., Finney, D. J. and Goodwin, L. G.

(1950). *Biological standardisation*, 2nd ed. London.

D'Arcy, P. F. and Griffin, J. P. (1972). *Iatrogenic diseases*, Oxford.

Danes, D. M. (ed.) (1977). *A textbook of adverse drug reactions*, Oxford.

Finney, D. J. (1964). *Statistical methods in biological assay*, 2nd ed., London.

Fisher, R. A. (1964). *Statistical methods for research workers*, Edinburgh.

Gaddum, J. H. (1933). *Spec. Rep. Ser. med. Res. Coun.* (*Lond.*) No 183, HMSO, London.

Garb, S. (1971). *Clinical guide to undesirable drug interactions and interferences*, London.

Goldstein, A. (1964). *Biostatistics*, London.

Goldstein, A., Aronow, L., and Kalman, S. M. (1974). *Principles of drug action*, New York.

Hill, A. B. (1967). *Principles of medical statistics*, 8th ed., London.

Hill, A. B. (ed.) (1965). *Controlled clinical trials*, Oxford.

Laurence, D. R. (1973). *Clinical pharmacology*, 4th ed., Edinburgh.

Laurence, D. R. (ed.) (1959). *Quantitative methods in human pharmacology*, Oxford.

Laurence, D. R. and Bacharach, A. L. (eds.) (1964). *Evaluation of drug activities: pharmacometrics*, New York.

Melmon, K. L. and Morelli, H. F. (eds.) (1972). *Clinical pharmacology: basic principles in therapeutics*, New York.

Wolstenholme, G. E. W. and Porter, R. (eds.) (1967). *Drug responses in man*, London.

Zaimis, E. (ed.) (1965). *Evaluation of new drugs in man*, Oxford.

ADDITIONAL GENERAL READING IN PHARMACOLOGY

Albert, A. (1973). *Selective toxicity*. 5th ed., London.

Ariëns, E. J., and Rossum, J. M. van (1964). *Molecular pharmacology*, London.

Barlow, R. B. (1964). *Chemical pharmacology*, 2nd ed., London.

Bovet, D., and Bovet-Nitti, F. (1948). *Médicaments du système nerveux végétatifs*, Basle.

Burger, A. (ed.) (1970) *Medicinal chemistry*, 3rd ed., New York.

Goldstein, A., Aronow, L., and Kalman, S. M. (1974). *Principles of drug action* 2nd ed. New York.

Goodman, L. S., and Gilman, A. (1975). *The pharmacological basis of therapeutics*, 5th ed., London.

Gordon, M. (ed.) (1964). *Psychopharmacological agents*, Vol. 1; (1967). Vol. 2, New York.

Heffter, A. *Handbuch der experimentellen Pharmakologie*. An encyclopaedia of pharmacology with advanced authoritative specialist volumes mostly written in English.

Henry, T. A. (1949). *The plant alkaloids*, 4th ed., London.

Korolkovas, A. (1970). *Essentials of molecular pharmacology*, New York.

Laurence, D. R. (1973). *Clinical pharmacology*, 4th ed., London.

Laurence, D. R., and Bacharach, A. L. (eds.) (1964). *Evaluation of drug activities*, New York.

Marley, E. (1966). *Pharmacological and chemical synonyms*, Amsterdam.

Modell, W. (ed.) (1976–77). *Drugs of choice*, St. Louis.

Root, W. S., and Hofmann, F. G. (eds.) (1963–8). *Physiological pharmacology*, New York.

Schnitzer, R. J., and Hawking, F. (1963–7). *Experimental chemotherapy*, London.

Sollmann, T. (1957). *Manual of pharmacology*, 8th ed., Philadelphia.

Review articles on pharmacology

Pharmacological Reviews.
Advances in Pharmacology.
Advances in Drug Research.
Progress in Medicinal Chemistry.
Annual Review of Pharmacology.

Pharmacopoeias

Pharmacopoeias are official or semi-official publications giving accounts of preparations of drugs used therapeutically.

British Pharmacopoeia (1968).
British Pharmaceutical Codex (1968).
British Veterinary Cosdex (1965).
British National Formulary.
United States Dispensatory.
The Extra Pharmacopoeia (Martindale) (1972).
New and Non-Official Remedies.

UNITS OF MEASUREMENT

mega (M)	10^6	micro (μ)	10^{-6}
kilo (k)	10^3	nano (n)	10^{-9}
centi (c)	10^{-2}	pico (p)	10^{-12}
milli (m)	10^{-3}	femto (f)	10^{-15}

WEIGHTS

		ng	μg	mg	g	kg
1 nanogram (ng)	=	1	10^{-3}	10^{-6}	10^{-9}	10^{-12}
1 microgram (μg)	=	10^3	1	10^{-3}	10^{-6}	10^{-9}
1 milligram (mg)	=	10^6	10^3	1	10^{-3}	10^{-6}
1 gram (g)	=	10^9	10^6	10^3	1	10^{-3}
1 kilogram (kg)	=	10^{12}	10^9	10^6	10^3	1

VOLUME

		Å^3	μm^3	mm^3	cm^3	m^3
Å^3	=	1	10^{-12}	10^{-21}	10^{-24}	10^{-30}
μm^3	=	10^{12}	1	10^{-9}	10^{-12}	10^{-18}
mm^3	=	10^{21}	10^9	1	10^{-3}	10^{-9}
cm^3	=	10^{24}	10^{12}	10^3	1	10^{-6}
m^3	=	10^{39}	10^{18}	10^9	10^6	1

		μl	ml	l
μl	=	1	10^{-3}	10^{-6}
ml	=	10^3	1	10^{-3}
l	=	10^6	10^3	1

CHEMICAL UNITS OF MEASUREMENT

Mole (mol) ≡ molecular weight × grams.
Molarity (mol/1) ≡ Moles of substance in 1 litre of solution (0·1 M, 0·01 M, etc.)
Volume per cent (vol %) ≡ ml of solute in 100 ml of solution.
Grams per cent weight/volume ≡ grams per cent w/v = grams in 100 ml solution.

AQUEOUS SOLUTIONS

The following salts and glucose are dissolved in water to produce 100 ml of solution. Weights in grams.

	NaCl	KCl	$CaCl_2$ (anhyd.)	$MgCl_2$ (anhyd.)	NaH_2PO_4 (anhyd.)	Na_2CO_3	$NaHCO_3$	Glucose
Ringer (frog)	0.65	0.014	0.012	—	0.001	—	0.02	0.2
Ringer (mammalian)	0.9	0.042	0.024	—	—	—	0.02	0.2
de Jalon	0.9	0.042	0.006	0.0005	—	—	0.05	0.05
Tyrode	0.8	0.02	0.02	0.01	0.005	—	0.1	0.1
Sea water	3.0	0.09	0.11	0.51†	0.006	0.003	0.02	0.025
Krebs–Henseleit original Ringer bicarbonate*	0.68	0.035	0.028	0.029†	0.016‡	—	0.21	—
Krebs original Ringer phosphate	0.68	0.035	0.028	0.029†	§	—	—	—

* Gassed with 5% CO_2 in gas phase.

† $MgSO_4 . 7H_2O$.

‡ KH_2PO_4.

§ Use 16·4 ml of 0·1 M phosphate buffer (17·8 g $Na_2HPO_4 . 2H_2O$ + 20 ml. N-HCl diluted to 1 litre).

INDEX OF CHEMICAL RINGS

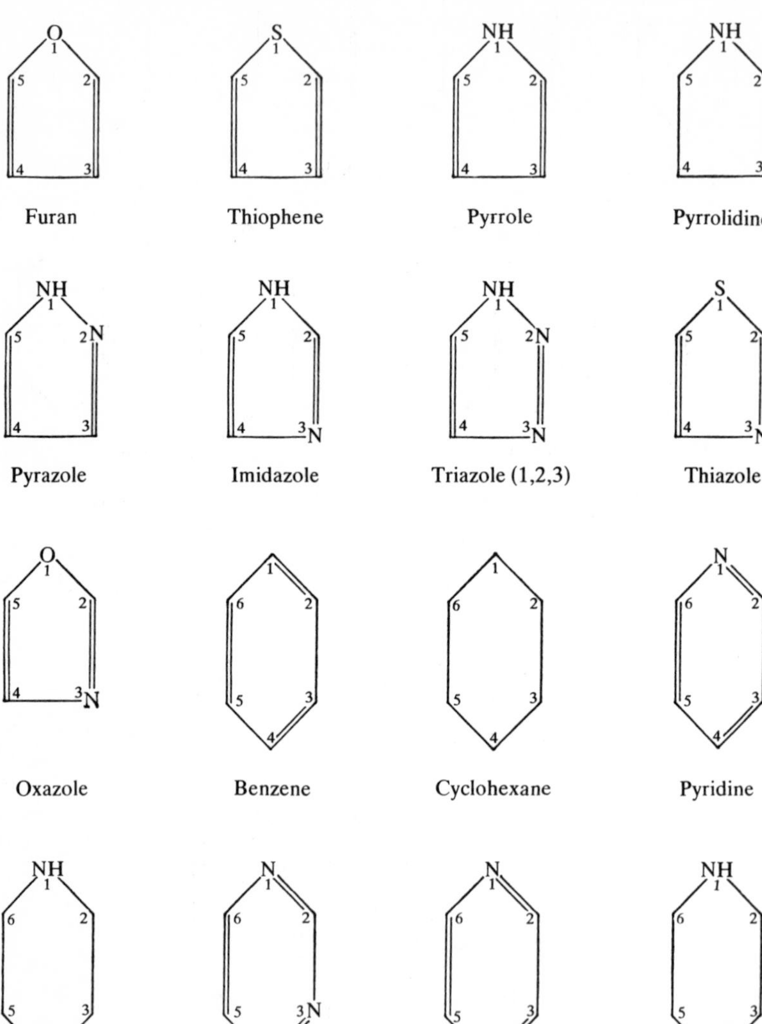

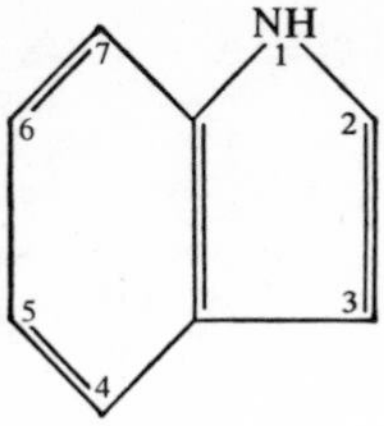

NH 1 2 3 4 5 6 7

Indole

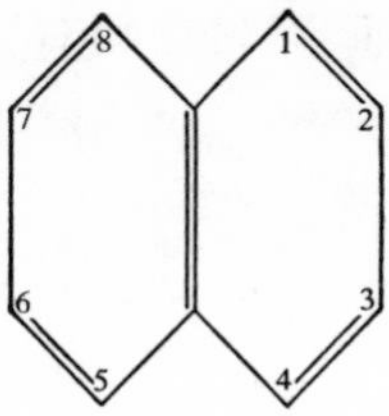

1 2 3 4 5 6 7 8

Naphthalene

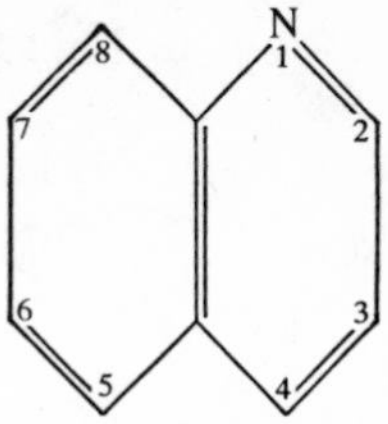

N 1 2 3 4 5 6 7 8

Quinoline

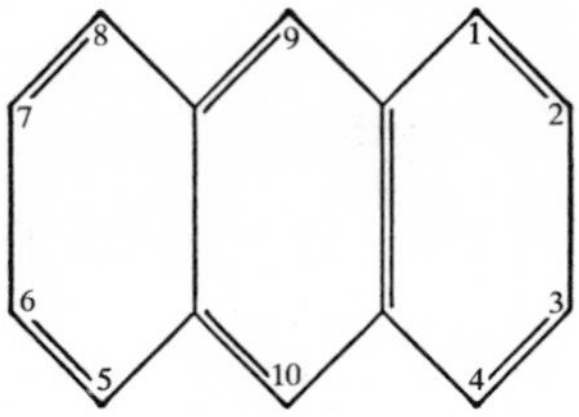

1 2 3 4 5 6 7 8 9 10

Anthracene

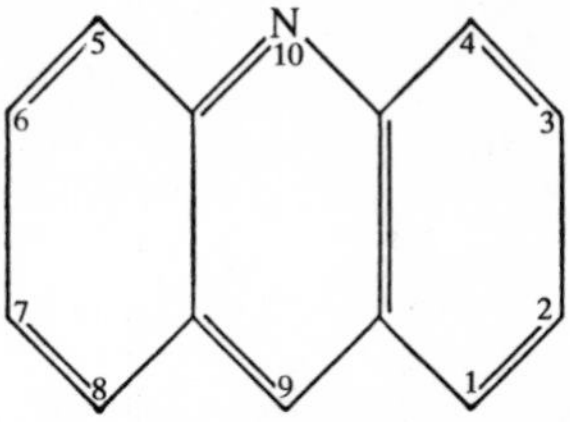

N 10 1 2 3 4 5 6 7 8 9

Acridine

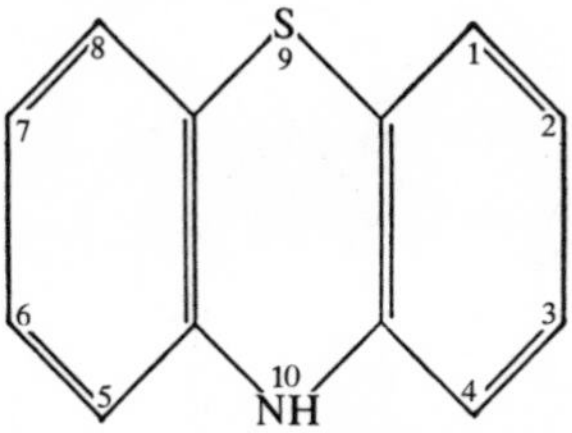

S 9 1 2 3 4 5 6 7 8 10 NH

Phenothiazine

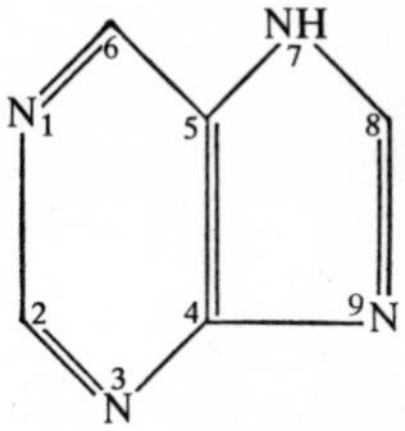

N 1 2 N 3 4 5 6 NH 7 8 9 N

Purine

1 2 3 4 5 6 7 8 9 10 11 12 13 14 15 16 17 A B C D

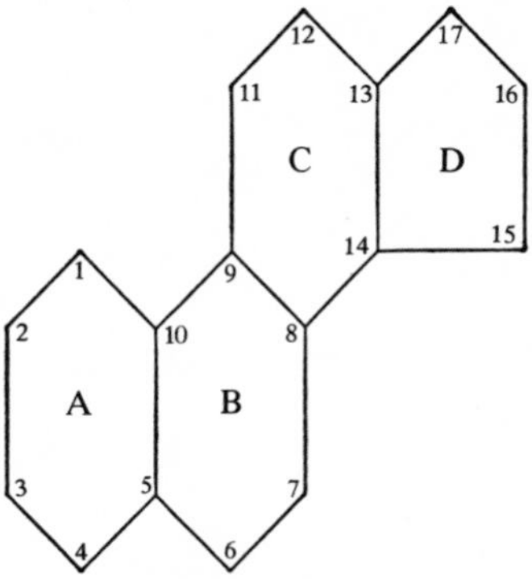

Steroid ring system

INDEX

ACTH, *see* corticotrophin
ADH, *see also* antidiuretic hormone; 81, 111, 189
ADP (adenosine diphosphate), 133
3′5′-AMP (adenosine monophosphate), 60
  cyclic, 31, 103, 304
ATP, (*see also* adenosine triphosphate), 103, 129, 133
ATPase 129
absorption of drugs, 13 *et seq.*
acacia, 143
accumulation of drugs, 22
acebutalol, 108
acenocoumarol, *see* nicoumalone
acetaminophen, *see* paracetamol
acetanilide, 21, 133–5
acetate, 172, 173
acetazolamide, 180, **190**, 193, 243
  and gout, 193
acetic acid, 20
acetylcholine, 2–9, 27–8, **72** *et seq.*, 91–2
  and adrenergic system, 96 *et seq.*
    ascaris, 217
    atropine, 7, 9
    autonomic ganglia, 91, 92
    choline, 149
    cholinergic nerve endings, 96 *et seq.*
    cholinesterase, 91, 92
    eserine, 89
    ether, 39
    gastrin, 137
    general anaesthesia, 34
    mixed receptor sites, 85–7
    morphine, 54
    muscarinic receptors, 83–5, 91–2
    nicotine, 80–2
    nicotinic receptors, 75–7
  assay of, 74, 234
  drugs which preserve, 79–80
  in qualitative analysis, 241
  structure, 3
acetylcholine esterase, 217
N-acetyldopamine, 161
N-acetylglucosamine, 201
N-acetylhistidine, 115
acetyl-β-methylcholine, 93
N-acetylmuramic acid, 201
acetylnorcholine, 92
acetylphenylhydrazine, 157
acetylsalicylic acid (aspirin), 133, **135**
  structure, 134
acidosis, 139, 190
acromegaly, 163
actinomycin, 161
action potential, 103
α-actions, **102** *et seq.*
β-actions, **102**, 124 *et seq.*
adamantine antiviral agents, 244
addiction (*see also* dependence)
  to amphetamine, 57
    cocaine, 70
    glutethimide, 44
    methadone, 55
    morphine, 54–5
    nicotine, 81
    pethidine, 55
    tobacco, 81
Addison's disease, 163, 172, 175, 192
  and ACTH, 172
    aldosterone, 192
adenine, 227
adenohypophysis, 162
adenosine, diphosphate, *see* ADP
3′,5′-adenosine monophosphate, 103
adenosine triphosphate (ATP) 103, 133, 147
adenyl cyclase, 29, 103, 104
adermine, *see* vitamin B_6
administration of drugs
  by inhalation, 18
  injection, 6
  mouth, 17
adrenal cortex, 171 *et seq.*, 234
  and aldosterone, 192
    androgens, 165
    assay of, 235
  insufficiency, 175
  steroids, 119, **171** *et seq.*
    and kidney, 192, 193
    biosynthesis of, 172, 173
adrenaline, 17, **96** *et seq.*, 140
  and β-blockers, 108
    circulation, 124
    cocaine, 70
    insulin, 170, 171
    nicotine, 82
    peristalsis, 140
    prostaglandins, 119–20
    salicylates, 135
    temperature, 133
  assay of, 234
  biosynthesis, 98
  structure, 98, 99
adrenergic nerves
  and cocaine, 70
  receptors, distribution of, 102
adrenocorticoids, 171 *et seq.*
adrenocortictrophic hormone, (*see also* corticotrophin), **163**, 171
adriamycin, 223, 224, **227**
adsorbents, 143
affinity constant, 9
agar, 141
aglycone, 128
agonist, **4–8,** 91, 92
agranulocytosis, 225
alcohol, 51–2
  and temperature, 133
  as anaesthetic, 33
  poisoning, 51
alcoholic neuritis, 147
alcoholics, vitamin B deficiency in, 148
alcoholism and pellagra, 148
aldocorten, 176
18-aldocorticosterone (*see also* aldosterone), 172, 173
aldophosphamide, 226
aldosterone, 172–4, 176, **192**
  and angiotensin, 112
aldosterone
  structure, 173
alflorone acetate, 176
alkaline phosphate, 163
alkalosis, 137, 138
  and diuretics, 190, 191
alkylators, 225–6
allantoin, 193
allergic reactions (*see also* allergy)
  and histamine, 115
    hypoglycaemic agents, 171
  and iron, 155
  states, vitamin P and, 147
allergy (*see also* allergic reactions)
  and antihistamines, 116
    corticosteroids, 176
    salicylates, 135
    sulphonylureas, 171
  in toxicity tests, 245
allobarbitone, 43
allopurinol, 194
aloes, 142–3
alphaxalone, 41
alprenolol, 108
althesin, 41
aluminium hydroxide, 139
  salts, 143
amantadine, 211
amenorrhoea, 178
amethocaine, 69, 70
amidase, 206
amiloride, 192
amines, sympathomimetic, structures, 104
2-aminoanthracene, 246

4-aminobenzene sulphonamide, 242
4-aminobenzoic acid (*see also* para-aminobenzoic acid), 146, 197, 199
γ-amino-butyric acid, *see* GABA
aminocephalosporanic acid, 207
aminoglycoside antibacterials, 208
aminoguanidine, 115
4-amino hippurate, 20
6-aminopenicillanic acid, 205
aminophylline, 225
aminopterin, 225
4-aminoquinoline, 216
8-aminoquinoline, 216
p-aminosalicylic acid (PAS), 209, 211
  structure, 210
amiphenazole, 64
  structure, 61
amitriptyline, 59
  and noradrenaline, 109
  structure, 58
ammonium chloride, 195
amobarbital, 43
amodiaquine, 214, **216**
amoebiasis, 209, 217
  structure of drugs used for, 217
amphenone B, 174
amphetamine, 104, **105**
  and temperature, 133
    urine pH, 20, 195
    structure, 104
amphotericin B, 201, **211,** 216
ampicillin, 204, **206**
  structure, 205
amyl nitrite, 127–128
amylobarbitone, 43
  and dexamphetamine, 57
  duration of action of, 43
amylopectin sulphate, 138
amytal, 43
anabolism, protein, and androgens, 186
anaemia
  macrocytic, 155
  megaloblastic, 149
  pernicious, 145, 155
    and liver extracts, 149
anaesthesia, block, 69, 70
  general, **33** *et seq.*
    and electroencephalogram, 36, 37
    and temperature, 133
    signs of, 36
    stages of, 36
  infiltration, 69
  local, **67** *et seq.*
  regional, 69, 70
  spinal, 69, 70
  theories of, 33–6
anaesthetic solutions, 40
anaesthetics, local, and bretylium, 101
  and noradrenaline, 109
    as antiarrhythmics, 131
    effect of pH on, 67
  metabolism of, 68
    structures, 68, 69
  volatile and gaseous, 37–40
anaesthetics, steroid, 40–1
analeptics, 60 *et seq.*,
  structures, 61
analgesia, local, 39
analgesics, **52–6**
  and temperature, 133
analysis, qualitative, 240–1
anaphylaxis and penicillin, 206
androgen-like properties, structures of drugs with, 185
androgens, **186,** 221
  and adrenal cortex, 163, 172
  as anti-oestrogens, 179
androstenedione, 184
androsterone, 184, 186
androteston, *see* testosterone propionate
aneurine, *see* Vitamin B_1
  and chronic alcoholism, 52
angina pectoris, 19, 127, 128
angiotensin, 20, **112**
  and aldosterone, 192
  I and II, 112, 174, 192
angiotensinogen, 112
ankylostoma, 217
Anovlar, 184
Antabuse, *see* disulphiram
antacids, 138–139
antagonist actions, 6 *et seq.*
antazoline, 140
anthelminthics, 118, **217**–19
anthracene purgatives, 142–3
anthraquinone, 142
anti-adrenergic drugs and glucagon, 171
antiarrhythmic drugs, 107–8, **130–1**
antibacterials, 196 *et seq.*
  activity of, 200
  choice of, 209
  combinations of, 203
antibiotics (*see also* antibacterials)
  as antineoplastics, 209
antibody formation and corticosteroids, 172, 175
  and glucocorticoids, 172
anticholinergic drugs and gastric secretion, 138
anticholinesterase, 74, 76–78, **79** *et seq.*, **92,** 217
  and acetylcholine, 74
    benzoquinonium, 88
    mixed receptor sites, 85
    muscarinic receptors, 83, 92
    procaine, 71
anticholinesterases, structures, 90
anticoagulant therapy, 157–60
anticonvulsants, 45–8
antidepressants, 57–60
antidiuretic hormone, 81, 161, 162, 164
antifungal agents, 211
antihistamines, 8, **116–17**
  as anti-emetics, 139
antimalarials
  resistance to, 215
  structures, 215
antimetabolites, 224–8
antimuscarines, 84
antimuscarinic compounds, *see* atropine-like compounds
anti-oestrogens, 179–185
antipyretic-analgesic group, **133** *et seq.*
  structures, 134
antipyrine, *see* phenazone
antiseptics, 212
antistin, *see* antazoline, 165
antithyroid drugs, 164, 165, **167–8**
antitoxins, assay of, 229
antitrypanosome drugs, 203
antitumour drugs, 221 *et seq.*
  and vomiting, 139
antivirus agents, 211–12
aplastic anaemia
  and chloramphenicol, 209
  troxidone, 47
apnoea and succinylcholine, 87
apoferritin, 154
apomorphine and vomiting, 139
aqueous solutions, 251
arabinose, 225
9-β-arabinosyladenosine, 212
arachidonic acid, 118
arecoline, 83, **92**
  structure, 4, 93
arginine, vasopressin, (*see also* AVP), 111
ariboflavinosis, 145
arsanilic acid, *see* atoxyl
arsenicals, 196, 197, 216
arsenoxides, 196, 242
arsphenamine, 196
  discovery of, 242
arterenol, 96
artificial kidney machines, 158
ascaris lumbricoides, 217
ascorbic acid (*see also* vitamin C), 144–5
  and corticotrophin, 163
  structure, 146
aspartic acid, 32
aspirin (acetylsalicylic acid), 133, **135**
  and bradykinin, 113
    thyroid, 166
assay, biological, **229** *et seq.*
  methods of, **232** *et seq.*
asthma and cromoglycate, 117–8
    ephedrine, 105
    prostaglandins, 119
astringents, 143
atoxyl, 196
atrial fibrillation, 131
    and digitalis, 131
  flutter, 131
atropa belladonna, 85
atropine, 7, 30, 37, **85–6**, 92, 94, 140

and acetylcholine, 84–85
anticholinesterases, 80
cardiac glycosides, 129
central nervous system, 86
histamine release, 115
muscarinic actions, 72, 74, **83–5,** 91
neostigmine, 89
peristalsis, 140
premedication, 37
in qualitative analysis, 241
poisoning, 85
structure, 7, 93
sulphate, 6
atropine-like actions and antihistamines, 116
compounds and muscarinic receptors, 84
Auerbach's plexus, 54, 63, 140, 141
'autocatalytic reaction', 157
autonomic ganglion, **80** *et seq.*
ganglia, drugs blocking transmission at, 90 *et seq.*
Avidin, 149
5-azacytidine, 225
azapetine, 106
azathioprine, 228
azide and nitrites, 127
aziridine, 223
of phenoxybenzamine, 106
azo-dyes, 196, 242

BCNU (carmustine), 227
BOL, *see* bromo-lysergic acid diethylamide
bacteria, resistant strains, 203–4
bacterial cell walls, 200–1, 221
bactericidal agents, **196** *et seq.*
bacteriostatic agents, 199
banthine, *see* methantheline
barbitone and urine pH, 195
duration of action of, 16, 43
barbiturate poisoning, 193
and bemegride, 64
ethamivan, 64
barbiturates, **42–5,** 57, 60
absorption of, 18
and dexamphetamine, 57
strychnine poisoning, 63
duration of action of, 43
effects of overdosage, 44, 60
for premedication, 37
tolerance to, 44
Basedow's disease, 167
basophil cells, 114, 115
and heparin, 157
belladonna plant, 1
bemegride 64
structure, 61
benadryl, *see* diphenhydramine
bendrofluazide, 190
structure, 191
bendroflumethiazide, *see* bendrofluazide.
benzalkonium, as antiseptic, 212
benzathine, penicillin, 206
benzerazide, 16
benzidine-azo dyes, 196
benzilylcholine mustard, 85, **94**
structure, 7, 93
benzocaine, structure, 69
benzodiazepines, 44, **50,** 244
benzoquinonium, 79, 88
3,4-benzpyrene, 21
benzthiadiazines, 190
benzylpenicillin, 205, 206
bephenium 217, 218
beriberi, 145, 147
beta rays, 167
betamethasone, 176
structure, 177
betel nut, 92
bethanidine, 101, **109**
and hypotension, 125
Bezold receptors, 126
reflex, 95
bicuculline, 27, **63**–4
structure, 61
biguanides, 171, **216**
bile, 140
bilein, 140
biliary colic and morphine, 54
pethidine, 55
binomial distribution, 231
bioavailability, 18
biological assay, **229** *et seq.*
of acetylcholine, 74
biotin, *see* vitamin H
bisacodyl, 141–2
bisonium compounds, 82
bisulphan, 227
black widow spider venom, 76
bladder and atropine, 85
muscarinic actions, 83
bleeding time, 158
bleomycin, 223, **227**
block anaesthesia, 69, 70
α-blockers, 102, **105–7**
structures, 106
β-blockers, 102 *et seq.*, **107** *et seq*, 125–131
structures, 108
blood–brain barrier, 85
and arsenicals, 216
blood coagulation, **157**–60
and corticosteroids, 175
factors, 160
dyscrasia and toxicity tests, 245
flow in various organs, 14
platelets, 120, 165
pressure and anaesthesia, 36
angiotensin, 112
corticosteroids, 175
ganglion blocks, 81–83
histamine, 115
nicotine, 81
nikethamide, 63
prostaglandins, 118
vasopressin, 110
red cells of, 154
sugar and ACTH, 163
insulin, 169–171
factors controlling, 169
vessels and muscarinic actions, 83
volume and corticosteroids, 175
bone and parathyroid, 168
rickets, 152
marrow
antineoplastics, 222–5
chloramphenicol, 209
botulinum toxin, 76
and acetylcholine, 80
bradycardia and anaesthesia, 37
heparin, 158
veratrine, 126
bradykinin, 113, 120, 134
and salicylates, 134
brain and cocaine, 70
serotonin, 30
xanthines, 60
blood flow in, 14
drug penetration, 15–16
bran, 141
bretylium, 101
brevital, 43
bromides, 45
bromobenzene, 21
bromo-lysergic acid diethylamide, and serotonin, 65
bronchi and atropine, 85
histamine, 115
prostaglandins, 119
bronchial irriatation and tobacco, 81
buccal mucosa, absorption by, 18
busulphan, 227
butazolidine (phenylbutazone), 134
butobarbitone, 43
butoxamine, 108, **109**
butyrophenol, 29
butyrylcholine, 3, 4, 8

CCNU (lomustrine), 227
C 10, *see* decamethonium
^{14}C, 96
COMT (*see also* catechol-O-methyl transferase), 104, 105
CRF, *see* corticotrophin releasing factor
caffeine, **59–60,** 104
and aspirin, 135
smooth muscle, 59
calciférol, *see* vitamin D_2
calcitonin, 168
calcium
and acetylcholine, 80
adrenergic system, 96
androgens, 186
cardiac glycosides, 129
catecholamines, 103
hyperthyroidism, 167
liquid paraffin, 141
parathyroid, 168
prothrombin, 157
vitamin D, 152
carbonate, 138

calcium (Contd)
permeability, 96
calomel, *see* mercurous chloride
cancer chemotherapy, 221 *et seq.*
candida, 204, 211
cannabis, 65
carbachol, 27, 83, 89, **90,** 92
carbamazepine, 46, **47**
carbenicillin, 206
structure, 205
carbenoxalone, 138
carbidopa, 30
carbimazole, 165
carbolic, 196
carbonic anhydrase, inhibitors, 190
carboxyphosphamide, 226
carbutamide, 165, 243
carcinogens, 221, 246
carcinoma of breast and oestrogens, 179, 184
lung, 81
prostate and oestrogens, 179
cardiac arrhythmia and halothane, 38
failure
frusemide, 191
organic mercurials, 191
glycosides, **128**–30, 139
and thiazides, 191
thyroid, 164
vomiting, 139
cardiovascular system and corticosteroids, 174
local anaesthetics, 68
drugs acting on, **124** *et seq.*
carmustine, 227
β-carotene, 151
carotene and liquid paraffin, 141
carotid-aortic pressor receptors, 122
cascara, 1, **142**–3, 241
castor oil, 142
catechol-O-methyl transferase, 98
catecholamines, 20, 38, 81, 124
and adrenergic system, **96** *et seq.*
anaesthesia, 37
antidepressants, 57
β-blockers, 108
circulation, 122
cocaine, 70
halothane, 38
causal prophylactics, 214
celestone, 176
cell membranes, bacterial, 200–1
general anaesthesia, 35
insulin, 169
urine pH, 194
potentials, 82,
walls, bacterial, **200**–1, 221
and penicillin, 221
cellular metabolism and xanthines, 60
cellulose, 141
central nervous system and
antitrypanosomal drugs, 216
imipramine, 59
iproniazid, 58
local anaesthetics, 68
cephaloridine, 207
cephalosporins, 207
cephalothin, 207
cerebral cortex and cocaine, 70
cetrimide, 212
cetyltrimethylammonium, 212
Chagas' disease, 216
chalk, 143
Ch'an su, 128
charcoal, activated, 143
chelators, 154
chemical rings, index of, 252–4
transmitters, assay of, 229
units of measurement, 250
chemotherapeutic action, principles of, 197 *et seq.*
spectra, 204
chloral hydrate, 44
chloraluric acid, 44
chlorambucil, 226
chloramphenicol, 20, 202, 203, 208, **209**
resistance to, 203
toxicity, 245
chlorcyclizine, 140
chlordiazepoxide, 45, **50,** 244
chlorhexidine, 212
chloride ions and adrenal steroids, 172
chlorinated xylenol, 212
chlorine as antiseptic, 212
chlormadinone, 183
chloroform, 33
chloroguanide, 214, 216, 242
L-*p*-chlorophenylalanine, 30
chloroquine, 209, 214–16
chlorotetracycline, 209
8-chlorotheophylline, 104
chlorothiazide, 130, **190–1,** 242
and digitalis, 130
structure, 191, 243
chlorotrianisene, 179, 181
chlorpromazine, 49, 50, 55, 65
and alcohol, 51
LSD, 29
temperature, 133, **139**
as anti-emetic, 139
chlorpropamide, 171
cholagogues, 140
cholecalciferol, *see* vitamin D
cholecystokinin, 140
cholesterol, 140, 152, 201
and adrenal steroids, 171, 173
cell membranes, 201–2
corticotrophin, 163
thyroid, 166
choline, 88, **92**
as vitamin, 145, 147, **149**
choline acetyltransferase, 75, 80, 86
ethylether, 5
cholinergic drugs, **87–8**
antagonists to, 87 *et seq.*
cholinergic link, 101
nerves, **72** *et seq.*
synapses, 86
cholinesterase, 20, **75** *et seq.*
'ageing of', 80
local anaesthetics, 71
nicotine, 81
chorionepithelioma, 225
chorionic gonadotrophins, 164
chromaffin cells, 96
chromatography, 241
chronotropic action, 124, 128–9
effect of noradrenaline, 124
chrysophanic acid, 143
cimetidine, 116, 117
cinchocaine, 69–70
cinchona alkaloids, 241
cis-vitamin A aldehyde, *see* retinene, 151
citric acid cycle, 34, 51
citrin, *see* vitamin P
clathrates, 34
claviceps purpurea, 114
clindamycin, 208
clinical trials, 241, 245–6
clomiphene, 179–80
clonidine, 125–6
clotting time, 158
cloxacillin, 206
cobalamin (*see also* vitamin B_{12}), 145, 155
structure, 155
cobamide, 149
cocaine, 69, **70,** 100
and
cerebral cortex, 70
'contact purgatives', 142
noradrenaline, 70, 109
temperature, 133
poisoning, 70
structure, 69
cod-liver oil, 151
codeine, 21, 53, **55**
and aspirin, 135
coeliac disease, 156
coenzyme A, 148
coenzyme B_{12}, 154, 156
colchicine, 227
coma, diabetic, 170
hypoglycaemic, 170
competitive inhibition, 6–8
conjugation of drugs, 21
'contact purgative', 142
contraceptives, oral, 180–2.
convulsants, **60** *et seq.*
structures, 61
convulsions, epileptic, 46
and amiphenazole, 64
atropine, 85
central nervous stimulants, 60 *et seq.*
cocaine, 70
pethidine, 55
strychnine, 63
temperature, 133
xanthines, 60

copper salts as astringents, 143
 sulphate, 139
corpus luteum, 180
  and contraceptives, 180
   menstrual cycle, 178
   prostaglandins, 120
corticosteroids, *see also* adrenal steroids, **171** *et seq.*, 227
 side-effects of, 175
corticosterone, 163, 174
 structure, 173
corticotrophin, 104, 162, **163**
 and prostaglandins, 119
 releasing factor, 162
cortisol (*see also* 17-hydroxycorticosterone, 163
cortisone, 235
 assay of, 235
 structure, 173
cortisone acetate (*see also* 11-dehydro-17-hydroxycorticosterone), 172, 176
corydalis, 63
cotrimazole, 207
coumarin group, 158–60
coupled beats and digitalis, 129
cretins, 166
cromoglycate (*see also* cromolyn), 18, 20, **117–8**
cross-over test, 237–238
cumulative action of barbiturates, 44
curare, 72, **78,** 82
curare-like compounds
 and acetylcholine, 76
 anticholinesterases, 80, 88
 ether, 39
 halothane, 39
Cushing's disease, 172, 175
cyanide and nitrites, 127
cyanocobalamin (*see also* vitamin B_{12}), 145, 147
 and macrocytic anaemia, 156
cyclic AMP (adenosine monophosphate), 29, 60, 120, 244
cyclobarbitone, 43
cyclo-oxygenase, 118
cyclopentane ring, 118
cyclophosphamide, 226-228
cyclopropane, 22, 37, **40**
 and procaine, 70
 partition coefficient of, 38
cycloserine, 201, 202, 211
cysteine, 20
cytarabine, 223, **225**
cytochrome P–450, 21
 oxidase, 144
cytosine arabinoside, 225

DBI, *see* phenformin
DCI, *see* dichloroisoprenaline
DDAVP (l-desimino-8-D-arginine vasopressin), 111
DDT, 15
DFP, *see* Dyflos and diisopropylfluorophosphonate
DHE, *see* dihydro-β-erythroidine
DMPP, *see* dimethyl-4-phenylpiperazium
DNA, 203, 210–12, 222 *et seq.*
DNOC, *see* 3,5-dinitro-*o*-cresol
DOCA (*see also* 11-deoxycorticosterone), 172–4
 structure, 173
DOPA (*see also* dihydroxyphenylalanine, 3-hydroxytyrosine), **96–8,** 161
 structure, 98
dactinomycin, 223, **227**
dapsone, 211, 216
dark adaptation, 151
daunomycin, 223, **227**
deadly nightshade, 85
decamethonium, 77, 78, **88**
 structure, 89
decarboxylases and pyridoxine, 148
dehydroascorbic acid, 144
  structure, 146
7-dehydrocholesterol (vitamin D_3), 150, 151
dehydrocholic acid, 140
dehydrocorticosterone, 235
11-dehydrocorticosterone, 172
11-dehydro-17-hydroxycorticosterone (cortisone acetate), 172
dehydrogenase, 22
delatestryl, *see* testosterone enanthate
delirium tremens, 51
 and chloral hydrate, 44
deltahydrocortisone, 176
demethylchlortetracycline, 209
demulcents, 143
deoxyadenosine, 156
11-deoxycorticoids (mineralocorticoids), 172
11-deoxycorticosterone, 172–4, 176
deoxycortone acetate, *see also* 11-deoxycorticosterone, 172–4, 176
deoxyhydrocortisone, 173, 174
dependence (*see also* addiction)
 on barbiturates, 44
  morphine, 54
  pethidine, 55
depolarizing block, 77
depot penicillin, 205
 preparations, 17
derazil, *see* chlorcyclizine
dermatitis, seborrhoeic and vitamin B_2, 147
desferrioxamine, 155
desipramine and noradrenaline, 100, 109
desmethylimipramine, 59
desoxycorticosterone acetate, *see* 11-deoxycorticosterone
Dettol, 212
 development of new drugs, 244–6
 deviation standard, 231–2
 dexamphetamine, 57
 dextran, 115
dexytal, *see* drinamyl
diabetes and salicylates, 133
 insipidus and thiazides, 191
   vasopressin, 111
 mellitus, 147, **168–70,** 193
  and thiazides, 191
diabetic coma, 170
dial, 43
diaminodiphenylsulphone, 216
diaminooxidase, 115
diamorphine (heroin), 53, **55**
4-diaminopyrimidine, 216, 242
'diastolic drift', 131
diazepam, 45, 46, **48,** 50
dibenamine, 94, 106, 107
dibenzazepine derivatives, 59
dibotin, *see* phenformin
dibozane, 106
dibucaine, *see* cinchocaine
dibutoline, **85,** 92
 structure, 93
dibutyryl cyclic AMP, 104
dichloralphenazone, 44
dichlormethotrexate, 225
dichloroisoprenaline, 102, **107**
 structure, 108
dichlorophen, 219
dichlorphenamide, 190
dichlorphenylaminoimidazoline, 125
dicophane, 15
dicoumarol, 158–160
 metabolism of, 22
dienoestrol, 179
 structure, 181
diethyl ether, 39
  partition coefficient of, 38
diethylaminoethanol, 71
diethylcarbamazine, 218, **219**
diethylstilboestrol, 179
diffusion, limited access, 14
digitalis, 128–30
 assay of, 233
 lanata, 130
 poisoning, 130
 purpurea, 130
digitoxigenin, 128
digitoxin, 128, 130
digitoxose, 130
digoxin, 130
di-homo-γ-linoleic acid, 118
dihydro-β-erythroidine, 27, 79, **88,** 89
dihydrofolate, 149, 224
dihydrofolic acid, 11, 199
  structure, 198
 reductase, 224, 225
dihydromorphinone, 53, **55**
dihydropteroic acid, 199
 structure, 198
2,5-dihydroxybenzoic acid, 135
dihydroxydihydroisoquinolines, 96
3,4-dihydroxymandelic acid, 99
3,4-dihydroxyphenylalanine, 3-hydroxytyrosine (*see also* DOPA), 96

diiodotyrosine, 165, 166
diisopropylfluorophosphonate, 79, **89–90**
dilantin, 131
diloxanide furoate, 217
dimenhydrinate, 140
dimethyl-4-phenyl piperazium, 82
3,5-dinitro-orthocresol, 133
2,4-dinitrophenol, 133
dioctyl sodium sulphosuccinate, 141
di-paralene, *see* chlorcyclizine
diphenhydramine, 116, **140**
  structure, 117
diphenylhydantoin, *see* phenytoin, 166
diphosphopyridine nucleotide, 148
dipyridamole, 128
discovery of new drugs, 241–4
distribution of drugs in tissues, 13 *et seq.*
disulfiram, 22, **52,** 97
diuresis and alcohol, 51
    posterior pituitary extract, 110, 111
diuretics, 189 *et seq.*
L-dopa, 30
dopadecarboxylase, 96, 97
dopamine (3-hydroxytyramine), 16, 28, **96**
  structure, 98
dopamine-β-hydroxylase, 97
dopamine-β-oxidase, 96, 105
dose
  assay, 235–6
  effect curve, 235
  effective (*see also* ED 50), 238
  individual effective (*see also* IED), 238
  lethal (*see also* LD), 233, 238
  mortality curve, 238
  ratio, 6
  response curve, 3–5, 221, 222
dracunculus, 217
dramamine, *see* dimenhydrinate
drinamyl, 57
dropsy and digitalis, 128
drug action, **1** *et seq.*
  combinations, 203
  excretion, 19–23
kinetics, **13** *et seq.*
  receptors, 6–12
drugs, delay of absorption, 13–15
  discovery of, **241** *et seq.*
'dual block', 88
durabolin, *see* nandrolone phenylpropionate
dydrogesterone, 182
dyes and chemotherapy, 196, 242
dyflos, *see* diisopropylfluorophosphonate
dysentery, amoebic, 217
ED, 50, 238
ecdysone, 161
edrophonium, 79, **88**
  structure, 90
effective dose, 238
Ehrlich, 196, 242
5,8,11,14-eicosatetragnoic acid, 120
eighth nerve
  and neomycin, 208
  streptomycin, 208
electroencephalogram
  and alcohol, 51
    anaesthesia, 36–37
    benzodiazepines, 50
    leptazol, 63
electrolyte excretion, 141, **190** *et seq.*
electrolytes
  and androgens, 186
  corticosteroids, 172, 174, 175
  digitalis, 129, 130
electro-shock therapy and phenytoin, 46
electron-spin resonance, 35
eledoisin, 113
emetics, 139
emetine, 217
emodine, 142–3
end-plate potentials, 78
endoperoxide, 118
  isomerase, 119
endorphins, **31,** 54
enemas, 141
enkephalin, 28, **31,** 54, 241
entamoeba histolytica, 217
enzyme system and general anaesthesia, 34
enzymes,
  in drug metabolism, 20–3
ephedrine, 104, **105**
epilepsy, 46
  and acetazolamide, 190
    bemegride, 64
    leptazol, 63
epinephrine, *see* adrenaline
ergocalciferol, *see* vitamin D_2
ergometrine, 114
ergonovine, *see* ergometrine
ergot, 106, **114**
  alkaloids, 105
ergotamine, 102
error in biological assay, 230 *et seq.* *seq.*
  limits of, 232, 234
erythromycin, 208
erythropoietin, 154
erythroxylon coca, 70
eserine, *see also* physostigmine, 89
  and peristalsis, 140
ethacrynic acid, 191–2
ethambutol, 210–11
ethamivan, 64
  structure, 61
ethamoxytriphetol, 179
ethanol, 22
  as antiseptic, 212
ether, anaesthetic, *see* diethyl ether
ethinyl estradiol, 179
ethinyloestradiol, 179, 242
  structure, 181
ethionamide, 211
ethisterone, 182
  structure, 183
ethosuximide, 46, **47**
ethyl chloride, 39
N-ethyl noradrenaline, 102
ethylene
  oxide as antiseptic, 212
ethyleneiminium, 94, 106
ethylstibamine, 216
ethynodiol diacetate, 184
    structure, 183
etiocholanolone, 184, 186
etorphine, 55
evipan, 43
exocrine glands and muscarinic actions, 83
excretion of drugs, 19–20
exophthalmic goitre, 167
exophthalmos producing substance, 163
eye and anticholinesterase, 80
    atropine, 85
    castor oil, 142
    chloroquine, 216
    dibutoline, 92
    homatropine, 92
    muscarinic actions, 83
    pilocarpine, 92
    vitamin A, 151

FSH, *see* follicle-stimulating hormone
fat, blood flow in, 14
fat-soluble vitamins, 150 *et seq.*
  structures of, 150
fatigue and xanthines, 60
Fehling's solution and chloral hydrate, 44
ferric ammonium citrate, 155
ferritin, 154
ferrous fumarate, 155
  gluconate, 155
  sulphate, 155
fever, 132–3
fibrin, 157
fibrinogen, 157–8
fibrinopeptide, 157
Fick method, 124
fiducial limits, 237
field of vision and strychnine, 63
filaria, 219
filipin, 201
filling pressure, 122
fish-liver oils, 15
flavine adenine dinucleotide, 147
flavonoids, 145
fludrocortisone, 176, 192
flufenamic acid, 136
5-fluorodeoxyuridylate, 225
9α-fluorohydrocortisone, 192
fluorouracil, 223, **225**
fluoroxene, 39
fluoxacillin, 206
fluoxymesterone, 186

structure, 185
flutenamic acid, 136
folate reductase 199, 200
inhibitors, 203
folates, 155, 199
folic acid, **145–9, 156–7,** 199
and erythrocyte formation, 156–7
gluten, 156
vitamin B complex, 148–9
antimetabolites of, 224
deficiency, 156
structure, 156
folic reductase, 157
folinic acid, 156, 157
follicle-stimulating hormone, 162, **163**
and contraception, 182
menstrual cycle, 178
formic acid, 22
formylcholine, 3
5-formyltetrahydrofolate, 225
N^5-formyltetrahydrofolinic acid, *see* folinic acid
foxglove, 128
frusemide, 191
Fuller's earth, 143
fungi and antibiotics, 201, 211

GABA, **27**, 28, 63–4.
GIF, *see* growth hormone release inhibiting factor
GMP, 31
GRF, *see* growth hormone releasing factor
gall-bladder, 140
and muscarinic actions, 83
gallamine, 9, **79, 88**
excretion of, 19
structure, 89
gamma
globulins, 163
rays, 167
ganglion blockers, **102** *et seq.*, 125–8
gastric juice, 137–9
motility and propantheline, 94
secretion
and heparin, 158
histamine, 116
insulin, 170
penicillin, 205
propantheline, 94
gastrin, 137, 138
I and II, 137
gentamicin, 20, 202, 208
gentisic acid, 135
gigantism and pituitary, 163
glaucoma, 89, 90
and acetazolamide, 190
pilocarpine, 92
globin zinc insulin injection, 170
globulin, 112
glossitis and vitamin B_1, 147
glucagon, 169, **171**
and insulin, 169

glucocorticoids, **172** *et seq.*, 227–8
gluconeogenesis, 172, 174
and corticosteroids, 174
glucose
and adrenal steroids, 172, 174
diuresis, 191
growth hormone, 163
insulin, **168**–70
glucuronic acid and thyroxine, 166
glutamate, 149
glutamic acid, 28, 32, 146, 149
dehydrogenase, 27
detoxylase, 27
structure, 146
glutaraldehyde, 212
glutathione, 144
gluten and folic acid, 156
glutethimide, 44–45
glycerin, 143
glyceryl trinitrate, **127,** 128
absorption of, 18
glycine, **27–29,** 62
glycogen, 104
and cortisone assay, 234
glucagon, 171
insulin, 168
salicylates, 135
cardiac, 128, 130
glycosides
glycuronic acid, 20
glycuronides, 135
goitre, 166
exophthalmic, 167
gonadotrophins, 162, **163–4**
and contraceptives, 180–184
assay of, 229
gonorrhoea, 209
gout, 191–194
and ethacrynic acid, 192
thiazides, 191
gramicidin, 201
Graves' disease, 167
griseofulvin, 211
growth
and thyroid, 166
vitamin A, 151
B_{12}, 149
hormone, **161–163**
release inhibiting factor, 162
releasing factor, 162
guanethidine, 101, **109,** 125
and hypotension, 109
guanine, 225
guanochlor, 109
guanoxan, 109
Gull's disease, 166
gums, 143

HC-3, *see* hemicholinium
5-HT, *see* serotonin
5-HTP, *see* 5-hydroxytryptophan
haemenzymes, 154
haemoglobin, 154
Hageman factor, 113
haldrone, 176

half-life of drugs, 23
halibut-liver oil, 151
hallucinogens, **64** *et seq.*
β-haloalkylamines, 94, 106
haloperidol, 29
halotestin, 186
halothane, 16, 37, **38–9**
partition coefficient of, 38
hashish, 33
hay fever and antihistamines, 116
cromoglycate, 117–18
heart
and digitalis, **128** *et seq.*
muscarinic actions, 83
blood flow in, 14
disease and thiazides, 191
heat regulating mechanisms, **132** *et seq.*
heavy metals and tannic acid, 143
helminthiasis, 217–219
hemicholinium, **75-6,** 80
heparin, **157**, 158
heroin, *see* diamorphine, 240
herpes, corneal, and idoxuridine, 212
hesperidin, *see* vitamin P
hexachlorophane, 212
hexadimethrine, 158
hexahydroazepinemethyleneamino-P, 206
hexamethonium, 27, 74, 80, **82–3,** 85, 125
absorption of, 17
and anticholinesterases, 80
excretion of, 19
structure, 91
hexitol, 193
hexobarbitone, 21, 42–43
hippurate, 193
histamine, 7, 8, **114–7**
gastric secretion, 137
heparin, 158
as central transmitter, 32
assay of, 234, 244
receptors, 107
structure, 117
histantin *see* chlorcyclizine
histidine, 114, 246
decarboxylase, 114
histostab, *see* antazoline
Hodgkin's disease, 224, 226
and vinblastine, 227
homatropine, **85,** 92
structure, 93
homologous series, 3
hookworms, 217–218
'hormone-releasing factors', 162
hormones, assay of, 229, 234
Huntingdon's chorea, 27
hycanthone, 219
hydralazine, 126
hydrazines, 58, 99
hydrochloric acid, 138, 195
hydrochlorothiazide, 190
structure, 191

hydrocortisone (*see also* 17-hydroxy-corticosterone), 161, 176
structure, 173
hydrolysis of drugs, 20
hydrostibamidine, 216
4-hydroxacetanilide, 21
hydroxocobalamin, 156
2-hydroxy-4-amino-6-hydroxy-methyl dihydropterin, 198
17-hydroxycorticosteroids, 172
17-hydroxycorticosterone, 172
17-hydroxy-11-deoxycortico-sterone, 172
hydroxydione, 41
6-hydroxydopamine, 100, 101
β-hydroxylase, 174
3′-hydroxypentobarbitone, 21
17-α-hydroxypregnenolone, 113
17-α-hydroxyprogesterone, 173
11-β-hydroxyprogesterone, 173
5-hydroxytryptamine (*see also* serotonin), 50
hallucinogens, 64–5
morphine, 54
3-hydroxytyramine, *see* dopamine
3-hydroxytyrosine, *see* DOPA
hyoscine, 85, **92**
and anaesthesia, 37
for motion sickness, 92, **139–40**
structure, 93
hyoscyamine, 85
hypercalcaemia, 168
corticosteroids, 175
hypercalciuria, 168
hyperchlorhydria, 138
hyperglycaemia and adrenal steroids, 174
insulin, 170–1
thiazides, 191
hyperpolarization, 84
hypersensitivity reaction (*see also* allergy), 21, 115
to methyldopa, 109
penicillin, 206
quinidine, 131
hypertension, 91
and ganglionic blocks, 81–2
iproniazid, 58
reserpine, 109
hyperthyroidism and β-blockers, 108
iodine, 167
hypervitaminosis D, 152
hypnotics, **42** *et seq.*
non-barbiturate, **44** *et seq.*
hypocalcaemia and corticosteroids, 175
hypoglycaemia, 170–171
hypoglycaemic agents, oral, 171
hypokalaemia, 190
and chlorothiazide, 130, 191
hypoparathyroidism, 168
hypotension, postural, 82
hypotensive drugs, **124** *et seq.*
hypothalamus and pituitary, 162
hypoxanthine and gout, 194
hypoxia and nitrous oxide, 39

^{131}I, 167
IED, 238, 240
IgE, 115
IPSP, *see* inhibitory postsynaptic potential, 63
idoxuridine, *see also* 5-iododeoxyuridine, 211–12
imipramine, 59
and noradrenaline, 109
structure, 58
immune reactions and corticosteroids, 175
immunosuppression, 228
inderal, *see* propanolol
indomethacin, 119, **136**
inflammation and adrenal steroids, 172, 175
inhalation of drugs, 18
inhibitors, ionic, of thyroid, 167
inhibitory postsynaptic potential, 62, 63
inotropic action, 128
insecticides, 79, 90
insulin, 1, 20, 104, 119, 161, **168** *et seq.*
and adrenal steroids, 175
biguanides, 171
cross-over test, 238
antagonists, 169
assay of, 229
preparations, 170
Intal, 117–8
interferons, 212
intestinal colic and atropine, 85
intestines and anticholinesterases, 92, 138
histamine, 115
morphine, 54
muscarinic action, 83
prostaglandins, 119
strychnine, 63
vitamin K, 153
intra-ocular tension
and acetazolamide, 190
dyflos, 90
pilocarpine, 92
intravascular clotting and contraceptives, 184
'intrinsic factor', 156
iodide, 167
iodine-131, 167
iodine and thyroid, 164–7
as antiseptic, 196, 212
radioactive, 167
iodotyrosine, 97, 164
ionic inhibitors of thyroid, 167
iproniazid, 58–9
iproveratrine, 102
iron, 154, **155**
and polycythaemia vera, 157
body requirement of, 154
deficiency, 154
dextrin, 155
dextran, 155
preparations, 154
as astringents, 143
sorbitol, 155
islets of Langerhans, 168
isocarboxazid, 58
isoniazid, 20, 115, **148,** 204, 211
structure, 210
isonicotinic acid hydrazide, *see also* isoniazid, 20, **148**
isophane, 170
isoprenaline, 102, 104–5, 107, **124**
absorption of, 18
and circulation, 124
structure, 104
isopropanol, 212
N-isopropyl noradrenaline, *see also* isoprenaline, 102
isoproterenol, *see also* isoprenaline, 124
isoricinoleic acid, 142
isoxsuprine, 104, **105**
structure, 104

kala-azar, 216
kallidin, 113
kallikrein, 113
kanamycin, 202, **208**
kaolin, 143
kemithal, 43
kenacort, 176
ketamine, 40
α-keto-glutaric acid, 147
ketonuria, 170
ketosis and adrenal steroids, 174
17-ketosteroids, 172, 174
and ACTH, 163
kidney, **188** *et seq.*
machines, 158
kidneys and vasopressin, 110
blood flow in, 14
kieselguhr, 143
kinase, 104
kinins, 112–13

LD 50, 238
LH, *see* luteinizing hormone
LRF, *see* luteinizing hormone releasing factor
LSD, *see also* lysergic acid diethylamide, **64–6,** 114
lachesine, 85, **94**
structure, 93
β-lactam ring, 203
lactic acid, 147
Lactobacillus casei, 148
lactis, 156
lactoflavin, *see* vitamin B_2
lanatocide C, 130
largactil, *see* chlorpromazine
lead salts as astringents, 143
lecithin, 140
leishmaniasis, 216
structures of drugs used for, 217

leprosy, 211
leptazol, 60, **63**
  structure, 61
lethal dose, 233, 238
leucovorin, 225
leukaemia, drugs used in, 224–8
leukopenia and antimetabolites, 225
    antithyroids, 165
    phenindione, 159
    sulphonamides, 207
levallorphan, 53, 56
  structure, 53
levamisole, **118,** 212, **217–18**
levodopa, 30
levorphanol, 53, **55**
lidocaine, *see* lignocaine
lignocaine, 68, **70**
  as antiarrhythmic, 131
  structure, 69
lincomycin, 208
lipid barriers and local anaesthetics, 67
  metabolism, 102
  solubility, 34
lipolysis and prostaglandins, 118
lipopolysaccharides, 133
lipoprotein lipase, 158
β-lipotrophin, 31
liquid paraffin, 141
    and vitamin K, 153
liver, blood flow in, 14
  damage and hydrazine derivatives, 58
  extracts, 149
lobelia, 64
lobeline, 64, **82**
  structure, 61
log-dose–effect, 235, 237
log-dose–response curve, 5–8
logarithmic probability paper, 238, 239
  scale, 4, 234–239
long-acting thyroid stimulator, 162–3
loop of Henle, 188, 190, 192
lumiflavme, 147
luminal, 43
lung infections and ampicillin, 206
luteinizing hormone, 162, **163**
    and contraceptives, 180
      menstrual cycle, 178
luteinizing hormone releasing factor, 162
lymphoma, 227
lysergic acid diethylamide, 64, 65, **66**
  structure, 114
lysol, 212

MAO, *see also* monoamine oxidase, 98–100, 104, 105, 109
MAO inhibitors, **58–9**
MER 25 (ethamoxytriphetol), 160
MSH, *see* melanocyte stimulating hormone
macrocytic anaemias, 155–7

magnesium
  and acetylcholine, 80
  carbonate, 138, 141
  hydroxide, 138
  oxide, 138, 141
  salts as purgatives, 141
  sulphate, 141
  trisilicate, 138, 143
magnetic resonance, 35
malaria, 214–16
  drugs used for, 215
maleic anhydride, 191
malonic acid, 42
malonylurea, 42
mammary carcinoma and oestrogens, 179, 184
mannitol, 193
marihuana, 65
mast cells, 114, 115
    and heparin, 157
      histamine, 115
measurement, units of, 250
mebendazole, **217,** 218
mecamylamine and autonomic ganglia, 83, 90, 125
    urine pH, 195
  as hypotensive, 83, **90**
  excretion of, 19
  structure, 91
mechlorethamine, *see* mustine, 226
mecillinam, 206
medrol, 176
medroxyprogesterone acetate, 182
    structure, 183
medulla and anaesthesia, 36
    strychnine, 62
  stimulants of, 60
mefenamic acid, 136
megaloblastic anaemia, 145, 149
    and phenytoin, 46
megestrol, 182
melanocyte stimulating hormone, 162
melanophore-stimulating hormone, 164
melarsonyl, 219
melarsoprol, 216
  structure, 217
melphalan, 226
membrane permeability, 83
    and local anaesthetics, 67
menadiol diphosphate, 159
menadione, *see* menaphthone
menaphthone, 153
  structure, 150
menstruation, 178
  and progesterone, 180
meperidine, *see* pethidine
mephenesin, 50
  and strychnine poisoning, 63
  carbamate, 50
mepps, 75, 76, 80
meprobamate, 50
  structure, 45
mepyramine, 8, **116**

  structure, 117
meralluride, 189
mercaptopurine, 223, **225,** 228
mercurials, organic, 189–190
mercuric chloride, 1, 196
    as emetic, 139
mercurophylline, 189
mercurous chloride, 142
merozoites, 214–215
mersalyl, 189
merthiolate, 212
mescaline, 65
messenger-RNA, 161
mestranol, 179
metabolism and corticosteroids, 174, 175
    sympathetic nerve stimulation, 96 *et seq.*
    temperature, 132
    thyroid, 166
  drug, 20–2
  sugar, 168–71
metals, heavy, as antibacterials, 196
metanephrine, 98, 99
metaraminol, 105
  and circulation, 124
methacholine, 83, 92
methadone, 55, 56
methaemoglobin and nitrites, 127
methallenoestril, 179
  structure, 181
methamphetamine, 105
  structure, 104
methanol, metabolism of, 22
methantheline, 85, **94**
methiacil, *see* methylthiouracil
methicillin, 206
methimazole, 165
methionine, 149
methisazone, 212
'method of least squares', 236
  'responses', 233
methohexitone, duration of action of, 41, 43
methonium, 77, 78
methotrexate, 200, 203, **223–5**
  and folic acid, 199
  structure, 200
methoxamine, 104, **105, 124**
methoxyflurane, 39
3-methoxy-4-hydroxy mandelic acid, 99
methoxyphenamine, 104, **105**
p-methoxyphenylethylmethylamine, 115
N-methylatropine, 9
p-methylcyclohexane, 226
methyl CCNU 227
methyl dilvasene, 5
  furmethide, 5
  lysergic butanolamide, 114
β-methyl xylocholine, 101
methyldopa, 97, **109,** 125
  as hypotensive, 125
  structure, 99

α-methyldopamine, 97, 99
3,3-methylene-bis-4-
  hydroxycoumarin, 158
4-methylhistamine, 116
methylmorphine, *see* codeine
6-methylmercaptopurineribo-
  nucleoside, 225
methyl nitrosamine, 225
α-methylnoradrenaline, 97, **109**
  structure, 99
n-methylphenobarbitone, 47
methylprednisolone, 176
  structure, 177
methyltestosterone, 186
  structure, 185
methylthiouracil, 165
α-methyltyrosine, 97
methylxanthines, 60
methyprylone, 44, 45
methysergide, 114
metopon, 53
metiamide, 116, 117
metronidazole, 217
metyrapone, 174
microcrystals of ice, 34
micro-electrophoresis, 62, 85, 86
migraine, 114, 126
milk expulsion and oxytocin, 111
mineral oil, *see* liquid paraffin.
mineralocorticoids, **172** *et seq.*, 193
  and spironolactone, 193
miniature end-plate potentials (mepps), **75**
mipafox, 90
mithramycin, 223
mitosis, 221, 222
mixed function oxidase, 20–1
  receptor sites, **85–7**
moniodotyrosine, 165, 166
monoamine oxidase, 57, 98–100
    inhibitors, **57–9,** 105, 109
monosodium urate, 193
'moon face', 175
morphine, 16, 52, **53–5,** 60, 63
    histamine release, 115
    temperature, 133
  antagonists, 56
  dependence and methadone, 55
  for premedication, 37
morphine-like compounds, 55
motion sickness, 116, **139–40**
    and hyoscine, 92
mucilages, 143
mucin, 140
mucopeptide, 201
muramyl peptides, 221
muscarine, **83,** 91
  and nicotine, 81
  structure, 93
muscarine-like drugs and atropine, 84, 85
muscarinic action, 27, **73–74**
    and gall-bladder, 140
      gastric secretion, 137
      peristalsis, 140
    of acetylcholine, 9
  receptors, 9, 11, **72** *et seq.*, 107
    agonists at, 91, 92
      structures, 93
    antagonists at, 92, 94
      structures, 93
    in Renshaw cells, 85
muscle action potential, 83
  blood flow in, 14
mustards, 223, **225–6**
mustargen, *see* mustine
mustine, 226
mutation, 221, 246
myasthenia gravis, 76
    and anticholinesterases, 80, 90
      edrophonium, 88
      neostigmine, 89
      tubocurarine, 79
myocardium and local anaesthetics, 68
    nikethamide, 63
    xanthines, 60
myoglobin, 154
mytolon, *see* benzoquinonium
myxoedema, 166–167

NAD (*see also* diphosphopyridine nucleotide), 148
NADP, *see also* triphosphopyridine nucleotide, 148
NAG (*see also* N-acetylglucosamine), 182
NAM, *see* N-acetylmuramic acid
N.E.D., *see* normal equivalent deviation
nalorphine, 53, 54
  in morphine dependence, 56
  structure, 53
nandrolone phenylpropionate, 186
naphthoquinone, 153
naproxen, 120
narceine, 53
narcotine, 53
necator, 217
nembutal, 43
neoarsphenamine
  discovery of, 242
neomercazole, *see* carbimazole
neomycin, 202, **208**
neopyrithiamine, 147
neostigmine, 79, 80, **88–9**
  structure, 90
nerve fibres, differential sensitivity of, 67
'nerve gases', 79, 90
nerve growth factor, 101–2
neuritis and vitamin B, 148
neurohypophysis, 162–**164**
neuromuscular
  junction and acetylcholine, **72** *et seq.*
  transmission, **24** *et seq.*
niacin, *see* nicotinamide
nialamide, 58
niclosamide, 218, **219**
nicotinamide, 145, **148**
nicotine, 27, **80–82,** 85, 87
  structure, 89
nicotinic acid, *see* nicotinamide, 147, 148
  receptors, 72, **74** *et seq.*
    and acetylcholine, 72 *et seq.*
    in Renshaw cells, 85
nicoumalone, 159
nicitating membrane, 80
nifurtimox, 216
nikethamide, **63,** 64
  structure, 61
Nilevar, *see* norethandrolone
niridazole, 219
nitrates, 126–8
nitrazepam, 44, 45, 46
nitrites, 126–28
nitrogen
    and ACTH, 163
      androgens, 186
  mustards, 107, **223–5**
  partition coefficient of, 38
nitrosoureas, 223, 226, **227**
nitrous oxide, 39–40
    and procaine, 71
    partition coefficient of, 38
noradrenaline, 28, **29–30,** 50, **96** *et seq.*, 107
  and
    circulation, 124
    cocaine, 70
    guanethidine, 101
    hypotensive drugs, 125
    imipramine, 59
    reserpine, 49, 96, 100
  release, drugs affecting, 109
  structure, 98
  uptake, inhibitors of, 109
nordefrin, *see* α-methyl-noradrenaline
norethandrolone, 186
  structure, 185
norethisterone, 182, 184
norethynodrel, 182, 184
  structure, 183
normal curve, 231
  equivalent deviation, 238
  frequency curve, 238
normetanephrine, 98
nortriptyline, 109
nuclear magnetic resonance, 35
nucleic acid
    synthesis, 149, **199–203,** 224
nystatin, 201, 204, 211

obesity, 105
occupancy, 9
octopamine (*see also* Synephrin), 104, 105
  structure, 99
oestradiol, 178–80
oestriol, 178–80
oestrogens, 161, **178** *et seq.*, 221, 245, 246

and adrenal cortex, 172
thyroid, 166
structures, 180
oestrone, 178, 180
onchocerca, 219
opium, **53,** 241
as anaesthetic, 33
opsin, 151
organic arsenicals, **196–97,** 216
mercurials, 189–190
organophosphorus compounds, 79
orinase, *see* tolbutamide
ornithine cycle, 195
osmotic diuresis, 193
gradient, 193
osteomalacia, 152
osteoporosis and androgens, 186
ouabain, 130
ovary
and menstrual cycle, 178
ovomucoid, 115
ovulation and gonadotrophins, 178–80
progesterone, 180
oxacillin, 206
structure, 205
oxamniquine, 219
oxamycin, see cyclosterine
7-oxa-13, 14-prostynoic acid, 120
oxidation of drugs in body, 20–2
oximes, 79
oxotremorine, 4
oxprenolol, 108
11-oxycorticoids, *see* glucocorticoids.
oxygen consumption and thyroid, 166
3′-oxyhexobarbitone, 21
oxyntic acid, 137
oxytetracycline, 209
oxythiamine, 147
oxytocin, 20, **110–2**, 162, 164
and milk expulsion, 111

P-2-AM, *see* pralidoxime
PABA, *see* 4-aminobenzoic acid
PAM, *see* pralidoxime
PAS, *see* *p*-aminosalicylic acid
PIF, *see* prolactin release inhibiting factor
PLPA, *see* L-*p*-chlorophenyl alanine
PSF, *see* prolactin releasing factor
PTP, *see* post-tetanic potentiation
Paget's disease of the bone, 168
pancreas, **168** *et seq.*
pancytopenia and hydralazine, 126
pantothenic acid, 145, 147, **148**
structure, 146
papaver somniferum, 53
papaveretum for premedication, 37
papaverine, 29, 53
para-aminobenzoic acid (*see also p*-aminobenzoic acid), 69, 71, 148
structure, 146
paracetamol, **133**, 135, 136
structure, 134
paraffin, liquid, 141, 153
parallel quantitative tests, 236
paramethasone, acetate, 176
structure, 177
parathormone, 104
parathyroid, 168
'Park peptide', 201
paromomycin, 208, **217**
partition coefficients, 38
pellagra, 145, 148
pempidine, 83, 91
as hypotensive, 125
structure, 91
penicillenyl derivatives, 206
penicillin, 1, 197, 201, **205–7**
and cell walls, 201, 221
discovery of, 197
excretion of, 19, 20
resistance to, 203
ristocetin and, 203
structure, 205
G, 205
V, 206
penicillinase, 203, 206, 207
penicillium, 212
penicilloic acid, 203
penicilloyl, 206
pentaerythritol tetranitrate, 127, 128
pentamethonium, 83, 90
structure, 91
pentamidine, 216–17
pentapeptides, 31
pentobarbital, 43
pentobarbitone, 21, 43
pentolinium, 83, 90
structure, 91
pentothal, 43
pentyl trimethylammonium, 4
pentylenetetrazol, *see* leptazol
pepsin, 137, 138
peptic ulcers, 137, 138
peptides, vasoactive, **110** *et seq.*
perchlorate, 164
and thyroid, 167
peristalsis, 140
permeability, ionic, 10
of cell membranes, 83, 96
permease, 11
pernicious anaemia, 145
and liver extracts, 149
peroxidase group, 118, 119
peruvian bark, 196
pethidine, 35, **55**, 56
for premedication, 37
petit mal, 46
phaeochromocytoma, 107, 108
phanodorm, *see* cyclobarbitone
pharmacokinetics, **13** *et seq.*
pharmacological analysis, qualitative, 240–1
phenacemide, 46, **47**
phenacetin, 21, 133, **135**–6
structure, 134
phenazocine, 55
phenazone, 133, **136**
structure, 134
phenelzine, **58**, 99
phenethicillin, 206
phenformin, 171
phenindamine, 116, 117
phenindione, 159
pheniprazine, 58
phenobarbital, *see* phenobarbitone
phenobarbitone, 22, 42, 43, **46**–7
and folic acid, 157
duration of action of, 43
metabolism, 21
structure, 47
phenolphthalein, 141, **142**
phenols, polyhydric, 20
phenolic steroids, 20
phenothiazine,
derivatives, **49**–50, 133
for premedication, 37
structure, 49
tranquillizers, 49–50, 59
phenoxybenzamine, 100, 102, **107**
and noradrenaline, 109
aziridine of, 106
structure, 106
phenoxyethylpenicillin, 206
phenoxymethyl isoquinolines, 211
phenoxymethylpenicillin, 206
structure, 205
phentolamine, 102, **106**
phenylacetic acid, 205, 206
phenylbiguanide, 212
phenylbutazone, 133, 135, 136
structure, 134, 195
phenylethanolamine-N-methyl transferase, 96
phenylethylamine, 104
phenytoin, **46–7**, 131, 166
and folic acid, 157
structure, 47
pholcodine, 55, 240
phosphagen, 133
phosphatase, alkaline, 163
phosphates, 141
and vitamin D, 152
phosphatidylethanolamine, 149
phosphodiesterase, 20, 60, 103, 104
phospholine, 90
phospholipase, 115
phosphonoacetic acid, 212
phosphoramide mustard, 226
phosphorus and androgens, 186
and vitamin D, 152
radioactive, 157
phosphorylase, 104
phosphorylation, 104
phthallide-isoquinoline, 63
physalaemin, 113
physostigmine, **79**, 89–90
phytate, 154
picrotoxin, **63**, 64
structure, 61
picrotoxinin, 63

pilocarpine, 83, 92
muscarinic action, 83
structure, 93
pindolol, 108
pinworms, 217–18
piperazine, **217**, 218
piperocaine, 69
piperoxan, 106
structure, 106
pitressin, *see* antidiuretic hormone, 164
pituitary gland, **162** *et seq.* 169
and chlorotrianisene, 179
clomiphene, 179
contraceptives, 180
corticosteroids, 172, 174
anterior lobe, **162–4**, 178
and menstrual cycle, 180
posterior lobe, 162, **164** *et seq.*
assay of, 230, 234
pivmecillinam, 206
placebo, 240
placenta and oestrogens, 178
oxytocin, 111
progresterone, 180
prostaglandins, 119
passage of drugs across, 16
plasma level, 14
Plasmodium sp., 214 *et seq.*
platinum diammines, 227
polycythaemia vera, 157
polyethylene glycol, 143
polyhydric phenols, 164
polynitrate reductase, 127
polyvinylpyrrolidone, 115
poppy, oriental, 53
porphyrins, 156
post-synaptic membrane, **74** *et seq.*
post-tetanic potentiation, 46
postural hypotension, 82
potassium and ACTH, 163
androgens, 186
corticosteroids, 163
digitalis, 129
ions and kidney, 188, 190
salts and posterior pituitary extract, 230
practolol, 108, 131
pralidoxime, 79
structure, 90
prednisolone, 176
structure, 177
prednisone, 176, 223–4, 227–8
structure, 177
pregnancy and oestrogens, 178
tetracyclines, 209
thyroid, 166
pregnanedione, 41
pregnenolone, 173
premedication, 37, 84
presynaptic inhibition, 63
membrane, 75 *et seq.*
prilocaine, 70
structure, 69
primaquine, 214–16
probability scale, 238–9
pro-banthine, *see* propantheline
probenecid, 194, 205
structure, 195
probit, 238–9
procainamide, 131
procaine, 20, 67–9, **70**, 131
penicillin, 205
progestagen, 245
progesterone, 180, **182**
and adrenal cortex, 172, 173
as anti-oestrogen, 179, 180
structure, 183
proguanil, 215, **216**
prolactin, 162, **163**
releasing factor, 162
release inhibiting factor, 162
promazine, 49, 50, 59
promethazine, 55, 116, 117
for motion sickness, 116, 140
pronethalol, 107–108
prontosil, 196, 243
propanediol derivatives, 50
propanidid, **40**, 41
propantheline, 85
structure, 93
propionyl choline, 4–5
structure, 3
propranolol, 102, **107–8**, 128
as antiarrhythmic, 131
propylene glycol, 143
propylthiouracil, 165
prostacyclin, 120
prostaglandin synthesase, 118
prostaglandins, 113, **118–20**,
and contraceptives 183–4
as central transmitters, 32
prostate, cancer of, and sex hormones, 179
prostigmin, *see* neostigmine
protamine and heparin, 158
insulin injection, 170
protease, 166
protectives, 143
protein
anabolism and testosterone, 186
binding, 15
synthesis, 202–3, 208
prothrombin, 157
and vitamin K, 153
pseudocholinesterase, 77, 87, 92
psychoses and corticosteroids, 175
pteridine, 199
structure, 146
$2NH_2$-4-OH-pteridine, 148
pteroic synthetase, 203
pteroylmonoglutamic acid, *see* folic acid
pulmonary oedema and frusemide, 191
pulse and anaesthesia, 36
rate and thyroid, 167
pupils and anticholinesterases, 80, 90
general anaesthesia, 36
morphine, 53
purgatives, **140** *et seq.*
anthracene, 142–143
bulk, 141
'contact', 142
irritant, 141–2
lubricant, 141
puri-nethol, *see* mercaptopurine
purine analogues, 224, 225
metabolism, 193
purines, 149, 155, 224
and folic acid, 149
puromycin, 161, 166
'purple hearts', *see* drinamyl
pyrantelpamoate, **217**, 218
pyrazinamide, 211
pyrazole, 22, 252
pyridine, 147
ring, 252
pyridoxal, *see also* vitamin B_6, 146, 148
kinase, 148
phosphate, 148
pyridoxamine, *see also* vitamin B_6, 148
phosphate, 148
pyridoxine, *see* vitamin B_6, 148
pyrilamine, *see* mepyramine
pyrimethanine, 214–16, 242
pyrimidine analogues, 224, 242
pyrimidines, 155
pyrithiamine, *see* neopyrithiamine
pyrogallol, 99
pyrogen-free water, 133
pyrogens, 133
pyruvic acid, 147
pyrviniumpamoate, 218

QSAR, 244
qualitative pharmacological analysis, **240–1**
quantitative structure activity relationships, 244
quinalbarbitone, 42, 43
quinidine, 130, 131
quinine, 131, **216**
structure, 215
quinone coenzymes, 159

RNA, 161, 202, 210–12, 225–7
and hormones, 161
radioactive iodine, 167
rashes, *see also* skin
and hydralazine, 126
penicillin, 206
phenytoin, 46
sulphonamindes, 207
sulphonylureas, 171
thiouracil, 165
troxidone, 47
rat poison, 159
rauwolfia derivatives, 48, 49
receptor sites, mixed, **85–7**
receptors, drug, 9–11
muscarinic, 9, 11, **72** *et seq.*

nicotinic, 11, **74** *et seq.*
α-receptors, **102** *et seq.*, 124
β-receptors, **102** *et seq.*, 124
reductase inhibitors, 203
reflexes and anaesthetics, 36
strychnine, 62
releasing factors, 162
renal colic and atropine, 85
renin, 175
and aldosterone, 192
Renshaw cells, 63, 72, 85
reserpine, 96, 100, 106, **109**
and noradrenaline release, 100
as hypotensive, 125
tranquillizer, 49–50
structure, 45
resistance to antimalarials, 215–216
chemotherapeutic drugs, **203**–204
streptomycin, 209
transferable, 203
resistant strains of bacteria, 203–4
resorcinol, 164
structure, 165
responses, method of, 233
respiration and anaesthesia, 36
caffeine, 60
ethanivan, 64
nalorphine, 56
nikethamide, 63
picrotoxin, 63
salicylates, 135–136
respiratory centre and morphine, 53
distress of newborn, 64
infections and nicotine, 81
reticular formation and anaesthesia, 35
retinene, 151
retinopathy, chloroquine, 216
rhodopsin, 151
rhubarb, 142–3
ribavirin, 212
riboflavine, *see* vitamin B_2.
phosphate, 147
ribose, 147
ribosomes, 202, 208
ricinoleic acid, 142
rickets, 152
Rickettsiae, 208, 209
rifampicin, 210–11
rifampin, 210–11
rings, chemical, index of, 252–4
ringworm, 211
ristocetin, 201, 203
roundworms, 217, 218
rutin, *see* vitamin P

St. Anthony's fire, 114
salbutamol, 105
structure, 104
salicylate poisoning, 135–6
salicylates, **133–6**
and uric acid, 194
urine pH, 195
salicylazosulphapyridine, 207
salicylic acid, 134
structure, 195
salicyluric acid, 135
salix alba, 134
sampling, errors of, 230
sarin, 90
schistosomiasis, 219
schizophrenia and hallucinogens, 64
scopolamine, *see* hyoscine
screening, 4, 243–4
scurvy, 144–145
seborrhoeic dermatitis and vitamin B_2, 147
secobarbital, 43
seconal, 43
secretin, 140
secretions and atropine, 85
sedatives, **42** *et seq.*
non-barbiturate, 44–5
selective action, 1
antagonists, 9, 10
chemotherapy, 197
semustine, 227
senna, 142–3
senses, special, and strychnine, 62–3
sequential analysis, 240
sera, assay of, 229
serotonin, 28, **30**
and Bezold receptors, 126
kinins, 113
LSD, 64
reserpine, 49, 109
sex hormones, **175** *et seq.*
sexual changes and corticosteroids, 175
side actions of drugs, 1
sigmoid curve, 238, 240
silicic acid, 138
silver nitrate, 143, 196
Simmonds' disease, 162
skeleton, blood flow in, 14
skin, *see also* rashes
and vitamin B, 148, 149
blood flow in, 14
sleep, 42
sleeping sickness, 216
smallpox and methisazone, 212
snake venom, 101–2, 112
sodium, and ACTH, 163
androgens, 186
corticosteroids, 172, 174, 175
ions and kidney, 188 *et seq.*
permeability and catecholamines, 103
veratrine alkaloids, 126
sodium antimony dimercaptosuccinate, 219
bicarbonate, **138**
and urine pH, 195
citrate and urine pH, 195
hypochlorite, 212
iodide (^{131}I), 167
nitrite, 127
salicylate, 135
stibogluconate, 216, 219
sulphate as diuretic, 193
purgative, 141
tauroglycocholate, 140
thiopental, *see* thiopentone sodium
valporate, 47
soluble insulin injection, 170
solutions, aqueous, 251
soneryl, 43
sotalol, 108
specific selectivity, 1
sphincter of Oddi, 55
spinal anaesthesia, 69–70
cord, 85–6
strychnine, 62
spirochaetes and antibiotics, 205
spironolactone, 174, 192–193
sprue, 145, 156
S-shaped curve, 5, **238**–240
standard deviation, 231–2
error, 232
preparations, 230
staphylococci and penicillin, 205
starch, 143
statolon, 212
steroids, anaesthetics, 40–1
synthetic, structures, 177
stibamine, 217
stibophen, 219
stilbamidine and histamine release, 115
stilboestrol, 179
structure, 181
stimulants of central nervous system, **57** *et seq.*
Stokes–Adams syndrome, 124
strepococci and penicillen, 205
Streptomyces sp., 155, 156, 208
streptomycin, 1, 202–4, **208–11**
excretion, 19, 20
resistance to, 203–4, 209
structure, 210
stroke output, 122
curve, 123
strophanthin G, *see* ouabain
strophanthus, 128
gratus, 130
strychnine, 62–3
poisoning, 63
structure, 61
substance P, 28, **30–1**, **113**
substrate competition, 100
succinylcholine, *see* suxamethonium
succinylsulpha pyridine, 207
sugar metabolism and insulin, **168** *et seq.*
suicidal tendencies and reserpine, 49
sulfamethoxazole, 207
sulphadiazine, 201, 242
sulphadoxine, 216
sulphalene, 216
sulphamethoxazole *see* sulfamethoxazole
sulphanilamide, 197, 199, 242
structure, 165, 198, 243

sulphanilamidoisopropylthiadiazide, 242, 243
sulphasalazine, 207, 208
sulphated polysaccharides, 158
O,N,-sulphatoglycosaminoglucuronate, 158
sulphinpyrazone, 194
 structure, 195
sulphonamides, **197**–204, 216
 and cotrimazole, 207
 and procaine, 71
  resistance, 203–4
  trimethoprim, 203
 antithyroid action, 164
 as carbonic anhydrase inhibitors, 190
 discovery of, 242
 excretion, 19
 toxic effects of, 207
sulphonyl ureas, 242
sulphuric acid and thyroxine, 166
sulphydryl groups, 191
sulthiame, 46, **47**
suramin, 216, **219**
suxamethonium, 20, 77, **87–8**
 and halothane, 39
 structure, 89
sympathetic block, 125
 nerve stimulation, effects of, **102** *et seq.*
  and circulation, 122
   peristalsis, 140
sympathomimetic substances, 100–2, **104**
  structures, 104
synephrine, 98
syphilis, 205, 209

TEA, *see* tetraethylammonium
TEC, *see* triethylcholine
TEPP, *see* tetraethylpyrophosphate
TFA, *see* tetrahydrofolic acid
TM10, *see* xylocholine
TMA, *see* tetramethylammonium
TP, *see* 2-mercaptopropionic acid
TRF, *see* thyrotrophin releasing factor
TSH, *see* thyrotrophin
tachycardia and iron, 155
tachyphylaxis, 100
tannic acid, 143
tannin, 143
tapazole, *see* methimazole
tapeworms, 217–18
tartrates, 141
taurine, 32
teichoic acid, 201
tensilon, *see* edrophonium
teratogenicity, 212
testes and oestrogen, 178
testosterone, 161, **179**
 cypionate injection, 186
  structure, 185
 enanthate, 186
 propionate injection, 186
  structure, 184, 185
tetanus and tubocurarine, 79
tetany and calcium deficiency, 168
  parathyroid, 168
tetracaine, *see* amethocaine
tetracyclines, 1, 202–4, **208–9**, 216
 and resistance, 201–2
 absorption of, 19
 excretion of, 19
 structures, 209
tetraethylammonium, 27, 82, **85**
 structure, 27
tetraethylpyrophosphate, 90
tetraethylthiuram disulphide, 52
tetrahydrocannabinol, 65
tetrahydrofolate, 149, 154, 224
tetrahydrofolic acid, 157, 199
  structure, 198
β-tetrahydronaphthylamine and temperature, 133
tetramethylammonium, 5, 80, **82**
 structure, 4, 91
thalidomide, 245
thebane, 53
theobromine, 59–60
theophylline, 29, **59–60**, 103–4
thermodynamic activity, 35
thiabendazole, 217, 218
thialbarbitone, 43
thiamine *see* vitamin B_1
 pyrophosphate, 147
thiazides, 190–1
thimecil, *see* methylthiouracil
thioamides, 164
thiobarbiturates, 143
thiocyanate, 164, 167
thioguanine, 223, **225**
thiomersal, 212
thiopentol, 43
thiopentone, 16
 and methoxyflurane, 39, 42, 43
 sodium, 40, 41
thiosemicarbazone, 212
thiouracil, 165
thiourea, 164
 structure, 165
threadworms, 217–18
threshold dose, method of, 233
thrombin, 157
thrombocytopenia, 207
thromboplastin, 157–8
thrombosis and contraceptives, 184, 245
thromboxanes, 120
thymidine, 149
thymidylate synthetase, 225
thyrocalcitonin, 168
thyroglobulin, 164
thyroid, **164** *et seq.*
 and TSH, 162, 167
 binding proteins, 166
 deficiency, 166–7
 hormones, structures, 165
 hyperactivity, 167
 inhibitors, 167
 stimulator, long-acting, 162–3
thyrotoxic goitre and radioactive iodine, 167
thyrotrophin, **162**, 166, 167
 releasing factor, 162
thyroxine, 161, 162, **164–8**
  temperature, 133
tobacco, 81, 82
tocopherols, *see also* vitamin E, 152
tolamolol, 108
tolazoline, 106
tolbutamide, 171
tolerance to barbiturates, 44
  cocaine, 70
  morphine, 54
  nitrites, 127
tolnaftate, 211
toluidine blue, 157
toxicity tests, 238
toxins, assay of, 229
tragacanth, 143
tranquillizing drugs, **48** *et seq.*
transferrin, 154
transmitter release, 34
trans-retinene, 151
trans-vitamin A, 151
tranylcypromine, 59
 structure, 58
trasylol and bradykinin, 113
treponema pallidum, 205
trial, clinical, 245–6
triamcinolone, 176
triamterene, 192
 structure, 191
trichlorethylalcohol, 44
trichlorethylene, **217**, 218
 and procaine, 70
 partition coefficient of, 38
trichomonas, 216, 217
tricyclic group (*see also* dibenzazepine derivatives) and noradrenaline, 109
triethanolamine nitrate, 127, 128
triethylcholine, **76**, 80
trifluoperazine, 49, 50
triflupromazine, 49
3,4,6-trihydroxyphenylethylamine, 100
triiodothyronine, 164–6
trimelarsan, 219
trimethadione, *see* troxidone
trimethoprim, 199, 200
 and sulphamethoxazole, 207
 and sulphonamides, 207
triphosphopyridine nucleotide, 148
triple response, 115–6
tritium, 96, 100
trolnitrate, *see* triethanolamine
trophozoites, 214–15
troxidone, 46, **47**
trypan blue, 196
 red, 196
trypanosomiasis, 216
tryparsamide, 196, **216**–17
tuberculosis, chemotherapy of, **209–11**

tubocurarine, 9, **78–9**, 85, 88
  and histamine release, 115
  excretion, 19
  structure, 89
D-tubocurarine, 74
tubulin, 227
tumours, chemotherapy of, **211** *et seq.*
typhoid and ampicillin, 206
tyramine, 100, **105**
  and monoamine oxidase inhibitors, 100, 104
    noradrenaline, 98
  structure, 99
tyrosine, 96, 97, 137
  hydroxylase, 96
  structure, 98
tyrothricin, 201

ubiquinones, 159
ultraviolet irradiation and vitamin D, 151–52
unit, definition of, 229
urea stibamine, 216
uric acid and ACTH, 163
    xanthines, 60
  excretion, 193–4
    drugs affecting, 191, **193**–4
  structure, 194
uricase, 193
uricosuric drugs, 194
  structures, 195
urine pH alterants, 194–5
urochloralic acid, 44
uterus and ergometrine, 114
    menstrual cycle, 178
    oxytocin, 111
    prostaglandins, 119
    vasopressin, 111

vagus, 137, 140
  and atropine, 85
    cardiac glycosides, 129
    gastric secretion, 138
    peristalsis, 140
valerylcholine, 3–4, 7–8
vancomycin, 201
vanillic acid, 64
variance, 232
vasoconstriction and cocaine, 70
    ergot alkaloids, 105–7
    nicotine, 81
vasodilatation and bradykinin, 113
    local anaesthetics, 68
    nicotinic acid, 148
    procaine, 71
vasomotor centres and xanthines, 60
vasopressin (*see also* antidiuretic hormone) 20, **110–2**, 164
vasotocin, 111
ventricular fibrillation, 129, 130
    and cocaine, 70
veratridine, 126
veratrin alkaloids, **126**, 139
veronal, 43
vidarabine, 212
vinblastine, 224, **227**, 228
vinca alkaloids, 223, 224, **227**
vincristine, 227
viomycin, 211
vision (*see also* eye)
  and strychnine, 63
  and vitamin A, 151
vitamin A, 151
    structure, 150
  B_1, 145, **147**
    structure, 146
  B_2, 145, **147**
    structure, 146
  B_6, 145, **147–8**
    structure, 146
  B_{12}, 145, **149**
    structure, 146
  B complex, **147** *et seq.*
  C, 144–145
    structure, 146
  D, **151**–2, 168
    and liquid paraffin, 141
      tetany, 152
    deficiency, 152
  D_2, calciferol
    structure, 150
  E, 152
    structure, 150
  H, 145, 147, **149**
    structure, 146
  K, 153
    and dicoumarol, 158–9
      liquid paraffin, 141, 153
  K_1 and K_2, 153
      structures, 150
  M, 148
  P, 145–7
vitamins, assay of, 229, 234
  fat soluble, **150** *et seq.*
    structures, 150
  water soluble, **144** *et seq.*
    structures, 146
volatile and gaseous anaesthetics, 38–40
volume, units of, 250
vomiting, 139–140
    and digitalis, 130
    iron, 155
    morphine, 53
    nicotine, 81
    oestrogens, 179
    sulphonamides, 207
    veratrin alkaloids, 126

warfarin, 159
water-soluble vitamins, **144** *et seq.*
weight gain and corticosteroids, 175
weights, units of, 250
whipworm, 218
willow bark, 134
withdrawal symptoms of morphine, 54
Withering, William, 128
worms, 217–219
Wuchereria bancrofti, 219

xanthine derivatives, **59**–60, 104, 194
    and gout, 194
xylenol, 212
xylocholine, 101

yohimbine, 106

zinc oxide, 143
  sulphate, 139
  suspension insulin injections, 170
'zone of inexcitability', 78